Butterworths International Medical Reviews

Neurology 1

Clinical Neurophysiology

Butterworths International Medical Reviews

Neurology 1

Editorial Board
A. K. Asbury
M. L. Dyken
S. Fahn
R. W. Gilliatt
M. J. G. Harrison
C. D. Marsden
E. Stålberg
R. R. Young

Future volumes to include

Movement Disorders

Cerebral Vascular Disease

Peripheral Nerves

Butterworths
International
Medical
Reviews

Neurology 1

Clinical
Neurophysiology

Edited by
Erik Stålberg, MD
Associate Professor,
Department of Clinical Neurophysiology,
University Hospital,
Uppsala, Sweden

and

Robert R. Young, MD
Associate Professor,
Department of Neurology,
Harvard Medical School,
Boston, Massachusetts, USA

Butterworths
London Boston
Sydney Wellington Durban Toronto

First published 1981

© Butterworth & Co (Publishers) Ltd. 1981

British Library Cataloguing in Publication Data
Neurology.
    Vol. 1: Clinical neurophysiology – (Butterworths
international medical reviews ISSN 0260–0137).
    1. Neurology
    1. Stålberg, Erik II. Young, Robert R.
    616.8   RC346   80–42166

ISBN 0–407–02294–5

Photoset by Butterworths Litho Preparation Department
Printed and bound in England by Hartnoll Print Ltd., Bodmin,
Cornwall.

Preface

This volume is the first in a new international series of critical reviews of topics in Neurology aimed at the fully-fledged clinician and the postgraduate trainee. This book is therefore *not* a textbook in clinical neurophysiology covering background knowledge in EEG and EMG and it is *not* primarily designed for specialized clinical neurophysiologists. It presents new data, trends and major advances in clinical neurophysiology of interest to clinicians who use these neurophysiological services in their routine practice.

We therefore, in this limited space, highlight a few topics in the widening field of clinical neurophysiology. Within these, we sought to provide wide coverage of all views including those which are controversial. Emphasis has been placed upon clinical relevance – even chapters which, at first glance, appear non-clinical, will provide, upon study, new insights into common medical problems. By presenting certain new results, we hope to provide further understanding of the pathophysiology in these disorders. By presenting some of the new techniques, we hope to create an increasing interest in clinical neurophysiology.

We wish to thank the publishers for inviting us to prepare this volume, the authors for their timely cooperation and our associates for their advice and help including our secretaries Lisbeth Grydén and Barbara Marino for retyping some of the manuscripts, sometimes more than once. Both of us have learned a great deal about the topics covered in this volume as we played an active role in its production.

Not only have we chosen authors and topics but we have interacted with the authors about matters of fact, points of interpretation and areas of emphasis. We therefore share equally any responsibility for errors, omissions or misinterpretations.

Erik Stålberg
Robert R. Young

List of contributors

Linda Y. Buchwald, MD
Chief of Neurology, Mt. Auburn Hospital, Cambridge,
Massachusetts, USA

Keith H. Chiappa, MD
Director, EEG and Evoked Potential Unit, Clinical Neurophysiology
Laboratory, and Assistant Neurologist, Massachusetts General
Hospital; Assistant Professor of Neurology, Harvard Medical School,
Boston, Massachusetts, USA

Jasper R. Daube, MD
Head of Section of Electroencephalography, Department of
Neurology, Mayo Clinic and Mayo Foundation, Associate Professor of
Neurology, Mayo Medical School, Rochester, Minnesota, USA

Volker Dietz, MD
Assistant Medical Director, Department of Clinical Neurology and
Neurophysiology, University of Freiburg, D–7800 Freiburg i. Br.,
GFR

Lennart Grimby, MD
Associate Professor, Department of Neurology, Karolinska Hospital,
Stockholm, Sweden

Christian Guilleminault, MD
Associate Professor of Psychiatry and Behavioral Sciences, Sleep
Disorders Clinic and Research Center, Stanford University Medical
School, Stanford, California, USA

A. M. Halliday, B SC, MB, CH B, FBCS
Consultant in Clinical Neurophysiology, Medical Research Council,
Institute of Neurology, National Hospital, London, UK

List of contributors

Jan Hannerz, MD
Associate Professor, Department of Neurology, Karolinska Hospital,
Stockholm, Sweden

Ulf Lindblom, MD
Professor and Chairman of Neurology, Karolinska Institute,
Karolinska Hospital, Stockholm, Sweden

Lars Lindström, PH D
Research Engineer, Department of Clinical Neurophysiology,
Sahlgren Hospital, Göteborg, Sweden

W. I. McDonald, PH D, FRCP
Professor, Institute of Neurology, National Hospital, London, UK

K. G. Ingemar Petersén, MD, PH D
Professor of Clinical Neurophysiology, Head of the Department of
Clinical Neurophysiology, University of Göteborg, Sahlgren Hospital,
Göteborg, Sweden

Pamela F. Prior, MD
Consultant Clinical Neurophysiologist, Department of Neurological
Sciences, St. Bartholomew's Hospital, London and Scientific Officer,
Medical Research Council Laboratories, Carshalton, UK

Donald B. Sanders, MD
Professor, Division of Neurology, Duke University Medical Center,
Durham, North Carolina, USA

Stefan C. Schatzki, MD
Assistant Clinical Professor of Radiology, Harvard Medical School
and Chief, Department of Radiology, Mt. Auburn Hospital,
Cambridge, Massachusetts, USA

E. M. Sedgwick, B SC, MD
Consultant and Senior Lecturer in Clinical Neurophysiology, Wessex
Neurological Centre, Southampton General Hospital, Southampton,
UK

Ulla Selldén, MD, PH D
Associate Professor, Department of Clinical Neurophysiology,
University of Göteborg, Sahlgren Hospital, Göteborg, Sweden

Bhagwan T. Shahani, MD, D PHIL (OXON.)
Director, EMG and Motor Control Unit, Clinical Neurophysiology
Laboratory, and Associate Neurologist, Massachusetts General
Hospital; Associate Professor of Neurology, Harvard Medical School,
Boston, Massachusetts, USA

Erik Stålberg, MD
Associate Professor, Department of Clinical Neurophysiology,
University Hospital, Uppsala, Sweden

Austin J. Sumner, MD
Associate Professor of Neurology and Director, Neurodiagnostic
Laboratory, Department of Neurology, Hospital of the University of
Pennsylvania, Philadelphia, Pennsylvania, USA

B. Gunnar Wallin, MD
Associate Professor, Department of Clinical Neurophysiology,
University Hospital, Uppsala, Sweden

Edward R. Wolpow, MD
Assistant Clinical Professor of Neurology, Harvard Medical School
and Director, Electromyography Laboratory, Mt. Auburn Hospital,
Cambridge, Massachusetts, USA

Robert R. Young, MD
Director of Clinical Neurophysiology Laboratory and Movement
Disorder Clinic, and Associate Neurologist, Massachusetts General
Hospital; Associate Professor of Neurology, Harvard Medical School,
Boston, Massachusetts, USA

Contents

Contents

1
What is clinical neurophysiology?

Erik Stålberg and Robert R. Young

Electroencephalography and electromyography arose, at least in the English-speaking world, from experiments in the physiology laboratory where Lord Adrian and his colleagues – Bronk, Forbes, Matthews and others – exploited new electronic techniques, such as vacuum tube amplifiers, for the study of electrical activity from brain and muscle of humans and other animals. Starting more than 40 years ago, first EEG, then EMG laboratories developed in hospitals for the physiological investigation of patients. In some countries, EEG and EMG were grouped together in more or less autonomous departments of clinical neurophysiology, but in others, including the USA, they developed within different specialties. Advances in neuroscience and medicine have permitted rapid growth in this field, which now requires full time physiological, medical and technical specialists. Although they study patients with different types of disorders, electroencephalographers and electromyographers have always employed essentially similar techniques and scientific understanding. With the advent of microprocessors, minicomputers and other means for recording evoked potentials, boundaries between EEG and EMG techniques have become even less distinct. Where EEG and EMG laboratories have hitherto been separate in many countries, largely for administrative reasons, they should now be combined under the term 'clinical neurophysiology'.

Originally, investigations were limited to EEG and EMG. These methods have proved useful for detection, registration and quantification of various disturbances of function in the central or peripheral nervous systems and neuromuscular apparatus. They are the electrophysiological counterparts to morphological techniques provided in neuropathology laboratories by autopsy or biopsy, and radiology departments, including CT scans. In this important respect, clinical

1

neurophysiology forms one of the bases of 'quantitative neurology', providing the clinician with objective information to aid his clinical assessment.

As indicated in this volume, modern trends in clinical neurophysiology have developed for two fundamental reasons. On the one hand, new questions have been formulated on the basis of general advances in neuroscience. Certain of the techniques used to collect the new data and concepts described below (sleep, motor control) have been available for many years. On the other hand, recent considerable technological advances have been of the utmost importance for the expansion of the field. For example, newly improved methods are available for EEG telemetry, sleep studies, tremor analysis and automatic data processing of various physiological parameters, including EEG, EMG, respiration and arterial or intracranial pressures. Entirely new techniques have been introduced to study evoked potentials, movement disorders, autonomic dysfunction, motor unit microphysiology and quantitative sensibility. Most of these are routinely available, at least in larger laboratories, and have increased the demand for, and potential value of, clinical neurophysiology.

Tentative solutions to important questions arising in the clinic – for example, 'does excess fusimotor drive account for the hyper-reflexia in spasticity?' – previously required investigators to design animal experiments. These questions can now often be tackled directly in the clinical neurophysiology laboratory. Such approaches are more satisfying, coming as they do from the specific patients in question. They are also more precise, since animal studies are, at best, indirect and may sometimes be misleading. Exact animal models of human disease states are typically either very difficult or impossible to produce. A new and important aspect has been the application of sophisticated techniques to the understanding of normal physiology in man. An example of this is the introduction of various microelectrode recording techniques which now allow us to tackle basic physiological problems concerning sensory, motor and autonomic functions which previously could only be studied in animals.

Clinical neurophysiology provides quantitative data which enables the clinician to reach a diagnosis necessary for appropriate management and therapy. Proper use of the latter depends not only upon precise diagnosis but also upon objective evaluation of neuropharmacological, medical, surgical and physical therapies. It is now possible to assess accurately neurophysiological function following various treatments or the passage of time. In this context, clinical neurophysiology facilitates monitoring of patients during neurological rehabilitation. The specialty has also expanded beyond its customary role in neurology, neurosurgery or physical medicine departments into other areas. It participates outside the hospital in occupational medicine, including ergonomic studies of muscular activity, EEG monitoring during shift work and toxicological screening. It is used in sports medicine and for monitoring subjects in specific situations such as school, aeroplanes or underwater work.

For the future, continued use of EEG can be foreseen in the evaluation of patients with disturbances of consciousness whether paroxysmal, e.g. during seizures, or more chronic, e.g. in metabolic encephalopathies. Now that CT scans are available, the clinical utility of EEG has been more clearly defined. It remains useful for physiological, rather than anatomical, evaluations and CT scans often permit excellent short-term physiological–pathological correlations. Its future use should become more apparent in monitoring patients during sleep, actual or impending coma, anaesthesia or possible seizures. Evoked potential techniques are still improving in terms of recording, analysis and interpretation. The same applies to nerve conduction studies where F waves are proving useful. EMG will further advance its essential role with new recording and analytical techniques. Similarly, measurements applied to reflexes, normal or abnormal motor control, sensation and autonomic disturbances are already broadening the scope of the specialty.

In summary, clinical neurophysiology will consolidate its position as a provider of quantitative data in the field of neurology. As such, it will, to an increasing extent, contribute to various therapies, monitor dynamic changes and both suggest principles and provide means such as activation of prostheses – orthoses and biofeedback in rehabilitation. It will also provide new insights into fundamental neurobiological processes and pose clearly-defined problems which will attract the interest of non-clinical neurophysiologists.

Clinical neurophysiology today requires a broader definition than simply EEG plus EMG. It includes the neurophysiological investigation of normal human function and diseases which affect either central or peripheral nervous systems, including the autonomic, and the neuromuscular apparatus.

2

The electrophysiological differentiation of motor units in man

Lennart Grimby and Jan Hannerz

Experiments on animals have demonstrated that motor units are differentiated as regards axonal conduction velocity[26], contraction time[16, 32], motoneuronal after-hyperpolarization[22] which partially controls the firing rate, histochemical muscle fibre type[25], fatiguability of the peripheral mechanisms[13, 14, 69] and finally input resistance[55] and synaptic supply[17, 53, 54] which determine the thresholds.

Histochemical differentiation in man is the same as in animals and it is probable that these physiological parameters are also similarly differentiated. The present review concerns physiological methods applicable to man for studies of single motor unit parameters, as well as knowledge of the physiological differentiation of single motor units in man and in particular, their voluntary use.

Contractile properties of single human motor units

Methods

With electrical stimulation of a whole motor nerve, a single α-axon is occasionally activated thus permitting study of contraction time and twitch tension of its muscle unit[81]. However, threshold differences between axons are small and there is a risk that more than one axon may have the same threshold. Further, tetanic tension cannot be studied since greater threshold differences are needed to obtain single motor unit responses with repetitive stimulation.

The disadvantages mentioned can be partly avoided by stimulation of the terminal nerve twigs at the motor point[11, 12]. Taylor and Stephens[88] have described techniques for intramuscular stimulation of single motor units by means of bipolar needle electrodes with small surfaces and a small interelectrode distance (e.g. Medelec type E/NDL) permitting studies not only of contraction time and twitch tension of single human motor units but also of their tetanic tension,

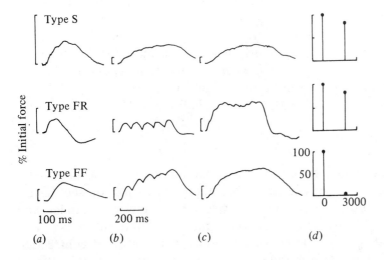

Figure 2.1 Examples of three motor unit types found in human medial gastrocnemius. (*a*) Isometric twitch (to the left calibration 10 g). (*b*) Isometric tetanus 10 pulses per second. (*c*) Isometric tetanus 20 pulses per second. (*d*) Fatigue test, control and after 3000 stimuli, expressed as percentage of initial isometric tension. (From Garnett *et al.*[31], courtesy of the Editor and publisher, *Journal of Physiology*)

fatiguability and even histochemical profiles, i.e. studies that are comparable to animal studies (*Figure 2.1*). However, these techniques are laborious and only a limited number of experimental findings have been published[31]. It should also be borne in mind that fatiguability of a motor unit during selective artificial stimulation is not the same as its fatiguability during natural activation when other motor units within the muscle participate, affecting the blood supply; central fatigue mechanisms are also involved in the latter case (*see* p. 16).

Milner-Brown, Stein and Yemm[65] have shown that twitch tension curves of single motor units can be obtained by averaging the increase in tension related to the single motor unit potential during maintained voluntary contraction. As well as providing unique opportunities for relating the contractile properties of single motor units to their firing properties this method is not too time-consuming. However, it can only be used when tension produced by the test unit has not 'fused' and when the unit fires at random in relation to other motor units in that muscle. Unless great care is taken, together with the special precautions observed by Milner-Brown, Stein and Yemm[65], such a test unit curve will be contaminated by other motor units. This will have serious consequences particularly when weak motor units are being studied. Unfortunately, even when all these precautions are *not* observed, this method still produces tension curves.

Contraction time

Animal experiments have shown that contraction times of the slowest motor units in a muscle are more than twice that of the fastest ones[16, 32]. Absolute contraction times differ between muscles and species, e.g. 15–90 ms in cat gastrocnemius, 50–110 in cat soleus[13] and 15–45 in rat soleus[57]. There is a bimodal distribution of contraction times at least in some muscles[13, 90]. There are, however, transitional forms[58] so that any dividing line between a slow and a fast twitch population is arbitrary.

In man reported contraction times of single motor units range from 30 to 110 ms in distal extremity muscles: Buchthal and Schmalbruch[11] found 40–80 ms in the anterior tibial muscle; Sica and McComas[81] 35–100 ms in short toe extensor; Milner-Brown, Stein and Yemm[66] 30–100 ms in first interosseus muscle in the hand; Burke, Skuse and Lethlean[12] 40–100 ms in abductor digiti minimi in the hand; and Garnett *et al.*[31] 30–110 ms in gastrocnemius muscle. All human studies indicate a continuum between the extremes noted. Burke, Skuse and Lethlean[12] found unimodal, while Sica and McComas[81] and Garnett *et al.*[31] found bimodal distribution of contraction times with a major peak below 80 ms and a small peak above 90 ms. This discrepancy and the suprisingly small slow twitch population may be due to the fact that slow twitch motor units are so weak their tension curves are difficult to record.

Tension

Animal experiments have shown that tensions produced by single motor units in a muscle are distributed over a wide range and tension is inversely correlated with contraction time[13, 14]. All slow twitch units produce low tension. The fast twitch population is, however, heterogenous: some fast units produce high tension but others low tension[76].

A number of authors have studied twitch tensions and their relation to contraction time in man. Sica and McComas[81] found twitch tensions between 2 and 14 g in short toe extensor muscle but estimated the real tensions to be three times higher because of disadvantageous insertion of the tendon. Milner-Brown, Stein and Yemm[66] found tensions between 1 and 50 g in first interosseus muscle and Garnett et al.[31] found tensions between 1.5 and 203 g in gastrocnemius. In interosseus and gastrocnemius muscles slow twitch units produced low tensions; there was also a tendency to an inverse relationship between twitch tensions and contraction time among fast twitch units, as has been found in animals. In short toe extensors, however, there was no significant relationship, possibly due to collateral sprouting present in this muscle which is also found in normal subjects[36, 51].

Peripheral fatigue

Fatiguability of peripheral mechanisms of single motor units during tetanic contraction has been intensively studied in animals[13, 14, 69]. The slow twitch population (S) is resistant to fatigue. However, the fast twitch population is very heterogenous, – a fast resistant group (FR), a fast fatiguable group (FF) and a fast intermediate group (Fint) have been distinguished[14]. It has been shown, however, that there is a continuum of intermediate forms[58]. Although classification of motor units into groups may be arbitrary, it facilitates their description and our comprehension of laboratory findings.

In man fatigue of different types of motor units during tetanic contraction have been studied by Garnett et al.[31] (*Figure 2.2*) in gastrocnemius with microstimulation at the motor point. Motor units with contraction times above 99 ms were classified as slow twitch units, and those with contraction times below 85 ms as fast twitch units, on the basis of a bimodal distribution of contraction times. The slow

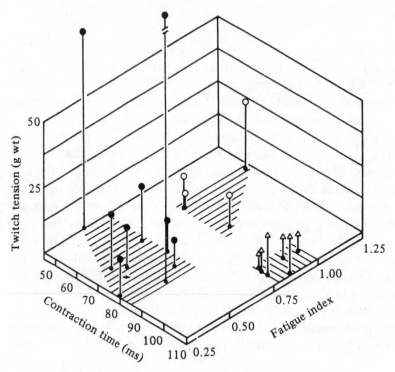

Figure 2.2 Three-dimensional graph relating twitch tension, twitch contraction time and fatigue index for 18 medial gastrocnemius motor units. Six type S (△), four type FR (○) and eight type FF (●). (From Garnett *et al.*[31], courtesy of the Editor and publisher, *Journal of Physiology*)

twitch population was homogenous and relatively fatigue-resistant. The fast twitch population, however, comprised one fatigue-resistant group and one fatiguable group, i.e. one S, one FR and one FF group could be distinguished as found in animals. Five motor units were also studied using the glycogen depletion technique[25]. Three S-units were found to have type I muscle fibres, one FR-unit also had type I fibres and one FF-unit had type IIb fibres. However, the authors emphasized that their material is limited because of the laborious techniques involved. Gydikov *et al.*[39] also reported one S, one FR and one FF group of motor units in man but their techniques cannot be evaluated so readily.

The axonal conduction properties of single human motor units

Methods

Electromyographic recording techniques have been useful for determination of axonal conduction velocity. In conventional studies of α-motor axons, the conduction velocity of only the fastest axons (MCV) is obtained[47]. Using a collision technique described by Hopf[49] or F waves[77, 80], the conduction velocity of the slowest axons can also be calculated (*see also* Chapter 6). Studies of single motor units, however, require selective recordings.

In normal muscles the *latency* of a single motor unit potential, after electrical nerve stimulation, can be measured for those motor units whose axons happen to be located so close to the electrode that they are activated at a low stimulus voltage without interference activity from other motor units. Latency is probably related to axonal conduction velocity of normal motor units but no exact information about axonal conduction velocity is obtained. Furthermore 'sprouted' motor units with an abnormal distal delay also occur in normal muscles[36, 51], and there may be a bias towards selection of such motor units since their potentials are more easily identified in the electromyogram. This risk of error decreases, however, with conduction distance and may be insignificant using F-waves.

Measurements of *axonal conduction velocity* of single motor units require identification of their potentials after proximal and distal nerve stimulation. There is a limited chance of an axon being located close to both stimulating electrodes in nerves of muscles having a normal number of motor units. In normal man, preparations with a sufficiently reduced number of motor units can be obtained in the following two ways. First, repeated lesions of terminal nerve twigs and consequent collateral sprouting decrease the number of motor units and increase muscle fibre density in the remaining ones[8]. Axonal conduction velocity in segments proximal to the induced lesions can then be studied without difficulty (*Figure 2.3*). However, a potential source of error is that distal nerve lesions may affect conduction velocity within proximal parts of these axons. Secondly, a few motor units in the short toe extensor muscle[60] and in the interosseus muscles of the hand[62] may be innervated by accessory nerves. After blockade of the main motor nerve with lidocaine (lignocaine), high selectivity in electromyographic recordings can easily be obtained[8]. A source of error involved

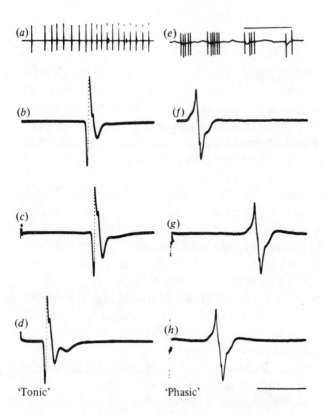

Figure 2.3 The axonal conduction velocity of one 'tonic' and one 'phasic' short toe extensor unit in a subject with previous lesions to the terminal nerve twigs distal to the stimulation points and consequent collateral sprouting. (*a*) and (*e*) attempts at continuous voluntary discharge. Time bar in (*a*) and (*e*) 100 ms. (*b*) and (*f*) test unit potential with voluntary contraction. (*c*) and (*g*) proximal supramaximal nerve stimulation. (*d*) and (*h*) distal stimulation. Time bar in (*b*), (*c*), (*d*) and (*f*), (*g*), (*h*) 10 ms. Distance between the stimulation points 38 cm. Latency difference 10 ms, i.e. axonal conduction velocity 38 m/s for the 'tonic' motor unit. Latency difference 7.5 ms and conduction velocity 51 m/s for the 'phasic' motor unit. (From Borg, Grimby and Hannerz[8], courtesy of the Editor and publisher, *Journal of Physiology*)

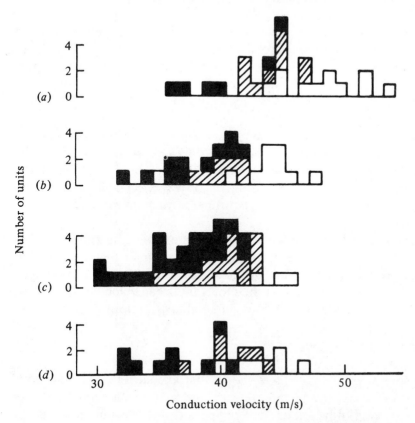

Figure 2.4 Axonal conduction velocities and voluntary discharge properties of 120 short toe extensor motor units. (*a*), (*b*) and (*c*) are three subjects with previous mechanical lesions to the terminal nerve twigs distal to the stimulation points and consequent collateral sprouting. (*d*) is 10 subjects with accessory nerve and main nerve blocked with lidocaine. 'Phasic' units (□), 'tonic' units (■), intermediates (▨). (From Borg, Grimby and Hannerz[8], courtesy of the Editor and publisher, *Journal of Physiology*)

in this type of preparation is that the exact length of the accessory nerves is not known. In the short toe extensor, there was good agreement between axonal conduction velocities obtained after collateral sprouting and those obtained after blockade of the main motor nerve (*Figure 2.4*) indicating that errors induced, being different for the two preparations, were of minor importance[8].

Axonal conduction velocity

Experiments on animals have shown that different α-motor axons to any one muscle have different conduction velocities[13, 14, 26, 63, 90]. In cats, velocities have been found to vary from 50 to 90 m/s (with most axons falling between 60 and 80 m/s) in the soleus[63], and from 50 to 110 m/s (with most axons falling between 80 and 100 m/s) in the gastrocnemius[90].

Hopf, in the first study to use collision techniques, found a minimum axonal conduction velocity in man only 4–7 m/s lower than the maximum velocity in the ulnar nerve[49]. After modifications of the Hopf technique, as well as using the F-wave, Shahani *et al.*[80] and Schiller, Stålberg and Hynninen[77] found a range more in accordance with that in the cat.

Only one study of conduction velocities of single human axons has been published[8] and some of its findings are summarized in *Figure 2.4*. Axonal conduction velocities of short toe extensor motor units ranged from 30 to 55 m/s. About half the motor units had velocities from 40 to 45 m/s and there was no obvious bimodal distribution.

Axonal refractory period

Experiments on animals have shown that axonal refractory period is related to axonal conduction velocity. In man, when axonal conduction velocity is known, the refractory period of single human axons can be calculated using highly selective electromyographic recordings and Hopf's collision technique[49]. Under normal conditions the refractory period of an axon, at stimulus strength 10 per cent above its threshold, was 1.5–2 ms and there was an inverse relation to its conduction velocity[10]. Under most pathological conditions this relation remained, but there were pathological states where the refractory period was more affected than the conduction velocity and vice versa.

Voluntary discharge properties of single human motor units

Methods

Only electromyographic techniques have been found useful for studies of single motor unit activity during voluntary contraction in man. Recordings from single α-axons in motor nerves have only been possible during curarization when there was no interference from activity in muscle afferents[30]. Recordings from anterior roots or horns are impossible in man.

However, electromyographic single motor unit studies in normal muscles are limited by the interference activity from other motor units and by the displacement of the recording electrode. Technical problems are least in studies of tonic isometric contraction since electrode location can be continuously adjusted, enabling highly

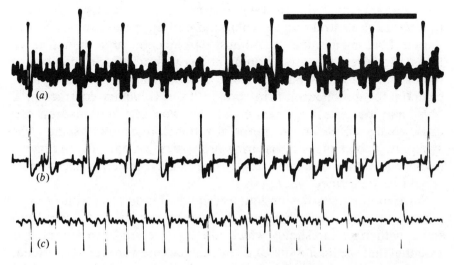

Figure 2.5 Three anterior tibial motor units discharging maximum sustained contraction. They fired seven times (*a*), 12 times (*b*) and 15 times (*c*) in 250 ms, i.e. at about 30 Hz (*a*), 50 Hz (*b*) and 60 Hz (*c*). Time bar 100 ms. (From Hannerz[42], courtesy of the Editor and publisher, *Acta Physiologica Scandinavica*)

selective electrodes, sensitive to displacement, to be used. Using single fibre electrodes contractions up to 30 per cent of the maximal muscle force can be studied[86]. Using a bipolar recording from two small electrode surfaces with a small interelectrode distance, single motor unit potentials can sometimes be followed up to 50–75 per cent of maximal muscle force[2, 3]. Using insulated wire electrodes in which small holes in the insulation have been made by an electric spark, equipped with a hook for fixation in the muscle, single motor unit potentials can sometimes be followed up to 100 per cent of maximal muscle force[41] (*Figure 2.5*).

Single motor unit studies during maximum phasic voluntary effort are difficult to interpret in normal muscles because each motor unit fires about 10 times in 100 ms, the different motor units tend to be synchronized, and because electrode displacement cannot be avoided with sudden maximal contraction of muscle, particularly under isotonic conditions. Systematic studies of phasic contraction require preparations with a reduced number of motor units as described above and illustrated in *Figure 2.3*. Such preparations are also required for fatigue studies where identification of single motor unit potentials, after supramaximal electrical nerve stimulation, is necessary in order to distinguish central fatigue from failure of electrical propagation at muscle fibre membrane, neuromuscular junction or terminal nerve twigs. However, the use of preparations with a reduced number of motor units may introduce errors. Inflow from muscle receptors, essential for motoneuron firing properties in voluntary contraction[40, 43, 91], may be disturbed. Lesions of the axon of a motoneuron can cause changes of its after-hyperpolarization[59], rejection of some of its synapses[7] and changes of its firing properties[23]. Control experiments involving normal muscles, e.g. using highly selective electrodes, should be performed where possible.

Since motor units having low thresholds during tonic contraction, which can more easily be studied, have properties that differ from those with high thresholds which are less accessible to study, it is essential that the limitations of the techniques used are clearly defined, that the quality of critical recordings is documented and that any bias in identification of one motor unit type is taken into consideration.

Firing rate and contraction time

In animal experiments, Eccles, Eccles and Lundberg[22] found that the after-hyperpolarization of a motoneuron, which tends to limit its maximum firing rate, is related to contraction time of the muscle fibres it innervates. Sréter *et al.*[83] showed that contractile properties of muscle fibres can be altered by long-term artificial stimulation of their motoneurons at particular rates. Lömo[61] has also altered contractile properties of denervated muscle fibres by stimulation. Thus the stimulation pattern influences contractile properties of muscle fibres.

The *minimum rates* for continuous firing in maintained voluntary contraction have been studied extensively since Adrian and Bronk[1]. Several authors[5, 71, 78, 79, 82] showed that low threshold motor units have minimum rates below 10 Hz, while motor units with higher thresholds have higher minimum rates. Tokizane and Shimazu[89] distinguished two groups of motor units, one with a minimum rate below 10 Hz, another with a minimum rate of about 15 Hz. However, later studies[42, 66, 72, 86] have not reproduced this finding but rather show a continuum of minimum rates from below 10 Hz up to above 30 Hz. Whether there is a bimodal or unimodal distribution of minimum rates cannot be decided because of selection bias involved in the use of electromyographic techniques.

Studies based on averaging techniques for determining contraction time[65] indicate that voluntary firing intervals and contraction time of individual motor units are matched, so that with slowly increasing voluntary effort a motor unit starts firing at regular intervals about the same time as its muscle fibres start fusing[37].

The literature on *maximum rates* during voluntary contraction in man is confusing due to differing periods of time used for calculation of firing rate; insufficient control of whether maximal tension within the muscle is actually attained voluntarily; and heterogeneity of motor units. Maximal muscle tension (defined as the tension obtained with electrical tetanization of the muscle) can only be maintained voluntarily for a period of time ranging from a few hundred milliseconds to a few seconds[38]. Obviously the maximal voluntary firing rates must be calculated from a limited number of discharges. On the other hand, quite misleading values are obtained if calculations are based on the shortest interval found, e.g. double discharges. Most human extremity muscles do not develop maximal tension with electrical tetanization below a rate of 50 Hz; this electrically evoked tension can also be attained voluntarily[6, 38, 64]. Thus, certain fast twitch motor units must have a maximal voluntary firing rate of 50 Hz or more. However, the longest contraction time in a muscle is more than double the shortest one (*see* p. 6) and 20 Hz should be sufficient for full fusion of certain slow twitch units.

A few studies of voluntary firing rates of single motor units have been made at maximal muscle tension. These indicate a range from about 30 to 65 Hz in anterior tibial muscle[42] as well as in short toe extensor muscle[36, 37] calculated on the basis of the maximal number of discharges within 250 ms (*Figure 2.5*). In these two muscles, maximal tension is attained with 50 Hz electrical tetanization and contraction times range from about 30 to 100 ms (*see* p. 6). With maximal voluntary effort each motor unit appears to fire at a slightly higher rate than that required for full fusion.

Recruitment and increase in frequency as mechanisms for increased tension

Tension can be increased not only by activation of new motor units – 'recruitment' – but also, since twitch tension is only about 20 per cent of tetanic tension, by an increase in firing frequency – 'frequency coding'[1]. The relative roles of recruitment and frequency coding in voluntary contraction have been discussed[1, 5, 15, 42, 67]. Some indications can be obtained from the basis of the distribution of contraction times (*see* p. 6) and the following findings: all participating motor units fire at about the same rate in weak or moderate tonic voluntary contractions; a motor unit is recruited when its minimum rate is attained by previously recruited motor units; differences in firing rate appear only with strong sustained contraction or phasic contraction[5, 15, 42, 78, 79, 87].Milner-Brown, Stein and Yemm[67] found evidence of recruitment mainly at low tension and concluded that frequency coding was the major mechanism at high tensions. Clamann[15], however, found recruitment up to 75 per cent and Hannerz[42] occasionally up to 90 per cent of maximal tension. Finally it must be emphasized that certain motor units have moderately high thresholds when the subject is thoroughly rested but very high thresholds after repeated prolonged contractions (*see* p. 22). The role of recruitment at high tensions depends on the level of fatigue[38, 42].

Central fatigue. 'Tonic' and 'phasic' motor units

There are many animal studies of fatigue of the peripheral mechanisms on artificial stimulation of the motoneuron or muscle fibres, but none of central fatigue with activation of motoneurons from supraspinal centres. Granit[33, 34] bases the terms 'tonic' and 'phasic' motor units on their response to tetanization of Ia afferents.

During maintained maximal voluntary effort in man, tension as well as electromyographic activity decrease[38, 50, 64, 75]. Under experimental conditions similar to those which might occur in everyday life, superimposed tetanization of the muscle nerve increases both tension and electrical activity, i.e. loss of tension is partially due to insufficient motoneuron activation[38, 50, 75]. By means of extraordinary motivation and training, however, tension response to superimposed stimulation may be eliminated while the increase in electrical response remains[64] even though some decrease is reported[84], i.e. the full capacity of the muscle may be used in spite of decreased motoneuron firing. The most likely explanation of the findings on extraordinary voluntary drive would be fatigue of the contractile mechanisms so that some motor units no longer produce significant tension and others no longer need high stimulation rates to fuse because of prolonged relaxation time.

Central fatigue of single anterior tibial and short toe extensor motor units during prolonged maximal voluntary effort has been studied in ordinarily motivated and trained subjects using superimposed supra-maximal electrical nerve stimulation to minimize confusion between central fatigue and failure of the peripheral electrical propagation[38]. All motor units fired, at rates ranging from 30 to 65 Hz, as long as voluntary effort resulted in maximal tension of the muscle (defined as the tension evoked by supramaximal tetanization at 50 Hz superimposed on voluntary contraction).

Firing rates as well as proportion of firing motor units decreased as the percentage of maximal tension that could be voluntarily maintained decreased. Firing rates of 50 Hz, required for maximal tension in rested fast twitch motor units, could usually be maintained for less than a second. Certain motor units ceased to respond tonically to maintained voluntary effort after only a few seconds and thereafter responded mainly phasically to sudden increases of effort. The more protracted the contraction, the greater the proportion of such motor units (*Figures 2.6*). Motor units with a limited tonic capacity had

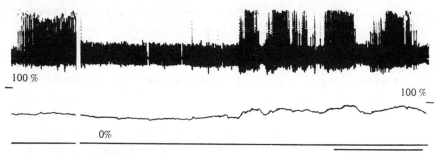

Figure 2.6 Firing properties of a 'phasic' short big toe extensor motor unit. After a long period of rest the unit fires tonically with moderate effort (*left*). After 30 seconds of maximal voluntary contraction, however, the unit does not respond to maintained maximal effort and fires only phasically on temporary increases of the voluntary drive (*right*). One hundred per cent of the maximal tension of the muscle obtained by supramaximal tetanization of the nerve to the muscle at 50 Hz immediately before the experiment (*left*) and after (*right*) is denoted. Note that the recruitment tension of the unit in relation to the maximal tension of the muscle is higher with fatigue than after rest. Time bar 10 s.

axonal conduction velocities[8] between 45 and 55 m/s and contraction times[37] between 40 and 60 ms. Thus, during prolonged voluntary effort, certain fast twitch muscle fibres are protected from exhaustion by central mechanisms (cf. also p. 22).

On the other hand, a steady state was reached after one or a few minutes when about half the remaining maximal tension could be maintained voluntarily and when the remaining active motor units had stable firing rates of 15–20 Hz. These continuously firing motor units had axonal conduction velocities[8] ranging from 30 to 45 m/s and contraction times[37] ranging from 60 to 90 ms. Those with the longest contraction times should fuse completely at firing rates noted above. Thus, during prolonged voluntary effort, certain slow twitch muscle fibres are not protected from exhaustion by central mechanisms. It must be emphasized, however, that there was a continuum of motor units between the two extremes described.

Size principle

In experiments on decerebrate cat, Henneman, Somjen and Carpenter[44, 45] found that the order of recruitment of motoneurons was very consistent so that a motoneuron with a small axon was recruited before a motoneuron with a large axon following a wide variety of inputs. They advanced the hypothesis that thresholds of motoneurons are determined by their size and that a particular cell receives the same proportion of its total input from each of the systems which is afferent to it. The term 'size' requires a comment. On the basis of physiological studies, axonal diameter has generally been considered to be an index of the size of the cell body. However, later morphological studies have shown only small differences to exist between the size of the cell bodies of motoneurons with small and large axons, though there is a large difference in dendrite volume and membrane surface (Kellerth, personal communication).

A great number of studies of maintained voluntary contraction in several different human muscles have shown an orderly recruitment of motor units[5, 28, 29, 42, 46, 66, 72, 78, 79, 82, 87] in accordance with the size principle. Desmedt and Godaux also studied isometric[19, 20] and isotonic[21] twitches of successively increasing magnitude and found the same recruitment order as in maintained contraction but a lower recruitment tension (*Figure 2.7*). However, twitch tension is only about 20 per cent of tetanic tension and with rapid acceleration the

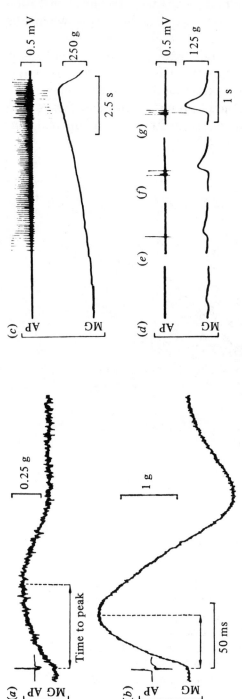

Figure 2.7 Recruitment order and force threshold of two motor units in the first interosseous muscle. Normal subject, 28 years old. The selective recording electrode allowed the action potentials of these two units to be clearly isolated from background activities. The isometric twitch of each unit was extracted by spike-triggered averaging of 512 discharge samples and presents a contraction time (time-to-peak) of 65 ms (*a*) and 39 ms (*b*) respectively. The peak forces are 0.3 g (*a*) and 1.5 g (*b*). The corresponding averaged action potentials, AP, are shown on the same time scale above the myogram MG. (*c*) Voluntary contraction of the interosseous muscle as the subject is tracking a slowly rising force ramp which reaches 300 g in about 10 s. The slower motor unit, illustrated in (*a*), starts discharging when the ramp force reaches 20 g while the other motor unit, which can easily be identified by its action potential waveform presenting a larger positive-going (downward) component (*see b*, 'AP'), only starts discharging later, when the ramp contraction reaches 280 g. (*d–g*) Ballistic voluntary contractions recorded during the same experiment. The isometric peak forces are 10 g (*d*), 20 g (*e*), 50 g (*f*) and 110 g (*g*) respectively. The contraction in (*e*) just exceeds the ballistic force threshold of the slower motor unit studied. The ballistic contraction in (*g*) also recruits the faster motor unit. (From Desmedt and Godaux[20], reprinted by permission from *Nature*, **267**, 717–719. Copyright © 1977 Macmillan Journals Limited.

recruitment tension of a motor unit varies with the level of fusion attained by motor units with lower thresholds even when the recruitment order is constant.

Quite a few studies have also shown that small, slowly conducting, and slowly contracting motor units are usually recruited before large, rapidly conducting, and rapidly contracting units, in accordance with the size principle. Freund, Wita and Sprung[28] found that motor units with low thresholds for maintained voluntary contraction had long

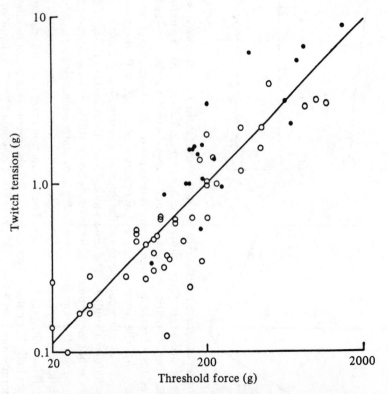

Figure 2.8 Twitch tensions produced by single motor units in one subject as a function of the force at which the motor units were recruited. (●) Measurements from single experiments in different subjects. (○) Measurements in a number of experiments in the same subject. The computed best-fitting straight line shown on this log–log plot had a slope close to unity, indicating a nearly linear relation between these two variables. From Milner-Brown, Stein and Yemm[66], courtesy of the Editor and publisher, *Journal of Physiology*)

latencies with electrical nerve stimulation indicating low axonal conduction velocity, while high threshold units had short latency indicating high conduction velocity. Milner-Brown, Stein and Yemm[66] found that a motor unit with a lower twitch tension was recruited before one with a higher tension in maintained voluntary contractions, i.e. an organization optimal for regulation of strength (*Figure 2.8*). Stålberg also found larger EMG potentials for high threshold than for low threshold units, using the so-called Macro EMG technique (personal communication). Milner-Brown *et al.*[66] found a relationship between threshold and contraction time in maintained voluntary contractions, as did Desmedt and Godaux[20] in twitch contractions.

Flexibility of recruitment order

As mentioned above, the size principle implies that each motoneuron receives the same proportion of its total input from each of the systems which are afferent to it. However, in the cat, there are great differences in synaptic distribution between motoneurons innervating slow and fast twitch muscle fibres[17,53,54]. There are also animal experiments defining inputs which result in predominant facilitation of fast twitch motor units[18,48,52,56]. Whether this alternative recruitment has any functional significance is in question[52]. However, if a cat's paw is suddenly wet the animal shakes it at 20 Hz to get it dry (unpublished observation). Motor units with contraction times above 25 ms, i.e. the whole slow twitch population, counteract 20 Hz alternating movements.

In human voluntary contraction considerable instability of recruitment order appears in abnormal states[35]. The recruitment order in tonic voluntary contraction in normal man can be changed by blockade of the afferent inflow[43]. Stephens, Garnett and Buller[31a,85] showed that the recruitment order of single motor units in the first interosseous muscle can be markedly changed simply by electrical stimulation of cutaneous afferents from the index finger in normal man.

The authors have found flexibility of the recruitment order with a change in mode of voluntary contraction[36,37,38,42]. Motor units with apparently unlimited tonic discharge, having low axonal conduction velocities, were compared with motor units with mainly phasic discharge during fatigue, having high axonal conduction velocities thus conforming with the experiments of Henneman, Somjen and Carpenter[44,45]. The authors concentrated on prolonged contraction, in which motor units with high axonal conduction velocities and low resistance to fatigue should be protected, and on rapidly reversed movements in which motor units with high axonal conduction velocities and short contraction times should, from a teleological viewpoint, be preferentially used.

In *prolonged voluntary contraction* the tension at which 'tonic' motor units were recruited remained constant or decreased with decreased maximal muscle tension (defined as the tension evoked by supramaximal tetanization at 50 Hz). 'Phasic' motor units, however, had successively increasing recruitment tensions in relation to the remaining tension as shown in *Figure 2.7*. This finding can only partly be explained as a result of a selective peripheral fatigue of high threshold units[38]. The harder the muscle was driven, the greater was the proportion of such 'adapting' motor units. Simultaneous recordings of one 'tonic' and one 'phasic' motor unit showed the 'phasic' motor unit was recruited after the 'tonic' one, but during prolonged contraction the 'phasic' motor unit could cease to fire when the 'tonic' motor unit fired at an increased rate.

Major changes of the recruitment were obtained on changing from maintained voluntary contraction to *rapidly reversed voluntary movement*. As mentioned above, a cat is capable of shaking its paw at 20 Hz and at such a high rate, contraction times of recruited motor units might be the limiting factor. Man is capable of waggling his toes at only 3 Hz and at such a low rate, central factors and not contraction time must be the limiting factor. However, human subjects occasionally succeed in terminating toe dorsiflexion within 100 ms after initiation and it is then that contraction times of recruited motor units may play a part. In a series of such twitches, selective or predominant activation of 'phasic' motor units occurred, i.e. the order of recruitment could be reversed. However, training was necessary before the subject was capable of such selective activation and in a series of trials only a minority were successful.

Reversal occurred only when great effort was used to elicit the twitch. In fact, when 'phasic' motor units fired in a burst, 'tonic' ones were more often inactive than when 'phasic' motor units fired just once. Inhibitory effects on small motoneurons may play some part in reversal. It is known from animal experiments that stimulation of motor cortex under certain conditions causes such an inhibition[74] and that Renshaw inhibition acts more strongly on tonic than on phasic[24] motoneurons. Reversal did not occur when the pre-existing level of facilitation of the motoneuron pool was high, e.g. with passive stretch of the muscle or subliminal voluntary facilitation. This fact, and the finding that reversal was favoured if contraction was aimed to stop immediately, indicate that 'programming' prior to contraction is of great importance in recruitment order.

Reversal of recruitment order was, however, also seen in other ballistic contractions than those stopped immediately after onset, provided that great effort was used to elicit the contraction (*Figure 2.9*). The discrepancy between the findings of Desmedt and Godaux

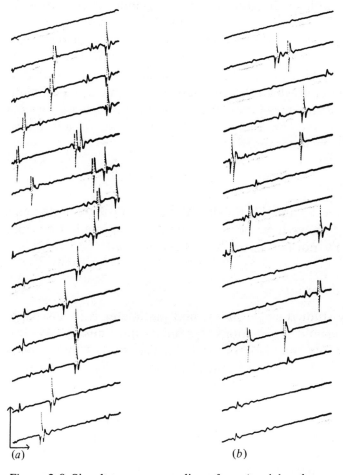

(a)   (b)

Figure 2.9 Simultaneous recording of one 'tonic' and one 'phasic' short big toe extensor motor unit. Continuous recording, each sweep 50 ms. The figure should be read as shown by the arrows. In slowly increasing isometric voluntary contraction (*a*) the 'tonic' motor unit fires at 20 Hz before the 'phasic' motor unit is recruited. In ballistic isotonic contraction (*b*), the 'phasic' motor unit fires selectively for the first 150 ms

illustrated in *Figure 2.7* and those illustrated in *Figure 2.9* may be due to differences in effort, 'programming' and the fact that they mainly studied motor units with thresholds below 30 per cent while the authors studied the mutual recruitment order of motor units with thresholds up to 90 per cent.

To conclude, it is generally agreed that most inputs are organized so that motor units with small axons, low tension, long contraction time and high resistance to fatigue are recruited before motor units with large axons, high tension, short contraction time and poor resistance to fatigue, but there *are* synaptic mechanisms for reversal of recruitment order. However, no one yet has found, or been able to study, any situation in which the alternative recruitment is systematically used. New techniques permitting studies of subjects performing athletic exercises may be required before the role of alternative recruitment can be determined.

Pathological states

More sophisticated techniques for the physiological single motor unit studies described above have been developed during the last decade, but so far mainly normal states have been studied.

Central motor disorders

The most easily studied single motor unit parameter is its discharge pattern with threshold contractions (*see* 'minimum rates', p. 14–15), and a considerable number of pathological studies have been published[2, 27, 73, 79, 93]. Studies of central motor disorders are the ones with greatest potential clinical value since peripheral disorders are already so accessible to electrophysiological study. Freund and Wita[27] found a decreased ability of motoneurons to produce constant intervals between discharges in almost any central motor disorder. Andreassen[2] and Andreassen and Rosenfalck[4] as well as Young and Shahani[92] used inconstancy of discharge intervals to analyse spasticity. Young and Shahani[93] also found different activation patterns of single motor units in different types of tremor. However, as yet only Petajan, Jarcho and Thurman[73] have reported a clinical implication. They found defective single motor unit control in relatives of patients with Huntington's chorea and suggested that such evaluation may constitute a valid presymptomatic test. (For further discussion, *see also* Chapter 9, this volume.)

Neuromuscular disorders

As mentioned above, motor units with a low threshold for maintained voluntary contraction have longer contraction times, lower twitch tension, better resistance to fatigue, smaller potentials and lower axonal conduction velocity than motor units with high threshold. Most probably there are also other electrophysiological differences. It must be emphasized that in normal muscles only low threshold units are available for systematic study using conventional electromyographic techniques, and normal values for action potential characteristics are obtained from such motor units. In abnormal muscles without a major reduction in the number of motor units, mainly low threshold units are studied here also, i.e. available normal values are sufficient but pathology restricted to high threshold units is not so easily detected. In abnormal muscles with a major reduction in motor units or a major increase in fibre density of the remaining motor units, high threshold units are also studied and a risk of error exists because there are no normal values for these action potential characteristics.

It would be advantageous to relate electromyographic findings to the original motor unit type. However, there is no motor unit parameter which can safely be said to be unaffected by the pathological process thus preventing its use in classification[9]. Motoneuron firing patterns are dependent on proprioceptive inflow[40, 43, 91] and are disturbed in neuromuscular disease[9]. Contraction time is dependent on the motoneuron firing pattern[61, 83]. Twitch tension is altered by disease and by compensatory collateral sprouting[68]. Axonal conduction velocity decreases in most neuropathies and only high axonal conduction velocities can be used to indicate that a unit was originally a high threshold unit.

Normal values for potentials of high threshold motor units could be obtained from muscles with an accessory innervation where a major reduction in the number of motor units can be attained by blocking the main nerve to the muscle. However, collecting a statistically representative number of motor units would be laborious.

Summary

It is known how the motor units of a normal muscle are differentiated as regards histological and histochemical properties, contraction time, tension, fatigue, axonal conduction velocity and voluntary discharge properties. It is not yet known, however, how these parameters are influenced by various pathological processes.

References

1 ADRIAN, E. D. and BRONK, D. W. The discharge of impulses in motor nerve fibres. Part II. The frequency of discharge in reflex and voluntary contractions. *Journal of Physiology*, **67**, 131–151 (1929)

2 ANDREASSEN, S. Single motor unit recording. In *Spasticity: Disordered Motor Control*, edited by R. G. Feldman, R. R. Young, and W. P. Koella, 205–218. Chicago, Year Book Medical Publishers (1980)

3 ANDREASSEN, S. and ROSENFALCK, A. Recording from a single motor unit during strong effort. *Electroencephalography and Clinical Neurophysiology*, **43**, 593 (1977)

4 ANDREASSEN, S. and ROSENFALCK, A. Impaired regulation of the firing pattern of single motor units. *Muscle and Nerve*, **1**, 416–418 (1978)

5 BIGLAND, B. and LIPPOLD, O. C. J. Motor unit activity in the voluntary contraction of human muscle. *Journal of Physiology*, **125**, 322–335 (1954)

6 BIGLAND-RITCHIE, B., JONES, D. A. and WOODS, J. J. Excitation frequency and muscle fatigue: Electrical responses during human voluntary and stimulated contractions. *Experimental Neurology*, **64**, 414–427 (1979)

7 BLINZINGER, K. and KREUTZBERG, G. Displacement of synaptic terminals from regenerating motoneurons by microglial cell. *Zeitschrift für Zellforschung*, **85**, 145–157 (1968)

8 BORG, J., GRIMBY, L. and HANNERZ, J. Axonal conduction velocity and voluntary discharge properties of individual short toe extensor motor units in man. *Journal of Physiology*, **277**, 143–152 (1978)

9 BORG, J., GRIMBY, L. and HANNERZ, J. Motor neuron firing range, axonal conduction velocity and muscle fiber histochemistry in neuromuscular diseases. *Muscle and Nerve*, **2**, 423–430 (1979)

10 BORG, J. Axonal refractory period of single short toe extensor motor units in man. *Journal of Neurology, Neurosurgery and Psychiatry*, **43**, 917–924 (1980)

11 BUCHTHAL, F. and SCHMALBRUCH, H. Contraction times and fibre types in intact human muscle. *Acta Physiologica Scandinavica*, **79**, 435–452 (1970)

12 BURKE, D., SKUSE, N. F. and LETHLEAN, A. K. Isometric contraction of the abductor digiti minimi muscle in man. *Journal of Neurology, Neurosurgery and Psychiatry*, **37**, 825–834 (1974)

13 BURKE, R. E. Motor unit types of cat triceps surae muscle. Journal of Physiology, **193**, 141–160 (1967)

14 BURKE, R. E., LEVINE, D. N., TSAIRIS, P. and ZAJAC, F. E. Physiological types and histochemical profiles of motor units in the cat gastrocnemius. *Journal of Physiology*, **234**, 723–748 (1973)

15 CLAMANN, H. P. Activity of single motor units during isometric tension. *Neurology* (Minneapolis), **20**, 254–260 (1970)

16 CLOSE, R. Properties of motor units in fast and slow skeletal muscles of the rat. *Journal of Physiology*, **193**, 45–55 (1967)

17 CONRADI, S., KELLERTH, J-O., BERTHOLD, C.-H. and HAMMARBERG, C. Electron microscopic studies of serially sectioned cat spinal α-motoneurons. *Journal of Comparative Neurology*, **184**, 769–782 (1979)

18 CREED, R. S., DENNY-BROWN, D., ECCLES, J. C., LIDDEL, E. G. T. and SHERRINGTON, C.S. *Reflex Activity of the Spinal Cord*. London, Humphrey Milford (1932)

19 DESMEDT, J. E. and GODAUX, E. Ballistic contractions in man: Characteristic recruitment pattern of single motor units of the tibialis anterior muscle. *Journal of Physiology*, **264**, 673–693 (1977)

20 DESMEDT, J. E. and GODAUX, E. Fast motor units are not preferentially activated in rapid voluntary contractions in man. *Nature*, **267**, 717–719 (1977)

21 DESMEDT, J. E. and GODAUX, E. Voluntary motor commands in human ballistic movements. *Annals of Neurology*, **5**, 415–421 (1979)

22 ECCLES, J. C., ECCLES, R. M. and LUNDBERG, A. Action potentials of alpha motoneurons supplying fast and slow muscles. *Journal of Physiology*, **142**, 461–478 (1958)

23 ECCLES, J. C., LIBET, B. and YOUNG, R. R. The behaviour of chromatolysed motoneurones studied by intracellular recording. *Journal of Physiology*, **143**, 11–40 (1958)

24 ECCLES, J. C., ECCLES, R. M., IGGO, A. and LUNDBERG, A. Electrophysiological investigations on Renshaw cells. *Journal of Physiology*, **159**, 461–478 (1961)

25 EDSTRÖM, L. and KUGELBERG, E. Histochemical composition, distribution of fibres and fatiguability of single motor units. *Journal of Neurology, Neurosurgery and Psychiatry*, **31**, 424–433 (1968)

26 ERLANGER, J. and GASSER, H. S. *Electrical Signs of Nervous Activity*, Philadelphia, University of Pennsylvania Press (1937)

27 FREUND, H. J. and WITA, C. W. Computeranalyse des Intervallmusters einzelner motorischer Einheiten bei Gesunden und Patienten mit supraspinalen motorischen Störungen. *Archiv für Psychiatrie und Nervenkrankheiten*, **214**, 56–71 (1971)

28 FREUND, H. J., WITA, C. W. and SPRUNG, C. Discharge properties and functional differentiation of single motor units in man. In *Neurophy-*

siological Studies in Man, edited by G. Somjen, Amsterdam, Excerpta Medica (1972)

29 FREUND, H. J., BÜDINGEN, H. J. and DIETZ, V. Activity of single motor units from human forearms muscles during voluntary isometric contractions. *Journal of Neurophysiology*, **38**, 933–946 (1975)

30 FREYSCHUSS, U. and KNUTSSON, E. Discharge patterns in motor nerve fibres during voluntary effort in man. *Acta Physiologica Scandinavica*, **83**, 278–279 (1971)

31 GARNETT, R. A. F., O'DONOVAN, M. J., STEPHENS, J. A. and TAYLOR A. Motor unit organization of human medial gastrocnemius. *Journal of Physiology*, **287**, 33–43 (1979)

31a GARNETT, R. and STEPHENS, J. A. Changes in the recruitment threshold of motor units produced by cutaneous stimulation in man. *Journal of Physiology*, **311**, 463–473 (1981)

32 GORDON, G. and PHILLIPS, C. G., Slow and rapid components in a flexor muscle. *Quarterly Journal of Experimental Neurology*, **38**, 35–54 (1953)

33 GRANIT, R. Reflex rebound by post-tetanic potentiation. Temporal summation-spasticity. *Journal of Physiology*, **131**, 32–51 (1956)

34 GRANIT, R., HENNATSCH, H. D. and STEG, G. Tonic and phasic ventral horn cells differentiated by post tetanic potentiation in cat extensors. *Acta Physiologica Scandinavica*, **37**, 114–126 (1956)

35 GRIMBY, L. and HANNERZ, J. Differences in recruitment order of motor units in phasic and tonic flexion reflex in 'spinal man'. *Journal of Neurology, Neurosurgery and Psychiatry*, **33**, 562–570 (1970)

36 GRIMBY, L. and HANNERZ, J. Firing rate and recruitment order of toe extensor motor units in different modes of voluntary contraction. *Journal of Physiology*, **264**, 865–879 (1977)

37 GRIMBY, L., HANNERZ, J. and HEDMAN, B. Contraction time and voluntary discharge properties of individual short toe extensor motor units in man. *Journal of Physiology*, **289**, 191–201 (1979)

38 GRIMBY, L., HANNERZ, J. and HEDMAN, B. Fatigue and voluntary discharge properties of single motor units in man. *Journal of Physiology* (In press)

39 GYDIKOV, A., DIMITROV, G., KOSAROV, D. and DIMITROVA, N. Functional differentiation of motor units in human opponens pollicis muscle. *Experimental Neurology*, **50**, 36–47 (1976)

40 HAGBARTH, K-E. and YOUNG, R. R. Participation of the stretch reflex in human physiological tremor. *Brain*, **102**, 509–526 (1979)

41 HANNERZ, J. An electrode for recording single motor unit activity during strong muscle contractions. *Electroencephalography and Clinical Neurophysiology*, **37**, 179–181 (1974)

42 HANNERZ, J. Discharge properties of motor units in relation to recruitment order in voluntary contraction. *Acta Physiologica Scandinavica*, **91**, 374–384 (1974)

43 HANNERZ, J. and GRIMBY, L. The afferent influence on the voluntary firing range of individual motor units in man. *Muscle and Nerve*, **2**, 414–422 (1979)

44 HENNEMAN, E., SOMJEN, G. and CARPENTER, D. O. Functional significance of cell size in spinal motoneurons. *Journal of Neurophysiology*, **28**, 560–580 (1965)

45 HENNEMAN, E., SOMJEN, G. and CARPENTER, D. O. Excitability and inhibitability of motoneurons of different sizes. *Journal of Neurophysiology*, **28**, 599–620 (1965)

46 HENNEMAN, E., SHAHANI, B. T. and YOUNG, R. R. Voluntary control of human motor units. *Neurology*, **25**, 368 (1975)

47 HODES, R., LARRABEE, M. G. and GERMAN, W. The human electromyogram in response to nerve stimulation and the conduction velocity of motor axons. *Archives of Neurology and Psychiatry*, **60**, 340–365 (1948)

48 HONGE, T., JANKOWSKA, E. and LUNDBERG, A. The rubrospinal tract. I. Effects on alpha motoneurons innervating hind limb muscles in cat. *Experimental Brain Research*, **7**, 344–364 (1969)

49 HOPF, H. C. Untersuchungen über die Unterschiede in der Leitgeschwindigkeit motorischer Nervenfasern beim Menschen. *Deutsche Zeitschrift für Nervenheilkunde*, **183**, 579–588 (1962)

50 IKAI, M., YABE, K. and ISCHII, K. Muskelkraft und muskuläre Ermüdung bei willkürlicher Anspannung und elektrischer Reizung des Muskels. *Sportarzt und Sportmedizin*, **5**, 197–204 (1967)

51 JENNEKENS, F. G. I., TOMLINSON, B. E. and WALTON, J. N. Histochemical aspects of five limb muscles in old age: an autopsy study. *Journal of Neurological Sciences*, **14**, 259–276 (1971)

52 KANDA, K., BURKE, R. E. and WALMSLEY B. Differential control of fast and slow twitch motor units in the decerebrate cat. *Experimental Brain Research*, **29**, 57–74 (1977)

53 KELLERTH, J-O., BERTHOLD, C-H. and CONRADI, S. Electron microscopic studies of serially sectioned cat spinal α-motoneurons. III. Motoneurons innervating fast-twitch (type FR) units of the gastrocnemius muscle. *Journal of Comparative Neurology*, **184**, 755–767 (1979)

54 KELLERTH, J-O., CONRADI, S. and BERTHOLD, C-H. (unpublished observations)

55 KERNELL, D. Input resistance, electrical excitability and size of ventral horn cells in the cat spinal cord. *Science*, **152**, 1637–1640 (1966)

56 KERNELL, D. and SJÖHOLM, H. Recruitment and firing rate modulation of motor unit tension in a small muscle of the cat's foot. *Brain Research*, **98**, 57–72 (1975)

57 KUGELBERG, E. Histochemical composition, contraction speed and fatiguability of rat soleus motor units. *Journal of the Neurological Sciences*, **20**, 177–198 (1973)

58 KUGELBERG, E. Adaptive transformation of rat soleus motor units during growth. *Journal of the Neurological Sciences*, **20**, 177–198 (1976)

59 KUNO, M., MIYATA, Y. and MUÑOZ-MARTINEZ, E. J. Differential reaction of fast and slow α-motoneurons to axotomy. *Journal of Physiology*, **240**, 725–739 (1974)

60 LAMBERT, E. H. The accessory deep peroneal nerve. A common variation in innervation of extensor digitorum brevis. *Neurology (Minneapolis)* **19**, 1169–1176 (1969)

61 LÖMO, T., WESTGAARD, R. H. and ENGELBRETSEN, L. Different stimulation patterns affect contractile properties of denervated red soleus muscle. In *Plasticity of Muscle*, edited by D. Pette, 297–310. Berlin, Walter de Gruyter (1980)

62 MARSDEN, C. D., MEADOWS, J. C. and MERTON, P. A. Isolated single motor units in human muscles and their rates of discharge during maximal voluntary effort. *Journal of Physiology*, **217**, 12–13 (1971)

63 McPHEDRAN, A. M., WUERKER, R. B. and HENNEMAN, E. Properties of motor units in a homogenous red muscle (soleus) of the cat. *Journal of Neurophysiology*, **28**, 71–84 (1965)

64 MERTON, P. A., Voluntary strength and fatigue. *Journal of Physiology*, **123**, 553–564 (1954)

65 MILNER-BROWN, H. S., STEIN, R. B. and YEMM, R. The contractile properties of human motor units during voluntary isometric contractions. *Journal of Physiology*, **228**, 285–306 (1973)

66 MILNER-BROWN, H. S., STEIN, R. B. and YEMM, R. The orderly recruitment of human motor units during voluntary isometric contractions. *Journal of Physiology*, **230**, 359–370 (1973)

67 MILNER-BROWN, H. S., STEIN, R. B. and YEMM, R. Changes in firing rate of human motor units during linearly changing voluntary contractions. *Journal of Physiology*, **230**, 371–390 (1973)

68 MILNER-BROWN, H. S., STEIN, R. B. and LEE, R. G. Contractile and electrical properties of human motor units in neuropathies and motor neurone disease. *Journal of Neurology, Neurosurgery and Psychiatry*, **37**, 670–676 (1974)

69 OLSON, C. B. and SWETT, C. P. Effect of prior activity on properties of different types of motor units. *Journal of Neurophysiology*, **34**, 1–16 (1971)

70 PAINTAL, A. S. Conduction in mammalian nerve fibres. In *New Developments in Electromyography and Clinical Neurophysiology*, edited by J. E. Desmedt, **2**, 19–41. Basel, S. Karger (1973)

71 PERSON, R. S. and KUDINA, L. P. Discharge frequency and discharge pattern of human motor units during voluntary contraction of muscle. *Electroencephalography and Clinical Neurophysiology*, **32**, 471–483 (1972)

72 PETAJAN, J. H. and PHILIP, B. A. Frequency control of motor unit action potentials. *Electroencephalography and Clinical Neurophysiology*, **27**, 66–72 (1969)

73 PETAJAN, J. H., JARCHO, L. W. and THURMAN, D. J. Motor unit control in Huntington's disease: A possible presymptomatic test. *Advances in Neurology*, **23**, 163–175 (1979)

74 PRESTON, J. B. and WHITLOCK, D. G. A comparison of motor cortex effects on slow and fast muscle innervations in the monkey. *Experimental Neurology*, **7**, 327–341 (1963)

75 REID, CH. The mechanism of voluntary muscular fatigue. *Quarterly Journal of Experimental Physiology*, **19**, 17–42 (1928)

76 REINKING, R. M., STEPHENS, J. A. and STUART, D. G. The motor units of cat medial gastrocnemius: Problem of their categorisation on the basis of mechanical properties. *Experimental Brain Research*, **23**, 301–313 (1975)

77 SCHILLER, H., STÅLBERG, E. and HYNNINEN, P. Can the range of F waves latencies be used as a measure of conduction velocity spectrum of α-axons? In *Abstracts, Sixth International Congress of Electromyography* (Stockholm, Sweden 1979), edited by A. Persson, *Acta Neurologica Scandinavica*, **60** (supplement 73), 269. Copenhagen, Munksgaard (1979)

78 SEYFFARTH, H. The behaviour of motor units in voluntary contraction. *Skrifter fra den norske videnskapsakademi* (Oslo), 1–63 (1940)

79 SEYFFARTH, H. The behaviour of motor units in healthy and paretic muscles in man. *Acta Psychiatrica* (Copenhagen), **16**, 79–109 (1941)

80 SHAHANI, B. T., POTTS, F., JUGUILON, A. and YOUNG, R. R. Maximal-minimal motor nerve conduction and F response in normal subjects and patients with ulnar compression neuropathies. *Muscle and Nerve*, **3**, 182 (1980)

81 SICA, R. E. P. and McCOMAS, A. J. Fast and slow twitch units in a human muscle. *Journal of Neurology, Neurosurgery and Psychiatry*, **34**, 113–120 (1971)

82 SMITH, O. Action potentials from single motor units in voluntary contraction *American Journal of Physiology*, **108**, 629–638 (1934)

83 SRÉTER, F. A., GERGELY, J., SALMONS, S. and ROMANUL, F. C. A. Synthesis by fast muscle of myosin light chain characteristics of slow muscle in response to long-term stimulation. *Nature (New Biology)*, **241**, 17–19 (1973)

84 STEPHENS, J. A. and TAYLOR, A. Fatigue of maintained voluntary muscle contraction in man. *Journal of Physiology*, **220**, 1–18 (1972)

85 STEPHENS, J. A. GARNETT, R. and BULLER, N. P. Reversal of recruitment order of single motor units produced by cutaneous stimulation during voluntary muscle contraction in man. *Nature*, **272**, 362–364 (1978)

86 STÅLBERG, E. and THIELE, B. Discharge patterns of motoneurones in humans. In *New Developments in Electromyography and Clinical Neurophysiology*, edited by J. E. Desmedt, **3**, 234–241. Basel, S. Karger (1973)

87 TANJI, J. and KATO, M. Recruitment of motor units in voluntary contraction of a finger muscle in man. *Experimental Neurology*, **40**, 759–770 (1973)

88 TAYLOR, A. and STEPHENS, J. A. Study of human motor unit contractions by controlled intramuscular microstimulation. *Brain Research*, **117**, 331–335 (1976)

89 TOKIZANE, T. and SHIMAZU, H. *Functional Differentiation of Human Skeletal Muscle*. 1–62. Tokyo, University of Tokyo Press (1964)

90 WUERKER, R. B., McPHEDRAN, A. M. and HENNEMAN, E. Properties of motor units in a heterogenous pale muscle (m. gastrocnemius) of the cat. *Journal of Neurophysiology*, **28**, 85–99 (1965)

91 YOUNG, R. R. and HAGBARTH, K-E. Physiological tremor enhanced by manoeuvres affecting the segmental stretch reflex. *Journal of Neurology, Neurosurgery and Psychiatry*, **43**, 248–256 (1980)

92 YOUNG, R. R. and SHAHANI, B. T. Analysis of single motor unit discharge patterns in different types of tremor. In *Contemporary Clinical Neurophysiology*, edited by W. A. Cobb and H. Van Duijn, 527–528. Amsterdam, Elsevier (1978)

93 YOUNG, R. R. and SHAHANI, B. T. Analysis of single motor unit discharge patterns in different types of tremor. In *Contemporary Clinical Neurophysiology*, edited by W. A. Cobb and H. Van Duijn, 527–528. Amsterdam, Elsevier (1978)

94 YOUNG R. R. and SHAHANI, B. T. A clinical neurophysiological analysis of single motor unit discharge patterns in spasticity. In *Spasticity: Disordered Motor Control*, edited by R. G. Feldman, R. R. Young and W. P. Koella, 219–231. Chicago, Year Book Medical Publishers (1980)

3

Quantitative EMG in nerve–muscle disorders

Jasper R. Daube

Clinical electromyography (EMG) records the electrical activity from a muscle by means of surface or needle electrodes. Diseases of anterior horn cell, peripheral nerve, neuromuscular junction, or muscle produce changes in the EMG, and the study of these changes aids in clinical diagnosis. This assessment has usually been subjective, made by a physician trained through apprenticeship to recognize the patterns seen in different clinical entities. However, as long as 30 years ago, some workers began to quantitate the changes in motor unit potentials in disease by photographing individual motor unit potentials recorded during minimal voluntary contraction and by manually measuring the amplitude, duration, and number of phases[87]. This technique was effective in distinguishing a wide variety of myopathies from neurogenic disorders[15, 16, 111]. However, the method is relatively time-consuming and has not come into widespread clinical use. In recent years, the expanding use of EMG and the increasing knowledge of disorders of nerve and muscle have made greater use of quantitative methods necessary to improve reliability and reproducibility[109], both among different investigators and at different times[27]. A number of methods of quantitation have been developed in recent years to meet these needs and have provided additional useful information not found with standard techniques. The value of quantitation has been highlighted by Buchthal[14] and Hausmanowa-Petrusewicz[47] and discussed by Pinelli[89].

Spontaneous activity

Fibrillation potentials, the spontaneous discharges occurring in non-innervated muscle fibres, have been quantitated by frequency and pattern of discharge[17, 22]. They have been characterized by their slow frequency and regularity, but there is no evidence that these parameters are of clinical significance. Irregular fibrillation potentials are uncommon and are not a sign of a specific disorder. The rate of discharge of fasciculation potentials also has been quantitated[53, 107]; the frequency of fasciculations in progressive diseases, such as motor neuron disease, is significantly slower than when they occur without accompanying disease, so-called benign fasciculations. However, the difference in frequency is not sufficient to be diagnostic in individual cases. The frequency of myotonic discharges that occur with various membrane disorders also has been measured, but no attempts at using the frequency to distinguish disorders with myotonic discharges have been reported[13]. Myokymic discharges are a form of iterative discharge in which groups of potentials recur in a regular fashion; they are seen in brain stem neoplasms, multiple sclerosis, radiation damage, inflammatory polyradiculopathies, and rarely in other isolated disorders. Quantitative measurement of the pattern and frequency of firing of myokymic discharges provides no help in distinguishing the cause[2]. The electrical characteristics of bizarre repetitive potentials have been quantitated with single fibre EMG and have been shown to have very low jitter, a feature suggesting a synchronized activation of many muscle fibres by direct ephaptic activation[102]. Quantitative measurements of bizarre repetitive potentials have not been reported to distinguish those seen in disorders of the lower motor neuron from those in muscle disorders. They remain, therefore, a nonspecific finding, common to various chronic diseases of nerve and muscle[30, 103].

A final form of spontaneous activity that has been quantitated, although to only a limited extent, is the activity associated with the syndromes of continuous muscle fibre activity, which have been referred to as neuromyotonia or neurotonia[112]. Most studies have described the features of neurotonia without using quantitation either to help define the mechanism of the discharges or to separate different causes.

Voluntary activity

The major application of quantitative EMG has been in the study of electrical activity generated with voluntary activation of muscle, a summation of electrical potentials of motor units[19]. With minimal contraction, only single motor unit potentials occur within the recording area of the needle electrode. As additional motor units are recruited, multiple potentials appear in the EMG signal, until with strong contractions superimposition of motor unit potentials from multiple motor units results in a dense pattern of electrical activity in which the individual discharges are no longer identifiable – the interference pattern.

The EMG signal, whether recorded by standard concentric needle electrode, mono- or bipolar concentric needle electrode, macro electrode, surface electrode, or single fibre needle electrode, is in a volume conductor and therefore may be affected by distant electrical generators[90] (*Figure 3.1*). In each case, the configuration of the

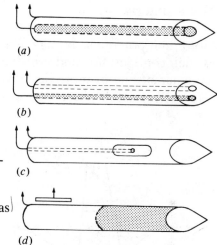

Figure 3.1 Recording electrodes for clinical electromyography. (*a*) Standard concentric; (*b*) bipolar concentric; (*c*) single fiber; and (*d*) macro. Shaded areas represent active electrode; unshaded areas represent reference electrode

recording electrode, its size, and the relative location of the active and the indifferent electrode enhance the activity near the active electrode while minimizing the activity at a distance. Each motor unit potential is generated by the muscle fibres in a motor unit within the recording area of the electrodes as they fire nearly synchronously[40, 41, 43]. The major negative components of motor unit potentials recorded with standard concentric or monopolar needle electrodes are produced by three to eight muscle fibres near the electrode[106].

Each type of the recording electrodes provides a somewhat different assessment of the changes in electrical activity in muscle with diseases of nerve and muscle. The standard concentric needle is most commonly used.

Single fibre EMG is a more recent development with less published data about the alterations in disease; but all reports on single fibre

EMG have been quantitative. Bipolar concentric electrodes have been applied primarily to quantitate firing patterns of motor unit potentials[3, 86] and only rarely to quantitation of motor unit potentials[4]. The macro electrode is a new development, and only a limited amount of information is available regarding its findings and clinical significance[99, 100]. Surface recordings have been used in estimating force[73], muscle fibre conduction velocity[114], local muscle fatigue (*see* Chapter 3) location of motor units[81, 82], and for kinesiologic studies (*see* Chapter 8).

Motor unit potentials

Motor unit potentials during voluntary activation can be characterized by their configuration and firing pattern[27]. The potential waveform is a sequence of one or more deviations from the baseline, called phases (*Figure 3.2*); each phase, the waveform between baseline crossings,

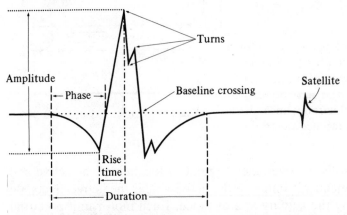

Figure 3.2 Schematic diagram of characteristics of motor unit potential. Each of the major parameters is indicated

has an amplitude, polarity, and sequence of occurrence. A reversal of polarity that does not cross the baseline during a phase is referred to as a turn. The time and the amplitude between turns define the slope or rate of rise of the potential. The slope of the major positive–negative inflection of a motor unit potential is primarily dependent on the distance of the nearest active muscle fibres from the recording electrode. A rise time of less than 500 μs indicates that the primary generator is less than 500 μm from the recording electrode. Individual

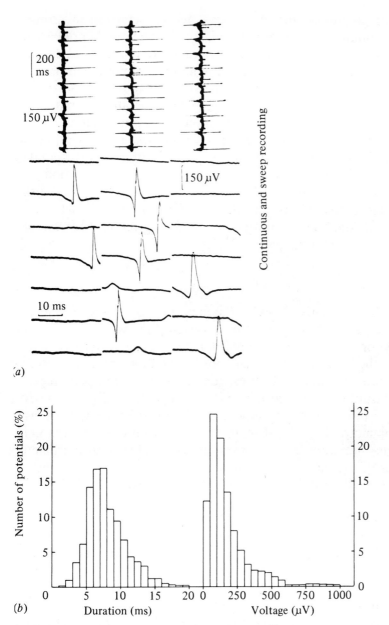

(a)

(b)

Figure 3.3(a) Single motor unit potentials recorded at slow and fast speeds. (*b*) Distribution of motor unit potential durations and amplitudes in normal human biceps muscle. (From Buchthal, F. *An Introduction to Electromyography*. Copenhagen, Gyldendalske Boghandel, Nordisk Forlag (1957), courtesy of the author and publisher)

motor unit potentials, therefore, may be characterized in terms of amplitude, timing and number of turns, timing and number of baseline crossings, slope of individual phases, duration of phases, and duration of the total potential (*Figure 3.3*). Since motor unit potentials have the same configuration during sequential discharges in normal muscle but vary in some diseases, stability of appearance is another parameter that may be quantitated in assessing motor unit potentials.

Each motor unit has its own typical threshold for activation and discharge frequency and pattern. As the effort and corresponding input to the anterior horn cell pool increase, each motor unit fires more rapidly and more motor units are recruited. The relationship between the thresholds of activation and the rates and patterns of firing of individual motor unit potentials during recruitment can also be used for their identification[20, 80, 86].

Quantitation

The goal of quantitative EMG is the identification of specific changes in electrical activity resulting from disease processes. Diseases may alter any one of the many determinants of the electrical signal, including the number of muscle fibres per unit area, diameter of muscle fibres, continuity of fibres, configuration of end-plate regions, character of transmission at the end-plate region, conduction in nerve terminals, number of motor units available for firing, firing patterns in individual motor units, and relative firing in different motor units. Pathologic alterations in any of these areas will change the parameters of the EMG signal.

The EMG is ordinarily assessed in one of two ways:

(1) evaluation of the amplitude, duration, configuration, and firing pattern of individual motor unit potentials; or
(2) evaluation of the interference pattern generated by a large number of the motor unit potentials.

EMG quantitation, especially automatic, has also used these two approaches. The most frequently used method is to isolate single motor unit potentials and measure changes in their parameters. The frequency components of the electrical activity during moderate or strong voluntary contraction have been studied by spectral analysis or by study of other parameters related to the frequency content in the signal.

Single motor unit potentials

Motor unit potentials can be readily identified and measured when only one is firing with minimal contraction, but often this recording situation is complicated by the repetitive occurrence of multiple potentials from other motor units represented within the recording area of the needle electrode. Various methods have been used to overcome this problem. Originally[15] one photographed a long enough sequence of motor unit potential discharges at standard amplification (100 µV/cm) to permit the visual identification of individual motor units by their recurrence. Manual measurements of 20 photographed motor unit potentials from muscles of normal subjects of different ages by Buchthal, Guld and Rosenfalck[15] provided extensive data that have proved to be of major value in testing for neuromuscular disease (*Table 3.1*). This technique applied to a wide range of diseases, has been reliable in distinguishing myopathies from neurogenic disorders[29, 35, 36, 61, 113] (*Figure 3.4*). The manual method has made this differentiation primarily on the basis of alterations in duration,

Table 3.1 Mean motor unit potential duration by patient age

Muscle	*Range of duration in normals (ms)*		
	Patient age (years)		
	5	*30*	*65*
Orbicularis oris	3.5–5.3	5.0–7.4	5.8–8.8
Masseter	5.0–7.4	6.6–9.8	6.7–10.1
Deltoid	7.4–11.0	9.8–14.6	12.2–18.4
Pectoralis	6.0–9.0	7.4–11.2	8.6–12.8
Biceps	6.4–9.6	7.9–11.9	10.0–15.0
Triceps	6.8–10.2	9.0–13.4	11.3–16.9
Extensor digitorum	5.5–8.3	7.4–11.0	9.2–13.8
First dorsal interosseous	6.8–10.2	8.5–12.7	9.8–14.6
Erector spinae	7.3–10.9	9.1–13.7	10.5–15.7
Vastus lateralis	8.6–12.8	10.7–16.1	12.3–18.5
Anterior tibial	7.5–11.3	9.8–14.8	12.4–18.6
Gastrocnemius	6.0–9.0	7.9–11.9	10.0–15.0

After Buchthal, Pinelli and Rosenfalck[16]

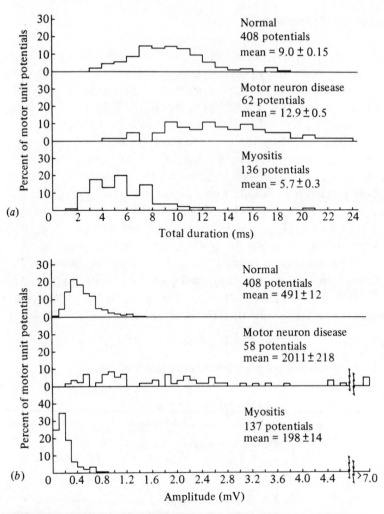

Figure 3.4 Distribution of duration (*a*) and amplitude, (*b*) of motor unit potentials in normal subjects and in patients with myopathy or neuropathy. Note that while mean values shift and long or short potentials are in excess, an overlap with normal remains

because amplitude is so much more variable. Random loss of muscle fibres from motor units in myopathies results in short-duration motor unit potentials; collateral sprouting after denervation in neurogenic disorders results in long-duration motor unit potentials. Loss of motor units, the primary change in a neuronal disease, is seen as poor recruitment, which has only rarely been quantitated[77].

Loss of synchronization of muscle fibre discharge, with slow conduction in nerve terminals or muscle fibres, dispersion of end-plate location, or longer nerve terminals, causes polyphasic potentials (more than four phases). Polyphasic motor unit potentials, which normally make up less than 10 per cent of potentials, are therefore increased in a number of disorders of nerve and muscle (a nonspecific finding) and do not help in identifying diseases, even when quantitated. The manual method not using signal-trigger and delay line is unable to recognize either 'satellite' potentials or the spike components in a motor unit potential that are isolated in time from the main components[62].

Accuracy and reliability of selection of a single motor unit potential, including late components, has been markedly enhanced in recent years by signal delay units[24, 25, 85, 98] which allow selection of a potential by amplitude and polarity criteria with superimposition of each recurrence (*Figure 3.5*). Comparison of these recurring potentials allows identification of a single motor unit by firing pattern and appearance. One can then assess stability and recognize variability of a recurrent motor unit potential with discharges. Photographic superimposition permits measurement of configurational parameters, including duration, amplitude, phases, turns and polarity. This method is most effective only when a single unit is firing; its effectiveness rapidly

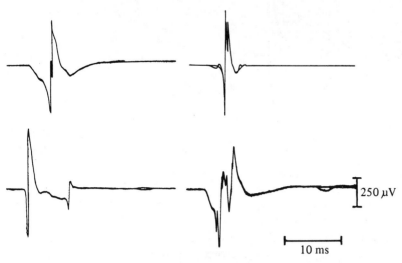

Figure 3.5 Single motor unit potentials superimposed with a signal delay unit permit more accurate identification and measurement of all components

deteriorates as more units are recruited[34]. The occurrence of multiple potentials with similar amplitudes makes selection of individual potentials difficult, but a combination amplitude–duration window can further enhance selection[5, 24]. These improvements in selection of motor unit potentials have increased speed and reliability but have not made more specific diagnosis possible[27]. Manual techniques, involving single motor unit measurement, do not provide a quantitative description of motor unit firing patterns or record high-threshold motor unit potentials.

An automated off-line interactive system basing motor unit potential identification on recurrence and measurement on subtraction of superimposed potentials has permitted study of motor units at higher frequencies, with a larger number of potentials present[91]. A faster on-line method combines recording with a 25 µm single fibre electrode with a standard recording surface; it facilitates selection of motor unit potentials during coactivation of many units[33, 66] (*Figure 3.6*) but has not been widely enough applied to assess its validity and accuracy.

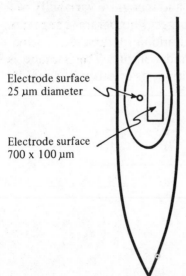

Electrode surface
25 µm diameter

Electrode surface
700 x 100 µm

Figure 3.6 Dual electrode for simultaneous recording from large and small surfaces. (After Stålberg and Trontelj[102])

However, it does allow averaging of other parameters, such as surface activity, twitch tensions and discharge patterns.

Selecting and photographing individual motor unit potentials, with or without a delay line, can be performed reliably without automation, but to improve accuracy and speed, the following three methods for automatic selection of single motor unit potentials have been used[11]: predetermined criterion, recurrence, and averaging.

Predetermined criterion

The simplest method of selecting individual potentials uses amplitude as the predetermined criterion[57, 65, 92, 93]. For example, in the system of Kopec and Hausmanowa-Petrusewicz[57], every period of electrical activity with a peak greater than a threshold value is considered a single motor unit potential and its duration, amplitude and number of phases are measured. When many motor units are active this method treats superimposed potentials as single potentials and measures a single motor unit potential many times, but nonetheless can reliably distinguish a myopathy from neurogenic disease. A variation of this method includes the additional criterion of rate of rise of potentials.

Recurrence

This approach automatically excludes potentials that are due to superimposition of multiple potentials by accepting only a potential that recurs with sufficient similarity to indicate that it is the discharge of a single motor unit[58, 76, 105]. An amplitude criterion has been added for initial selection of a period of electrical activity which is then compared with the next potential reaching the same amplitude. Comparisons of the two have been made by summed differences[58], least-squared differences[6, 7] or polarity reversals and baseline crossings[76]. If potentials are sufficiently similar, they are assumed to represent the same unit, and their amplitude, phases and duration are measured. If the second potential does not match, it is discarded and the search continues for an appropriate match. Similar techniques include rate of rise of maximal slope of the positive–negative inflection as a selection criterion[26]. Others select, by amplitude criteria, potentials that serve as templates for comparison with subsequent potentials by matched-filtering techniques[31].

Averaging

An amplitude or rate of rise criterion selects a potential, and any one that meets this criterion is arithmetically averaged[63, 69, 83]. The average potential is assumed to be the activity of a single motor unit potential even with surface recordings[72]. Other techniques use an amplitude–duration window or record the vector EMG of single motor units on the skin surface[45].

Each of these automated methods can distinguish neurogenic and myopathic disorders[4, 7, 10, 47, 58, 63, 75, 97, 104], but only infrequently can they add new information[62]. All methods focus on the most valuable parameter, potential duration, but different criteria are used to define duration. With manual measurement, one subjectively defines when the potential first leaves and finally returns to the baseline, *duration* being the interval between. With automatic methods, a threshold may be set and the potential is assumed to begin and end when the electrical activity rises above or falls below it for a specific period[6, 7, 57, 58, 64, 67, 76, 88]. In other automatic systems, either the operator selects the potential limits or sets the ratio of total duration to the duration of individual components. Amplitude, which is more variable because it is largely dependent on the distance between the recording electrode and the generating muscle fibres, has been used less than duration in manual measurement. However, when the rise time from maximal positive to negative inflection is less than 500 µs, amplitude can be useful. It may be measured either from baseline to peak or more commonly from peak to peak[6, 58]. Another method[57] summates the total negative-to-positive peaks within a motor unit potential. Clearly, each of these will give very different values and cannot be compared directly; each method involves determination of its own normal values. A third parameter, polarity change, has been measured as number of phases (baseline crossings minus one[15, 16, 76]) or as number of turns (fixed amplitude change after potential reversal[6, 57]). Multivariate analysis using all these parameters may further improve accuracy of diagnosis[10].

Other parameters of importance in motor unit characterization, such as variability of the motor unit potential during its recurrence or patterns of firing[77], are not presently being measured. The off-line method of motor unit potential subtraction provides information about firing pattern[91], but this and other techniques do not assess recruitment. The area over which a motor unit potential can be recorded with a sharp inflection (rise time less than 500 µs) has been assessed quantitatively in only a few studies[18], but has been of value in identifying neurogenic disorders.

Quantitation of the interference pattern

Another general method for quantitating EMG, assessment of the interference pattern, also has been in use for many years[94, 111], but with limited success[32, 42]. Many such methods have been tried on the basis of theoretical analyses similar to those used in EEG[28, 59, 93]. The interference pattern is the summation of activity of single muscle fibres[68], but the random superimposition of many of them[70, 71] effectively obscures individual motor unit potentials. Interference quantitation techniques are, therefore, based on analysis of features related to frequency of the waveforms or their components. The simplest measurement, that of total amplitude, has not been used alone in clinical diagnostic EMG, although it has been the basis of many attempts to assess activity in a muscle from surface recordings[23, 73, 78]. Surface recordings in assessment of force generated by a muscle have more commonly used integration of the signal[74, 79, 88]. Only one study integrated surface recordings to identify abnormalities due to disease, but without sufficient sensitivity to be of diagnostic value[67].

Interference pattern analysis with needle electrodes has been almost entirely with standard concentric or monopolar electrodes using turns or baseline crossings in some combination with amplitude. Willison's[113] method has been most widely applied. Initial studies used manual measurements but electronic devices have been developed to

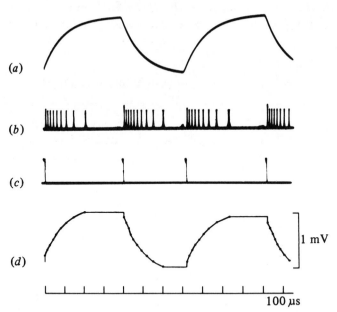

Figure 3.7 Conversion of a calibration signal to pulse trains by Willison's method[113]. One train represents amplitude; the other represents reversal of direction of signal (turns). (*a*) Analogue input; (*b*) amplitude pulses; (*c*) turns pulses; and (*d*) analogue calculated from (*a*) and (*b*)

do so more rapidly and accurately[48, 49, 50]. Electrical waveforms are converted into two trains of pulses that are counted to characterize the signal. Amplitude is represented by one train of pulses produced for fixed voltage changes, usually 100 μV; more rapid voltage changes are seen as higher frequency trains of pulses (*Figure 3.7*). The other train defines the direction (positive or negative) of signals, a pulse occurring whenever the direction reverses. Different sites in a muscle are sampled during a constant load, and these are compared with normal values for subjects in the same age range with the same load (*Table 3.2*). The requirement of a constant load has made this method somewhat unwieldy for routine clinical use. It can identify neurogenic and myopathic disorders in a reproducible fashion that can be followed over time[49, 50, 95]. Similar methods with computerized techniques have confirmed the validity of this method[21, 46, 51, 52, 57, 108]. The turns per unit time can be related to the frequency of waveforms in the signal and are therefore related to the duration of individual waveforms (*see* Chapter 3). Analog estimates of this duration can provide an index that differentiates neural from muscle diseases[83, 84].

With each method, changes occur as the individual spike components of the contributing motor unit potentials become shorter or as

Table 3.2 Normal values for interference analysis by Willison's method*

Muscle	Biceps	Triceps	Vastus medialis	Tibialis anterior
Number of subjects	24	25	27	20
Age range (years)	26–75	22–76	20–78	26–78
Number of areas (mean)	17.1	16.6	18.1	16.9
Load (kg)	2	2	5	2
Amplitude (mV)				
Mean	0.35	0.46	0.33	0.45
SD	0.07	0.10	0.05	0.09
Frequency (per second)				
Mean	371	392	263	307
SD	89	89	73	43

*Modified from Hayward and Willison[49]

the motor unit potentials become polyphasic with short-duration components. They are, therefore, accurate in the presence of myopathies with short-duration or polyphasic potentials or of neuropathies with long-duration potentials, but could be misleading if the polyphasic potentials were the result of re-innervation in neural disease (*Figure 3.8*). The major drawback to their use has been the need to monitor the force exerted.

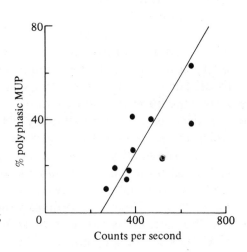

Figure 3.8 Comparison of percent polyphasic motor unit potentials measured by Buchthal's method[16] (single motor unit potential) and counts per second by Willison's method[113] (interference) in triceps muscles of 10 patients with various myopathies. (r = 0.77; slope = 6.31; intercept = 248.6)

Development of small computer systems for spectral analysis has re-opened the possibility of applying frequency analysis to the EMG signal[54] (*see further* Chapter 4). The summated EMG signal can be reproduced from the fast Fourier transforms of individual motor unit potentials when motor units are homogeneous[1], but accuracy with the heterogenous population of motor units in normal and abnormal human EMGs remains to be shown for surface recordings; most applications have been in physiologic studies[8, 44, 55, 56, 110]. Interpretation of spectral analysis is further complicated by the pattern of firing[60] (*see* Chapter 3) and type of electrodes[115] which alter the spectral components of the EMG signal. Variations of spectral analysis also have been applied to EMG; for instance, the recording of first and second derivatives of the interference pattern to assess the amount of high-frequency components[37, 38, 39]. Only Larsson's studies[64] have shown that frequency analysis can make the same distinctions between myopathy and neuropathy that arise from other methods and follow these changes during the course of a disease.

Single fibre electromyography

Single fibre EMG (SFEMG, *see further* Chapter 5) can record single muscle fibre action potentials of all types, including spontaneous activity such as fibrillation potentials and bizarre repetitive potentials[102]. Its principal clinical application has been in the recording of motor units activated by voluntary contraction. SFEMG enhances recording from a small number of muscle fibres near the electrode while suppressing the activity of more distant fibres by two means. First, a 500 Hz filter effectively eliminates contributions from fibres more than 0.5 mm distant, since intervening tissue acts as a low-pass filter, permitting only low frequencies to reach the recording electrode. Second, a small recording surface (25 µm), which reduces to one or two the number of muscle fibres in direct contact with the electrode and decreases to approximately 300 µm the effective distance over which the recordings from individual muscle fibres can be made.

The combination of these two factors permits recording from individual muscle fibres within 300 µm of the electrode as biphasic or triphasic potentials with a rise time of less than 300 µs and amplitudes up to 25 mV. Precise recordings from individual muscle fibres which can be accurately measured and quantitated constitute one of SFEMG's major advantages. The small size of the active recording electrode results in some disadvantages, especially the need for extremely precise localization and maintenance of the electrode in a specific location while a series of measurements is made. Reliable SFEMG is, therefore, highly dependent on the electromyographer's skill at manipulation of the needle electrode. This skill is much like that required for quantitation of motor unit potentials with standard concentric needle electrodes, and the electromyographer with the latter skill usually can readily perform SFEMG.

SFEMG recordings, derived from the same activity that comprises standard motor unit potentials, can be directly related to them, but include parameters not commonly assessed on standard needle electromyography: fibre density, jitter and blocking. Each is altered as standard motor unit potentials are, by various neuromuscular disorders and abnormalities can provide important clues in the identification of specific diseases.

An essential element in SFEMG is a method of isolating and displaying a series of sweeps from single potentials. This is most readily obtained with a trigger and signal delay unit, which was also later introduced for manual quantitation of motor unit potentials.

Single fibre potential measurement is facilitated by an automatic sweep counter because jitter measurements are made on a defined number of potentials.

Fibre density

Generally, in normal muscle, during mild voluntary activation, single fibre EMG will record an action potential from only one muscle fibre in a motor unit, with an amplitude exceeding 200 µV and with a rise time less than 300 µs. Such an action potential is generated by a muscle fibre within 300 µm from the recording electrodes. Approximately 60 percent of recording sites in normal muscle have such single potentials from one particular motor unit but the percentage varies with patient age and from muscle to muscle. At some locations, two single fibre potentials are recorded together, time locked to one another. Pairs of potentials are found at approximately 35 percent of electrode placements, while three or more time-locked potentials occur in the remaining small percentage of recording sites (*Figure 3.9*).

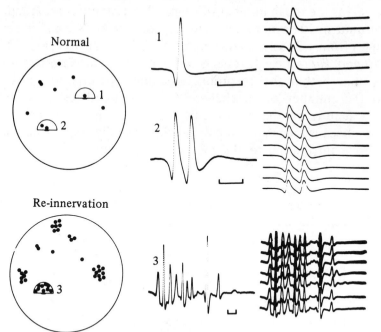

Figure 3.9 Single fibre EMG recordings with single, pairs, and multiple single fibre potentials recorded from one motor unit at one site. Time calibration 1 ms (From Stålberg and Trontelj[102], courtesy of the authors and publisher, *Single Fibre Electromyography*)

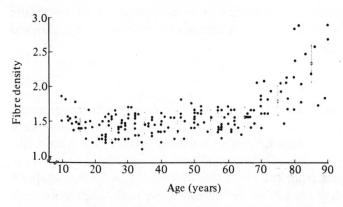

Figure 3.10 Fibre density in extensor digitorum communis muscle of persons of different ages. (From Stålberg and Trontelj[102], courtesy of the authors and publisher, *Single Fibre Electromyography*)

Fibre density is the mean number of single fibre potentials recorded from motor units in 20 or more different recording sites. Normal fibre density ranges from 1.3 to 1.8 in normal persons less than 70 years old (*Figure 3.10* and *Table 3.3*). It reflects the density of muscle fibres in one motor unit within the recording area and corresponds most directly to the number of notches seen on standard motor unit potentials, a feature of the motor unit potential sometimes called 'complexity', because each of these notches usually represents a separate fibre contributing to the motor unit potential.

Table 3.3 Normal fibre density values for single fibre EMG

Muscle	Fibre density (mean ± SD)		
	Patient age (years) 20–59	60–69	≥70
Extensor dig. communis	1.25–1.80 (1.48 ± 0.16)	1.25–1.90 (1.55 ± 0.14)	1.35–2.20 (1.78 ± 0.21)
Biceps	1.10–1.50 (1.30 ± 0.10)	1.20–1.50 (1.30 ± 0.10)	1.30–1.70 (1.50 ± 1.6)
Vastus lateralis	1.10–1.50 (1.30 ± 0.10)	1.30–1.70 (1.50 ± 0.10)	1.23–1.71 (1.48 ± 0.14)
Anterior tibial	1.20–2.0 (1.60 ± 0.20)	1.30–2.10 (1.70 ± 0.20)	No data

Fibre density will increase with any disorder that results in histologic grouping of muscle fibres. Grouping is most common in neurogenic disorders with re-innervation, and an increase in fibre density is, therefore, seen in any disorders of peripheral nerve or anterior horn cell. Density increase is particularly striking early during the course of re-innervation, when the differences in conduction along regenerating nerve terminals results in pronounced asynchrony of firing of newly re-innervated muscle fibres and in dispersion of the single fibre potentials. However, some grouping of muscle fibres also may be seen in myopathies as a result of fibre splitting or fibre regeneration after necrosis. Increases in fibre density, therefore, are also seen in a number of myopathies.

Jitter

When two or more single fibre potentials are recorded from a single motor unit, the interpotential interval between the two shows a small fluctuation referred to as jitter (*see* pp. 101–103).

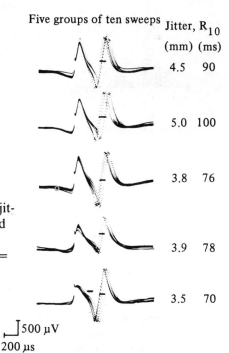

Five groups of ten sweeps

	Jitter, R_{10}	
	(mm)	(ms)
	4.5	90
	5.0	100
	3.8	76
	3.9	78
	3.5	70

Figure 3.11 Manual measurement of jitter by method of Stålberg, Ekstedt and Broman[101]. Mean R_{10} (range of 10) = 82.8 µs. Mean consecutive difference = $R_{10} \times 0.37 = 31.4$ µs

500 µV
200 µs

Jitter measures the variability of the interval between two single fibre potentials and this can be expressed as the standard deviation of the interpotential interval. Because occasionally there is a gradual change in the mean interpotential interval over time, jitter is more accurately measured using the mean consecutive difference (MCD):

$$MCD = \frac{|IPI_1 - IPI_2| + |IPI_2 - IPI_3| + \ldots + |IPI_{n-1} - IPI_n|}{n - 1}$$

in which IPI is the interpotential interval and n is the number of intervals measured.

The mean consecutive difference is calculated from 50 or more consecutive interpotential intervals, but it may also be derived from the mean-of-range in smaller groups by use of a conversion factor (*Figure 3.11*).

The normal muscle jitter, typically less than 50 μs, varies with age and muscle (*Figure 3.12*) (*Table 3.4*).

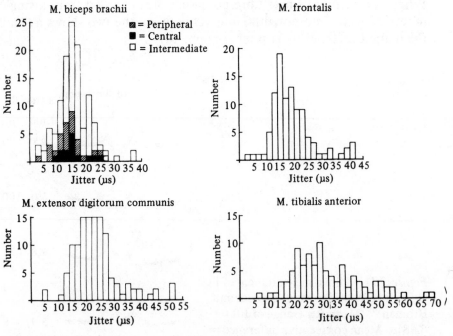

Figure 3.12 Jitter values in muscle fibre pairs in normal muscles. Biceps measurements include values from different sites in the muscle. (From Stålberg and Ekstedt, J. Single fibre EMG and microphysiology of the motor unit in normal and diseased human muscle. In *New Developments in Electromyography and Clinical Neurophysiology*, **1**, edited by J. E. Desmedt, 113–129. Basel, S. Karger (1973) courtesy of the authors and publisher)

Table 3.4 Normal jitter values (MCD) for single fibre EMG

Muscle	Range in μs (mean ± SD)		
	Patient age (years)		
	20–39	40–59	60–79
Extensor digitorum communis	16–34 (25.0 ± 4.2)	18–35 (26.3 ± 4.0)	25–43 (32.5 ± 5.6)
Deltoid	No data	19–35 (26.0 ± 4.0)	25–45 (35.0 ± 5.0)
Orbicularis oris	No data	18–38 (29.0 ± 5.0)	18–46 (32.0 ± 7.0)
Vastus lateralis	No data	25–46 (37.9 ± 5.7)	25–46 (37.9 ± 5.7)

In normal muscle, jitter is not identifiable with standard needle EMG but, if one records with a low frequency cut-off of 500 Hz and a sweep speed of 100 or 200 μs/cm, jitter can be identified with a standard concentric needle electrode[12] (*Figure 3.13*). Values of jitter using a standard concentric needle electrode are somewhat smaller than those recorded with a single fibre electrode.

Single fiber electrode   Standard concentric electrode

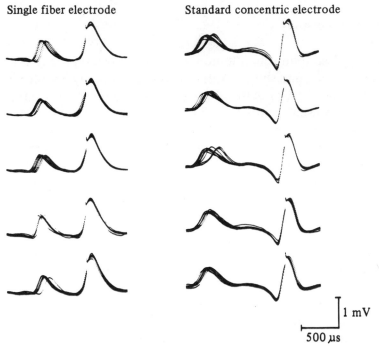

1 mV

500 μs

Figure 3.13 Jitter recordings in normal muscle with two types of electrode

The cause of the jitter, a variation in neuromuscular transmission time and its usefulness in detecting neuromuscular transmission disturbances is discussed in Chapter 5.

Blocking

In a normal muscle, an end-plate potential always reaches threshold and initiates a single fibre action potential; therefore, when multiple single fibre potentials are found, they occur with each discharge of the motor unit potential. However, if an end-plate potential does not reach threshold or if conduction fails in a nerve terminal, one or more single fibre potentials will be missing with some discharges of the motor unit. These potentials are blocked. Some normal elderly persons have occasional blocking in some muscles.

Blocking is most commonly seen in disorders such as myasthenia gravis[96, 102], and is evidence of a defect severe enough to be associated with weakness. It is also seen after re-innervation where the end-plate may be immature. Blocking is further discussed in Chapter 5.

Comparison of methods

Many authors describing quantitation of EMG have reported that their systems can distinguish neurogenic atrophies from myopathies in patients with clinically well-defined diseases, usually muscular dystrophy and spinal muscular atrophy. These systems make the same distinction that is usually readily made with subjective assessment, but they do so with improved speed and reproducibility of the quantitative measurement which has allowed more reliable serial assessment of change with disease as a patient is followed. Comparison has not shown clear superiority of one method over another, but suggests a combination of methods is needed for the greatest diagnostic accuracy[9, 14, 35, 74, 108]. In addition, all methods suffer from technical problems. Each technique depends heavily on monitoring by the electromyographer and on selecting the activity for input. Very different or incorrect values can be obtained if the input is not properly controlled. Few methods have adequately defined normal values in different muscles in different age groups, nor can many identify specific abnormalities heretofore not demonstrable by standard techniques. An exception to this is the measurement of jitter with SFEMG which can detect abnormalities at the neuromuscular junction that cannot be recognized with standard techniques. Prospective evaluation of these methods for predicting final diagnosis, as determined by clinical and biopsy criteria, is needed.

Summary

Quantitative electromyography is valuable in providing reliable, reproducible measurements of the abnormalities seen with diseases of nerve and muscle. It is important in characterizing unusual disorders and in defining the details of the abnormalities seen in experimental studies of disease of nerve and muscle. It also is helpful in following a course of evaluation of peripheral neuromuscular diseases and in identifying mild abnormalities. The technique can differentiate most myopathic and neurogenic disorders, although many of each disorder type do not produce measurable change, even with quantitative EMG. The major drawback of quantitation is the greater amount of time needed to make the measurements than are necessary for the experienced electromyographer to assess the EMG signal subjectively. In disorders in which multiple muscles need to be examined, this is a major drawback, and in the laboratory, attempting to serve many patients on a cost-effective basis also may be a disadvantage. Until both of these problems can be met, quantitative EMG probably will continue to be limited to the assessment of special problems.

References

1 AGARWAL, G. C. and GOTTLIEB, G. L. An analysis of the electromyogram by Fourier, simulation and experimental techniques. *IEEE Transactions on Biomedical Engineering*, **BME–22,** 225–229 (1975)

2 ALBERS, J. W., ALLEN, A. A., II, BASTRON, J. A. and DAUBE, J. R. Limb myokymia. *Muscle and Nerve* (In press)

3 ANDREASSEN, S. and ROSENFALCK, A. Recording from a single motor unit during strong effort. *IEEE Transactions on Biomedical Engineering*, **BME–25,** 501–508 (1978)

4 BAJADA, S., TOURAINE, A. and SAMSON-DOLLFUS, D. Quantitative E.M.G: a study of the biceps muscle in normal subjects and patients with neurogenic muscle disease (abstract). *Acta Neurologica Scandinavia*, Supplementum **73,** 298 (1979)

5 BAK, M. J. and SCHMIDT, E. M. An analog delay circuit for on-line visual confirmation of discriminated neuroelectric signals. *IEEE Transactions on Biomedical Engineering*, **BME–24,** 69–71 (1977)

6 BERGMANS, J. Computer-assisted measurement of the parameters of single motor unit potentials in human electromyography. In *New Developments in Electromyography and Clinical Neurophysiology*, **2,** edited by J. E. Desmedt, 482–488. Basel, S. Karger (1973)

7 BERGMANS, J. Clinical applications. Applications to EMG. In *EEG Informatics: A Didactic Review of Methods and Applications of EEG Data Processing*, edited by A. Rémond, 263–280. Amsterdam, Elsevier/North Holland Biomedical Press (1977)

8 BETTS, B. and SMITH, J. L. Period-amplitude analysis of EMG from slow and fast extensors of cat during locomotion and jumping. *Electroencephalography and Clinical Neurophysiology*, **47,** 571–581 (1979)

9 BLACK, J. T., BHATT, G. P., DEJESUS, P. V., SCHOTLAND, D. L. and ROWLAND, L. P. Diagnostic accuracy of clinical data, quantitative electromyography and histochemistry in neuromuscular disease: a study of 105 cases. *Journal of Neurological Sciences*, **21,** 59–70 (1974)

10 BLINOWSKA, K. J., HAUSMANOWA-PETRUSEWICZ, I., MILLER-LARSSON, and ZACHARA, J. Z. The analysis of single EMG potentials by means of multivariate methods. *Electromyography and Clinical Neurophysiology*, **20,** 105–123 (1980)

11 BOYD, D. C., BRATTY, P. J. A. and LAWRENCE, P. D. A review of the methods of automatic analysis in clinical electromyography. *Computers in Biology and Medicine*, **6,** 179–190 (1976)

12 BOYD, D. C., LAWRENCE, P. D. and BRATTY, P. J. A. The effect of electromyographic jitter on single motor unit EMG potentials. *IEEE Transactions on Biomedical Engineering*, **BME–26,** 471–478 (1979)

13 BRUMLIK, J., DRECHSLER, B. and VANNIN, T. M. The myotonic discharge in various neurological syndromes: a neurophysiological analysis. *Electromyography*, **10,** 369–383 (1970)

14 BUCHTHAL, F. Electrophysiological signs of myopathy as related with muscle biopsy. *Acta Neurologica (Napoli)*, **32,** 1–29 (1977)

15 BUCHTHAL, F., GULD, C. and ROSENFALCK, P. Action potential parameters in normal human muscle and their dependence on physical variables. *Acta Physiologica Scandinavica*, **32,** 200–218 (1954)

16 BUCHTHAL, F., PINELLI, P. and ROSENFALCK, P. Action potential parameters in normal human muscle and their physiological determinants. *Acta Physiologica Scandinavica*, **32,** 219–229 (1954)

17 BUCHTHAL, F. and ROSENFALCK, P. Spontaneous electrical activity of human muscle. *Electroencephalography and Clinical Neurophysiology*, **20**, 321–336 (1966)

18 BUCHTHAL, F., ROSENFALCK, P. and ERMINIO, F. Motor unit territory and fiber density in myopathies. *Neurology (Minneapolis)*, **10**, 398–408 (1960)

19 BUCHTHAL, F. and SCHMALBRUCH, H. Motor unit of mammalian muscle. *Physiological Reviews*, **60**, 90–142 (1980)

20 CLAMANN, H. P. Statistical analysis of motor unit firing patterns in a human skeletal muscle. *Biophysical Journal*, **9**, 1233–1251 (1969)

21 COLSTON, J. R. and FEARNLEY, M. E. Preliminary experience with an experimental action potential analyser in clinical electromyography. *Annals of Physical Medicine*, **9**, 127–138 (1967)

22 CONRAD, B., SINDERMANN, F. and PROCHAZKA, V. J. Interval analysis of repetitive denervation potentials of human skeletal muscle. *Journal of Neurology, Neurosurgery and Psychiatry*, **35**, 834–840 (1972)

23 CROSBY, P. A. Use of surface electromyogram as a measure of dynamic force in human limb muscles. *Medical and Biological Engineering and Computing*, **16**, 519–523, (1978)

24 CZEKAJEWSKI, J., EKSTEDT, J. and STÅLBERG, E. Oscilloscopic recording of muscle fibre action potentials. The window trigger and the delay unit. *Electroencephalography and Clinical Neurophysiology*, **27**, 536–539 (1969)

25 DAHL, K. and BUCHTHAL, F. Digital memory recorder in electromyography and nerve conduction studies. *Electroencephalography and Clinical Neurophysiology*, **45**, 538–544 (1978)

26 DAUBE, J. R. Comparison of methods of quantitating EMG. In *Fifth International Congress of Electromyography*. (Rochester, Minnesota, September 21–24, 1975), Omaha, Nebraska, International Federation of Societies for Electroencephalography and Clinical Neurophysiology (abstract)

27 DAUBE, J. R. The description of motor unit potentials in electromyography. *Neurology (Minneapolis)*, **28**, 623–625 (1978)

28 DE LUCA, C. J. and VAN DYK, E. J. Derivation of some parameters of myoelectric signals recorded during sustained constant force isometric contractions. *Biophysical Journal*, **15**, 1167–1180 (1975)

29 DO CARMO, R. J. Motor unit action potential parameters in human newborn infants. *Archives of Neurology*, **3**, 136–140 (1960)

30 EMERYK, B., HAUSMANOWA-PETRUSEWICZ, I. and NOWAK, T. Spontaneous volleys of bizarre high-frequency potentials (b.h.f.p.) in neuro-muscular diseases. Part II. An analysis of the morphology of spontaneous volleys of bizarre high-frequency potentials in neuro-

muscular diseases. *Electromyography and Clinical Neurophysiology*, **14**, 339–354 (1974)

31 ERB, K. and ESSLEN, E. Detection of single motor units in EMG-signals. *Biomedizinische Technik*, **21**, 283–284 (1976)

32 FEX, J. and KRAKAU, C. E. T. Some experiences with Walton's frequency analysis of the electromyogram. *Journal of Neurology, Neurosurgery and Psychiatry*, **20**, 178–184 (1957)

33 FOOTE, R. A., O'FALLON, W. M. and DAUBE, J. R. A comparison of single fiber and routine EMG in normal subjects and patients with inflammatory myopathy. *Bulletin of the Los Angeles Neurological Societies*, **43**, 95–103 (1978)

34 FUGLSANG-FREDERIKSEN, A. and MÅNSSON, A. Analysis of electrical activity of normal muscle in man at different degrees of voluntary effort. *Journal of Neurology, Neurosurgery and Psychiatry*, **38**, 683–694 (1975)

35 FUGLSANG-FREDERIKSEN, A., SCHEEL, U. and BUCHTHAL, F. Diagnostic yield of analysis of the pattern of electrical activity and of individual motor unit potentials in myopathy. *Journal of Neurology, Neurosurgery and Psychiatry*, **39**, 742–750 (1976)

36 FUGLSANG-FREDERIKSEN, A., SCHEEL, U. and BUCHTHAL, F. Diagnostic yield of the analysis of the pattern of electrical activity of muscle and of individual motor unit potentials in neurogenic involvement. *Journal of Neurology, Neurosurgery and Psychiatry*, **40**, 544–554 (1977)

37 FUSFELD, R. D. Analysis of electromyographic signals by measurement of wave duration. *Electroencephalography and Clinical Neurophysiology*, **30**, 337–344 (1971)

38 FUSFELD, R. D. A study of the differentiated electromyogram. *Electroencephalography and Clinical Neurophysiology*, **33**, 511–515 (1972)

39 FUSFELD, R. D. Instrument for quantitative analysis of the electromyogram. *Medical and Biological Engineering and Computing*, **16**, 290–295 (1978)

40 GATH, I and STALBERG, E. The calculated radial decline of the extracellular action potential compared with in situ measurements in the human brachial biceps. *Electroencephalography and Clinical Neurophysiology*, **44**, 547–552 (1978)

41 GATH, I. and STÅLBERG, E. Motor unit action potentials simulated through single muscle fibre action potentials (abstract). *Acta Neurologica Scandinavica*, Supplementum **73**, 150 (1979)

42 GERSTEN, J. W., CENKOVICH, F. S. and JONES, G. D. Harmonic analysis of normal and abnormal electromyograms. *American Journal of Physical Medicine*, **44,** 235–240 (1965)

43 GRIEP, P. A. M. The motor unit action potential: a model approach of the 'forward problem' based on histochemical and physiological methods. *Thesis*, University of Amsterdam, Netherlands (1979)

44 GRIEVE, D. W. and CAVANAGH, P. R. The quantitative analysis of phasic electromyograms. In *New Developments in Electromyography and Clinical Neurophysiology*, **2,** edited by J. E. Desmedt, 489–496. Basel, S. Karger (1973)

45 GYDIKOV, A., KOSAROV, D. and GERILOVSKY, L. Vectorelectromyographic investigations on motor units with short, inclined and curved muscle fibres. *Electromyography and Clinical Neurophysiology*, **17,** 127–141 (1977)

46 HARIDASAN, G., SANGHVI, S. H., JINDAL, G. D., JOSHI, V. M. and DESAI, A. D. Quantitative electromyography using automatic analysis: a comparative study with a fixed fraction of a subject's maximum effort and two levels of thresholds for analysis. *Journal of the Neurological Sciences*, **42,** 53–64 (1979)

47 HAUSMANOWA-PETRUSEWICZ, I. Diagnostic value of quantitative electromyography: its scope and limitations. *Electroencephalography and Clinical Neurophysiology*, Supplement **34,** 487–492 (1978)

48 HAYWARD, M. Automatic analysis of the electromyogram in healthy subjects of different ages. *Journal of the Neurological Sciences*, **33,** 397–413 (1977)

49 HAYWARD, M. and WILLISON, R. G. The recognition of myogenic and neurogenic lesions by quantitative EMG. In *New Developments in Electromyography and Clinical Neurophysiology*, **2,** edited by J. E. Desmedt, 448–453. Basel, S. Karger (1973)

50 HAYWARD, M. and WILLISON, R. G. Automatic analysis of the electromyogram in patients with chronic partial denervation. *Journal of the Neurological Sciences*, **33,** 415–423 (1977)

51 HIROSE, K., UONO, M. and SOBUE, I. Quantitative electromyography: comparison between manual values and computer ones on normal subjects. *Electromyography and Clinical Neurophysiology*, **14,** 315–320 (1974)

52 HIROSE, K., UONO, M. and SOBUE, I. Quantitative electromyography: difference between myopathic findings and neuropathic ones. *Electromyography and Clinical Neurophysiology*, **15,** 431–449 (1975)

53 HJORTH, R. J., WALSH, J. C. and WILLISON, R. G. The distribution and frequency of spontaneous fasciculations in motor neurone disease. *Journal of the Neurological Sciences*, **18**, 469–474 (1973)

54 HUBER, F. On-line power spectra on small computers. *Computers and Biomedical Research*, **7**, 1–6 (1974)

55 KADEFORS, R., KAISER, E. and PETERSÉN, I. Dynamic spectrum analysis of myo-potentials with special reference to muscle fatigue. *Electromyography*, **8**, 39–74 (1968)

56 KOMI, P. V. and TESCH, P. EMG frequency spectrum, muscle structure, and fatigue during dynamic contractions in man. *European Journal of Applied Physiology and Occupational Physiology*, **42**, 41–50 (1979)

57 KOPEĆ, J. and HAUSMANOWA-PETRUSEWICZ, I. On-line computer application in clinical quantitative electromyography. *Electromyography and Clinical Neurophysiology*, **16**, 49–64 (1976)

58 KUNZE, K. Quantitative EMG analysis in myogenic and neurogenic muscle diseases. In *New Developments in Electromyography and Clinical Neurophysiology*, **2**, edited by J. R. Desmedt, 469–476. Basel, S. Karger (1973)

59 KWATNY, E., THOMAS, D. H. and KWATNY, H. G. An application of signal processing techniques to the study of myoelectric signals. *IEEE Transactions on Biomedical Engineering*, **BME–17**, 303–312 (1970)

60 LAGO, P. and JONES, N. B. Effect of motor-unit firing time statistics on e.m.g. spectra. *Medical and Biological Engineering and Computing*, **15**, 648–655 (1977)

61 LAMBERT, E. H. and McMORRIS, R. O. Size of motor unit action potentials in neuromuscular disorders (abstract). *Federation Proceedings*, **12**, 81 (1953)

62 LANG, A. H. and PARTANEN, V. S. J. 'Satellite potentials' and the duration of motor unit potentials in normal, neuropathic and myopathic muscles. *Journal of the Neurological Sciences*, **27**, 513–524 (1976)

63 LANG, A. H. and TUOMOLA, G. The time parameters of motor unit potentials recorded with multi-electrodes and the summation technique. *Electromyography and Clinical Neurophysiology*, **14**, 513–525 (1974)

64 LARSSON, L.-E. On the relation between the EMG frequency spectrum and the duration of symptoms in lesions of the peripheral motor neuron. *Electroencephalography and Clinical Neurophysiology*, **38**, 69–78 (1975)

65 LEE, R. G. and WHITE, D. G. Computer analysis of motor unit action potentials in routine clinical electromyography. In *New Developments in Electromyography and Clinical Neurophysiology*, **2**, edited by J. E. Desmedt, 454–461. Basel, S. Karger (1973)

66 LEIFER, L. and PINELLI, P. Analysis of motor units by computer aided electromyography. *Third International Congress of Electrophysiological Kinesiology*, (Pavia, Italy, August 30–September 4, 1976)

67 LENMAN, J. A. R. Quantitative electromyographic changes associated with muscular weakness. *Journal of Neurology, Neurosurgery and Psychiatry*, **22**, 306–310 (1959)

68 LINDSTRÖM, L. H. and MAGNUSSON, R. I. Interpretation of myoelectric power spectra: a model and its applications. *Proceedings of the Institute of Electrical and Electronics Engineers*, **65**, 653–662 (1977)

69 MAGORA, A. and GONEN, B. A new technique for the extraction of the activity of single motor units from the electromyography of maximal contraction. *Electromyography*, **10**, 155–170 (1970)

70 MAGORA, A. and GONEN, B. Computer analysis of the relation between duration and degree of superposition of electromyographic spikes. *Electromyography and Clinical Neurophysiology*, **17**, 83–98 (1977)

71 MAGORA, A. and GONEN, B. Computer editing of electromyographic recordings. *Electromyography and Clinical Neurophysiology*, **18**, 35–43 (1978)

72 MARANZANA FIGINI, M., BESTETTI, G. and VALLI, G. Measuring motor unit action potential duration by means of surface electrode EMG. *Electromyography and Clinical Neurophysiology*, **18**, 45–56 (1978)

73 MARIANI, J., MATON, B. and BOUISSET, S. Force gradation and motor unit activity during voluntary movements in man. *Electroencephalography and Clinical Neurophysiology*, **48**, 573–582 (1980)

74 MATON, B. Motor unit differentiation and integrated surface EMG in voluntary isometric contraction. *European Journal of Applied Physiology and Occupational Physiology*, **35**, 149–157 (1976)

75 McCOMAS, A. J. and SICA, R. E. Automatic quantitative analysis of the electromyogram in partially denervated distal muscles: comparison with motor unit counting. *Canadian Journal of Neurological Sciences*, **5**, 377–383 (1978)

76 MECHELSE, K. and SCHIPPER, J. M. Measurement of motor unit potentials using a PDP 8 computer (abstract). *Electroencephalography and Clinical Neurophysiology*, **43**, 623–624 (1977)

77 MILLER, R. G. and SHERRATT, M. Firing rates of human motor units in partially denervated muscle. *Neurology (Minneapolis)*, **28,** 1241–1248 (1978)

78 MILNER-BROWN, H. S. and STEIN, R. B. The relation between the surface electromyogram and muscular force. *Journal of Physiology (London)*, **246,** 549–569 (1975)

79 MIYANO, H. and SADOYAMA, T. Theoretical analysis of surface EMG in voluntary isometric contraction. *European Journal of Applied Physiology and Occupational Physiology*, **40,** 155–164 (1979)

80 MONSTER, A. W. Two ranges in the firing rate response of volitionally activated low-threshold EDC motor units. *Electromyography and Clinical Neurophysiology*, **17,** 231–237 (1977)

81 MONSTER, A. W. and CHAN, H. Surface electromyogram potentials of motor units; relationship between potential size and unit location in a large human skeletal muscle. *Experimental Neurology*, **67,** 280 –297 (1980)

82 MONSTER, A. W., PITTORE, J. and BARRIE, W. A system for rapid acquisition of surface potential maps of human skeletal muscle motor units. *IEEE Transactions on Biomedical Engineering*, **BME–27,** 110–112 (1980)

83 MOOSA, A. and BROWN, B. H. Quantitative electromyography: a new analogue technique for detecting changes in action potential duration. *Journal of Neurology, Neurosurgery and Psychiatry*, **35,** 216–220 (1972)

84 MOOSA, A., BROWN, B. H. and DUBOWITZ, V. Quantitative electromyography: carrier detection in Duchenne type muscular dystrophy using a new automatic technique. *Journal of Neurology, Neurosurgery and Psychiatry*, **35,** 841–844 (1972)

85 NISSEN-PETERSEN, H., GULD, C. and BUCHTHAL, F. A delay line to record random action potentials. *Electroencephalography and Clinical Neurophysiology*, **26,** 100–106 (1969)

86 PETAJAN, J. H. Clinical electromyographic studies of diseases of the motor unit. *Electroencephalography and Clinical Neurophysiology*, **36,** 395–401 (1974)

87 PETERSÉN, I. and KUGELBERG, E. Duration and form of action potential in the normal human muscle. *Journal of Neurology, Neurosurgery and Psychiatry*, **12,** 124–128 (1949)

88 PETROFSKY, J. S. Frequency and amplitude analysis of the EMG during exercise on the bicycle ergometer. *European Journal of Applied Physiology and Occupational Physiology*, **41,** 1–15 (1979)

89 PINELLI, P. The value of motor unit parameter measurements. In *Current Concepts in Clinical Neurophysiology*. (Didactic Lectures of the Ninth International Congress of Electroencephalography and Clinical Neurophysiology. Amsterdam, September 1977), edited by H. van Duijn, D. N. J. Donker and A. C. van Huffelen, 111–122. The Hague, N. V. Drukkerij Trio, (1977)

90 PLONSEY, R. Action potential sources and their volume conductor fields. *Proceedings of the Institute of Electrical and Electronics Engineers*, **65**, 601–611 (1977)

91 PROCHAZKA, V. J., CONRAD, B. and SINDERMANN, F. Computerized single-unit interval analysis and its clinical application. In *New Developments in Electromyography and Clinical Neurophysiology*, **2**, edited by J. E. Desmedt, 462–468. Basel, S. Karger (1973)

92 RATHJEN, R., SIMONS, D. G. and PETERSON, C. R. Computer analysis of the duration of motor-unit potentials. *Archives of Physical Medicine and Rehabilitation*, **49**, 524–527 (1968)

93 REINKING, R. M. and STEPHENS, J. A. Interface unit for on-line measurements of motor unit properties with a small laboratory computer. *American Journal of Physical Medicine*, **54**, 186–193 (1975)

94 RICHARDSON, A. T. The analysis of muscle action potentials in the differential diagnosis of neuromuscular diseases. *Archives of Physical Medicine and Rehabilitation*, **32**, 199–206 (1951)

95 ROSE, A. L. and WILLISON, R. G. Quantitative electromyography using automatic analysis: studies in healthy subjects and patients with primary muscle disease. *Journal of Neurology, Neurosurgery and Psychiatry*, **30**, 403–410 (1967)

96 SANDERS, D. B., HOWARD, J. F., JR. and JOHNS, T. R. Single-fiber electromyography in myasthenia gravis. *Neurology (Minneapolis)*, **29**, 68–76 (1979)

97 SICA, R. E., McCOMAS, A. J. and FERREIRA, J. C. Evaluation of an automated method for analysing the electromyogram. *Canadian Journal of Neurological Sciences*, **5**, 275–281 (1978)

98 STÅLBERG, E. Propagation velocity in human muscle fibres in situ. *Acta Physiologica Scandinavica*, **70**, Supplement 287, 1–112 (1966)

99 STÅLBERG, E. Macro EMG: a new recording technique. *Journal of Neurology, Neurosurgery and Psychiatry*, **43**, 475–482 (1980)

100 STÅLBERG, E. and ANTONI, L. Electrophysiological cross section of the motor unit. *Journal of Neurology, Neurosurgery and Psychiatry*, **43**, 469–474 (1980)

101 STÅLBERG, E., EKSTEDT, J. and BROMAN, A. The electromyographic jitter in normal human muscles. *Electroencephalography and Clinical Neurophysiology*, **31**, 429–438 (1971)

102 STÅLBERG, E. and TRONTELJ, J. V. *Single Fibre Electromyography*. Old Woking, Surrey, UK, Miravalle Press (1979)

103 STOEHR, M. Low frequency bizarre discharges: a particular type of electromyographical spontaneous activity in paretic skeletal muscle. *Electromyography and Clinical Neurophysiology*, **18**, 147–156 (1978)

104 SULG, I. A., HOKKANEN, E., MATTILA, P. and TOIVAKKA, E. Quantitative multiparameter analysis of the EMG (abstract). *Acta Neurologica Scandinavica*, Supplementum **73**, 306 (1979)

105 TAGLIETTI, V., CINQUINI, G., MOGLIA, A. and ARRIGO, A. EMG automatic analysis of the tibialis anterior muscle in normal subjects. *Third International Congress of Electrophysiological Kinesiology*, (Pavia, Italy, August 30–September 4, 1976)

106 THIELE, B. and BOEHLE, A. Number of single muscle fibre action potentials contributing to the motor unit potential. *Fifth International Congress of Electromyography*, (Rochester, Minnesota, September 21–24, 1975), Omaha, Nebraska, International Federation of Societies for Electroencephalography and Clinical Neurophysiology (abstract)

107 TROJABORG, W. and BUCHTHAL, F. Malignant and benign fasciculations. *Acta Neurologica Scandinavica*, Supplementum **13**, 251–254 (1965)

108 TROUP, J. D. G. and CHAPMAN, A. E. Analysis of the waveform of the electromyograph using the analyser described by Fitch (1967). *Electromyography and Clinical Neurophysiology*, **12**, 325–346 (1972)

109 VIITASALO, J. H. T. and KOMI, P. V. Signal characteristics of EMG with special reference to reproducibility of measurements. *Acta Physiologica Scandinavica*, **93**, 531–539 (1975)

110 VISSER, S. L. and DE RIJKE, W. Automatic digital analysis of the EMG during standardized flexion and extension of the foot. *European Neurology*, **13**, 441–450 (1975)

111 WALTON, J. N. The electromyogram in myopathy: analysis with the audio-frequency spectrometer. *Journal of Neurology, Neurosurgery and Psychiatry*, **15**, 219–226 (1952)

112 WARMOLTS, J.R and MENDELL, J. R. Neurotonia: impulse-induced repetitive discharges in motor nerves in peripheral neuropathy. *Annals of Neurology*, **7**, 245–250 (1980)

113 WILLISON, R. G. Quantitative electromyography. In *Electrodiagnosis and Electromyography*, 3rd Edn., edited by S. Licht, 390–411. New Haven, Conn., USA, Elizabeth Licht (1971)

114 YEMM, R. The representation of motor-unit action-potentials on skin-surface electromyograms of the masseter and temporal muscles in man. *Archives of Oral Biology*, **22**, 201–205 (1977)

115 ZIPP, P. Effect of electrode parameters on the bandwidth of the surface e.m.g. power-density spectrum. *Medical and Biological Engineering and Computing*, **16**, 537–541 (1978)

4

Power spectra of myoelectric signals: motor unit activity and muscle fatigue

Lars Lindström and Ingemar Petersén

Introduction

Power spectrum analysis of myoelectric signals can be traced back to 1951 when Richardson[60] used a filter to divide the EMG spectrum into two parts which were used to give a measure of the spectral content. Clinical application of spectral analysis in the more standard sense of the word was probably first made by Walton in 1952[74]. Other early reports are those of Nightingale[51, 52] and Fex and Krakau[15]. During the last decade, with increased availability of electronic analyzers, in particular digital computers, numerous reports on myoelectric power spectra have emerged.

The power spectrum, illustrated in *Figure 4.1*, has been found[22, 28, 44, 51, 68, 74] to be peaked with a maximum in the frequency region between some 10 Hz and 100 Hz, if the signals are obtained with surface electrodes, and between 100 Hz or lower, and about 200 Hz, if intramuscular electrodes are used. Changes in the power spectrum are found in certain pathological states. In patients with primary myopathies, the spectral peak is displaced to frequencies as high as 400–600 Hz[15, 17, 32,34, 74], whereas in those with neuropathy, the high frequency content is lower than normal[32, 34, 69]. The observation that the power spectrum differs from normal in patients with changes in plasma electrolytes is also of interest from the clinical point of view[35]. It has also been found that, as a result of sustained contractions, the power density increases in the low frequencies[25, 28, 29, 64, 65]. This phenomenon, considered to be a sign of 'localized muscle fatigue'[6], will be discussed and analyzed.

Knowledge of the power spectrum and its relation to motor unit or single muscle fiber action potentials offers new possibilities for a

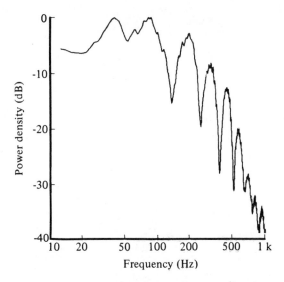

Figure 4.1 Power spectrum of a myoelectric
(EMG) signal with a predominant single motor
unit contribution led off with a bipolar surface
electrode from the biceps brachii muscle. On
the high frequency side of the spectrum are
seen multiple so-called 'dips' which are caused
by the electrode arrangement. From the position of these dips, propagation velocity of the
action potentials can be calculated

rational interpretation of myoelectric findings. The first part of this
chapter will deal with these aspects. The second part will discuss the
change in the myoelectric power spectrum found in connection with
forceful or prolonged muscular work. The aim of the second part is to
point out possible mechanisms for this change and to show that it can
be used as a parameter quantifying the influence of preceding muscle
work on the muscle itself.

Power spectrum shape in relation to EMG measures

The influence upon the spectrum of certain features of the signal –
especially those commonly used to characterize myoelectric signals –
will be expounded in this section. The power spectrum characteristics
are discussed in the case of many signal sources being active at the

68

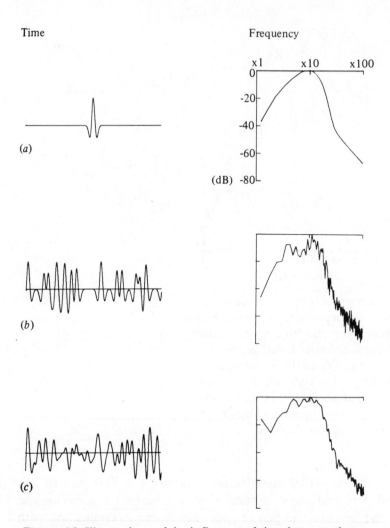

Figure 4.2 Illustrations of the influence of signal summation on
the observed power spectrum. The power spectra are plotted on
bi-logarithmic scales with a frequency axis covering two decades
and the vertical power–density axis having 20 dB per division.
(*a*) Original action potential and its spectrum. (*b*) Summated
signal of 13 identical contributions distributed randomly over
the observation interval. The power spectrum, although subject
to random variations, has the same overall shape as that of the
single potential. The number of computer calculated zero
crossings are 24 which is close to the expected number of 26.
(*c*) Summated signal with increased number of identical contributions: 220 randomly distributed action potentials with 34
zero crossings. The power spectrum has the same features as (*b*)

same time, as in EMG interference patterns obtained at moderate to strong contraction levels. Rather than giving a purely mathematical explanation, illustrations obtained from computer simulations are used. These simulations also bear a direct relation to the use of 'turn points' and 'zero crossings' (*see* Chapter 3) to characterize the composite myoelectric signal. It is emphasized that use of the word *frequency* in context with power spectra refers to the independent variable of the spectrum and is not equivalent to the repetition rate of, say, a motor unit signal.

Recruitment and signal repetition rate

A single motor unit action potential and its power spectrum is illustrated in *Figure 4.2(a)*. In this simulation the computer also calculates the number of zero crossings. In *Figure 4.2(b)*, an increased contraction level is simulated by adding a few action potentials occurring randomly during the observation time. The corresponding power spectrum suffers from fluctuations, but otherwise has the same shape as that of the individual contributions. The number of zero crossings have increased in relation to the intensity. Finally the number of contributions is increased to correspond with a high contraction level; even then, as shown in *Figure 4.2(c)*, the shape of the power spectrum is the same as that belonging to the single signal. The number of zero crossings, however, have not increased in relation to the increase in the intensity. It is therefore concluded that, for randomly added signals of the same configuration, properties of individual motor unit action potentials can still be extracted from the myoelectric interference signal by spectral analysis. For the EMG signal composed of motor unit potentials with different shapes, the observed power spectrum represents a weighted mean of the spectra from the contributing motor units.

Duration

One of the measures used to characterize myoelectric signals, duration, to a large extent determines the distribution of power over the frequency interval: pulses of short duration contain more high frequency energy than pulses of long duration. In *Figure 4.3(a)* and (*b*) this is illustrated for two pulses of identical shape but with different duration, caused by 'stretching' the time scale. An increase in duration moves the power spectrum towards lower frequencies but the relative shape of the spectral curve is preserved. The center frequency and the bandwidth are both diminished.

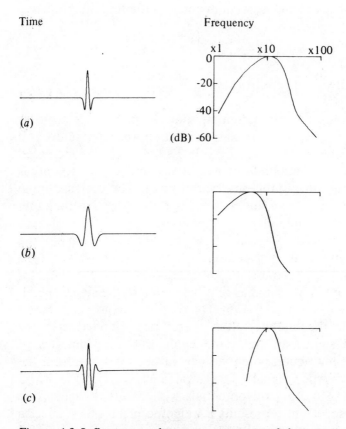

Figure 4.3 Influence on the power spectrum of changes in duration and number of phases of a simulated action potential. Axes as for *Figure 4.2*. (*a*) Original signal with spectrum. (*b*) Increased duration (caused by stretching the time scale) moves the spectrum towards lower frequencies with preserved relative shape. (*c*) Increasing the number of phases with constant duration of each phase causes the spectrum to be more peaked but to have essentially the same center frequency

Number of phases

The number of phases of a motor unit action potential strongly influences the power spectrum. However, this influence is intimately interwoven with that of the duration. For constant values of duration, an increase in the number of phases pushes the spectrum towards higher frequencies, whereas for durations increasing proportionally to the increase of phases, a more pronounced peak is found in the power spectrum. *Figure 4.3(c)* illustrates the influence of the number of phases on the power spectrum.

Turns and zeros

Earlier it was shown that the number of zero crossings of the myoelectric signal increased proportionally with the number of individual action potentials for low contraction levels and that this proportionality was lost at high contraction levels. If the simulation experiments are repeated with larger variations in intensity of individual contributions, curves of a kind shown in *Figure 4.4* are found.

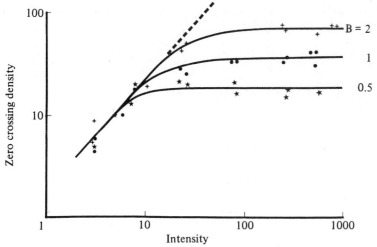

Figure 4.4 Zero crossing density as a function of signal source intensity. At low intensities, a proportionality exists which is lost when the summated signal attains the character of Gaussian random noise. This change occurs at different points depending on the spectral properties, here described by the relative values of the signal bandwidth B

This saturation of zero crossing density is an indication that the individual contributions can no longer be distinguished in the summated signal. It is now a Gaussian noise signal and the zero crossing density is entirely determined by spectral properties[59]. It is thus in general not an indication of action potential grouping when the zero crossing density is found to be lower than the value extrapolated from low signal intensities.

Since a very close relation exists between zero crossings and turn-points (a zero crossing of the signal's time derivative is equal to a turn-point), the same reasoning is also valid for this latter measure. It was therefore concluded[39] that the method of turn-point analysis[9] yields mixed information about spectral properties of individual action potentials, the number of active motor units and their repetition rates. The contraction level, if low to moderate, does strongly affect the output reading of turns. Occasionally, investigations of local muscle fatigue were found where turn-point analysis has shown decreased intensity of turns as fatigue develops, a finding which has been interpreted as increased synchronization. In view of the present analysis and in view of the fact that rather strong contractions are used experimentally to produce fatigue (high signal intensity with the character of Gaussian noise), a more likely interpretation is that these changes are caused by a spectral shift of the individual action potentials towards lower frequencies.

Amplitude and other measures of signal strength

Several measures are commonly used to characterize signal strength, e.g. amplitude, the full-wave rectified and averaged signal (FRA), and the root mean square of the signal (RMS). One should observe that these measures are created in different ways and thus reflect different properties of the signal. For example, with distinguishable action potentials, the FRA value is linearly proportional to both amplitude, duration and repetition rate, whereas the RMS value is linearly proportional to amplitude but is related by a square root dependence to duration and repetition rate. For noise signals, on the other hand, the FRA and RMS values are proportional regardless of the signal genesis. Of the various measures used, only the RMS value has an immediate relation to the power spectrum in that the total power of the signal is equal to the area under the spectral curve.

Propagation velocity

The power spectrum is strongly influenced by the geometrical arrangement of electrode plates. For bipolar electrodes with plates lined up parallel to the muscle fibers, the difference in arrival time of the signal at the two plates causes the filtering function of the electrode to alternate between maxima and zeros, the latter causing so-called dips in the observed power spectrum[36]. The positions of these dips are dependent only upon electrode plate separation and propagation velocity. Dip analysis can thus be used to measure this velocity with surface electrodes during voluntary contractions.

The propagation velocity of a single fiber action potential is an interesting parameter from the point of view of signal theory, because its influence will persist through all mathematical manipulations in situations where various processes are modelled. In all expressions describing the power spectrum, the velocity always appears together with the frequency as a quotient (frequency divided by velocity). This means that any velocity change can be seen as a shift of the spectral curve along the frequency axis[37, 42]. Fourier transformation of a potential of fixed geometrical shape also shows that the power spectrum density is inversely proportional to the squared value of the velocity[43]. A signal increase, in addition to a spectral shift, is therefore a necessity when the propagation velocity, for some reason, decreases. The observed signal strength is also dependent on the product of recruitment of motor units and their repetition rate. However, measures of signal strength will behave differently depending on whether the action potentials are separable, as is often the case with needle electrodes, or not, as with surface electrodes.

Changes in the myoelectric power spectrum during muscle work

One of the first attempts to quantify work-induced changes in frequency content of the myoelectric signal was made in 1960 by Kondo[31]. Using analogue filters he divided the signal spectrum into two parts (below and above 50 Hz) and used their power ratio as a measure of 'fatigue'. More detailed power spectrum analysis was first applied to fatigue studies in 1962 by Kogi and Hakamada[29] and by Kaiser and Petersén[28]. Using octave band filtering they found a decrease of power density in the high frequency region and an increase in the low frequency region during 'fatigue'. Subsequent investigations produced consistent results[25, 33, 45, 64, 65]. Explanations offered by these investigators are: dysfunction of muscle spindles; synchronization of motor unit signals; a combination of synchronization and asynchronization; re-recruitment of motor units; and motor unit signal changes.

The latter explanation was further elaborated in 1970 when Lindström, Magnusson and Petersén[43] verified in humans the occurrence of theoretically predicted[36] features of the myoelectric power spectrum. The underlying theory demonstrated that the observed changes were dependent almost entirely upon the propagation velocity of the action potentials. This agrees with earlier reports from measurements of propagation velocity in single muscle fibers[70] and intracellular measurements of action potential durations[21]. Alternative methods to measure the velocity, both directly[46] and indirectly[41] have since been developed.

Connections between spectral changes and the production and accumulation of acid metabolites have been verified. In 1970, Mortimer, Magnusson and Petersén[48] showed that reduced wash-out of anaerobic metabolites severely affected the propagation velocity, in contrast to the case with a lack of oxygen and preserved perfusion. They also showed that the velocity recovered to its original value within a couple of minutes, in agreement with other authors[4].

Implications of measurements

Experiments on EMG changes during forceful muscle work will be presented here. Most examples are from the authors' own laboratory; a few of them hitherto unpublished.

The shape of the myoelectric power spectrum remains essentially unaltered with various muscle loadings[30, 44] except for those of very low force[14]. A slight, consistent increase of the center frequency with load can be observed, however (*see Figure 4.5*).

During strong muscle contractions the power spectrum shows a decrease of high frequency power and an increase of low frequency power which can be expressed as a shift of the spectral curve (*Figure 4.6*). It has been shown with dip analysis that this shift is caused by a decrease in propagation velocity[43]. It has also been shown[41] that the center frequency of the power spectrum is proportional to velocity. Decreases in center frequency during isometric and isotonic contractions have been shown to follow approximately exponential curves characterized by their time constants.

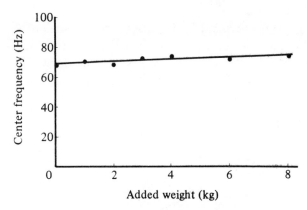

Figure 4.5 Weak dependence of the power spectrum, expressed as the center frequency, on muscle loading with fatigue effects removed. Signals obtained with surface electrodes from biceps brachii muscle with vertical upper arm and horizontal supinated forearm, load at the wrist

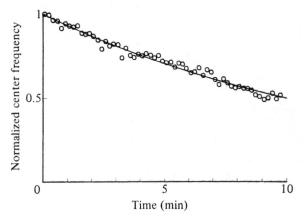

Figure 4.6 Dependence of the power spectrum on the developing fatigue. Signals from a masseter muscle under a constant biting force of 30 N

The subjective experience of a fatiguing contraction is closely related to these myoelectric changes[45]. Using the so-called RPE measure (rating scale of perceived exertion) originally developed to measure the influence of general fatigue[3], linear relationships were found between subjective symptoms of fatigue and spectral shifts of the myoelectric power, as illustrated in *Figure 4.7*. The initial RPE value and the rate of change were found to be proportional to the load.

For high loads, however, the spectral shift developed faster in relation to an RPE change than with lower loads. This indicates that some delaying process is present between the events reflected by the myoelectric signal and those producing the subjective experience.

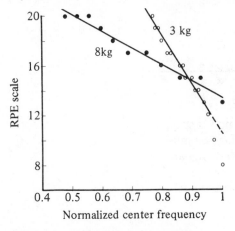

Figure 4.7 Subjective experience of muscle fatigue, expressed on a rating scale of perceived exertion, plotted versus the myoelectric spectral changes for two different loadings of the biceps brachii muscle. Measurements are made every 15 s

Linear regression analysis, performed on logarithmically-scaled data of spectral center frequencies, yields a regression coefficient which is the inverse of the time constant mentioned above and which characterizes the velocity decrease measured with dip analysis. The correlations described between myoelectric spectral changes and both subjective sensations of fatigue and impaired muscle performance have, in the authors' opinion, justified their use of the term 'EMG fatigue index' for the regression coefficient.

Plots of EMG fatigue index versus force yield detailed information concerning the development of fatigue at low forces. In a series of EMG experiments on masseter muscle fatigue, it was found that there exist critical force levels at 15–20 percent of maximum voluntary contraction, below which no fatigue could be detected by this myoelectric method[40]. These levels of fatigue-free force agree well with those arrived at in investigations using other methods and also with data on mechanical interference with blood flow[1, 10, 53].

When plotting fatigue time constants versus exerted force, curves are obtained which decrease with force and exhibit marked asymptotic values for low loads. Their striking resemblance to so-called 'strength-endurance' curves used in work physiology[61, 66] suggested the applicability of the EMG fatigue time constant as a predictor of endurance in isometric or isotonic muscular contractions. *Figure 4.8* shows a close

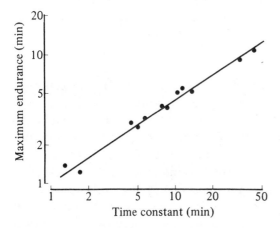

Figure 4.8 The relation between the EMG fatigue time constant, equal to the inverse value of the EMG fatigue index, during isometric isotonic contractions and maximal endurance. The slope of this bi-logarithmic curve is approximately two-thirds

relationship between these two quantities: endurance is proportional to the EMG time constant raised to the power of approximately two-thirds.

Assuming that maximal endurance (in highly motivated subjects performing non-dynamic contractions) is determined by the concentration of metabolites and the temperature in the interstitial spaces of a muscle, one can derive a theoretical relationship between endurance and EMG fatigue time constant which is in good agreement with experimental findings. Both heat and metabolites produced are transported to the extracellular space at a rate which is diffusion limited. With rapidly developing fatigue, intracellular concentrations will change considerably before the corresponding interstitial concentrations have reached certain critical values. On the other hand, with slowly developing fatigue, an almost equilibrated state is achieved, and the intracellular concentrations attain comparatively low levels with maximal endurance, i.e. EMG changes will be less with low loads than with high ones, in agreement with the findings presented in *Figure 4.7*.

Fatiguing, repetitive, dynamic work can be modelled as a succession of events where fatiguing contractions alternate with recovering relaxations. The parameters involved are force, period time and duty cycle (the work time in relation to period time). The center frequency of the power spectrum (or the velocity) decreases approximately exponentially with a time constant which is force-dependent during fatiguing contractions[43] and increases almost independently of force during relaxation[25]. Combining these two counteracting effects, one finds that the center frequency during periodic muscle loading tends to decrease exponentially at the beginning of the work but then stabilizes at a certain level below the initial value[38, 54]. The position of this level is dependent on the fatigue time constant and thus on the force. It is also dependent on the duty cycle; high values for the duty cycle push the plateau value towards that for steady loadings while low values, associated with very short work periods, only produce minor depressions. Of interest is that this dependence is strongly non-linear; duty cycles below 0.3–0.5 only give small changes. The period time, if much less than the time constants of fatigue and recovery, seems to have only a minor influence on the velocity changes.

Biological mechanisms of EMG findings in muscle fatigue

Today there seems to be a general agreement that the tension developed by a muscle impedes the bloodflow[1, 10, 71]. For a number of different muscles investigated, it has been found that forces greater than 20 per cent of maximum voluntary contraction (MVC) arrest the circulation. With a deficiency of oxygen, muscles must resort to anaerobic metabolism which produces acids in large amounts.

The accumulation of anaerobic metabolites lowers the pH[8]. According to theories of membrane excitability, hydrogen ions play an important role in the genesis of action potentials either through conformational changes of membrane proteins or through an electric field-dependent exchange mechanism, or both[2]. Experimental evidence from Tasaki, Singer and Takenaka[72] has shown membrane excitability to decrease strongly with decreasing intracellular pH.

Recent work[73] has also demonstrated that membrane excitability is far less influenced by extracellular than by intracellular pH. Interestingly enough, Nakamaru and Schwartz[50] have demonstrated that binding of calcium ions to proteins in the sarcoplasmic reticulum increases when pH in the incubated medium decreases: in other words, less calcium ions will be available to produce contraction when intracellular pH drops. Taken together, these findings strongly indicate the key role hydrogen ions have in membrane excitation; they also support the idea that hydrogen ions, or rather their absence, might be a mediator between electric phenomena in the membranes – the action potentials – and the release of calcium ions from the sarcoplasmic reticulum: the 'excitation–contraction' coupling.

Membrane excitability, of course, directly influences the propagation velocity of action potentials; high excitability means high velocity and vice versa. A decrease in velocity, observed as spectral changes in the myoelectric signal, can therefore be traced back to a decrease in membrane excitability and, in this context, to a lowered intracellular pH. Several investigators have tried in vain to correlate EMG changes with the metabolic state of muscle without making distinctions between intra- and extracellular compartments or, even worse, to the concentration of metabolites in arterial blood.

Excitability of membranes also depends strongly on temperature[7]. Since heat is produced by muscle contractions[11, 24], one would expect that the force and duration will affect the propagation velocity of action potentials. Edwards, Hill and Jones[12] found that the rate of muscle temperature rise is nearly linearly dependent upon the force (approximately $0.01°C$ per minute per % of MVC).

Frauendorf et al.[16] and Petrofsky[58] found that increased muscle temperature reduces signal strength and moves the power spectrum towards higher frequencies, while Sabbahi, DeLuca and Powers[63] found the reverse effect with cooling. These findings are in accordance with the expected influence of temperature on propagation velocity of action potentials.

We thus have two opposing factors influencing the membrane excitability: anaerobic metabolites and heat. Both have generation rates proportional to muscle force and both are essentially eliminated from the interior of the muscle fiber by diffusion. They will thus follow each other closely but with a dominating influence by the acid metabolites during contraction. Excess heat production found after fatiguing contractions[12, 13] might explain the overshoot of spectral changes found during the recovery phase[4, 25].

Applications of spectral analysis to muscle fatigue studies

Besides the application to basic physiology, three other disciplines have utilized myoelectric power spectrum analysis more systematically: clinical neurophysiology, ergonomics and respiratory physiology.

EMG technique has been used for some 30 years in occupational research, mostly with a kinesiological approach[5] but vocational EMG (or better, occupational EMG) was introduced in the early '70s[47, 57]. Quantitative descriptions in terms of myoelectric signal strength[20] and investigations using spectral analysis to detect localized muscle fatigue during occupational work are more recent[54].

Incidents of fatigue are common in heavy industrial work[26, 55]. In certain cases where a complicated interplay occurs between muscles – as in the shoulder region – myoelectric spectral methods have proved their ability to spot those muscles among several synergists which are highly fatigued[23]. Knowledge of differences in muscle response to external loading is of importance in occupational education[56] and design of working places. EMG including power spectrum analysis has proved to be a useful instrument in preventive medicine research which aims at increased knowledge of connections between muscular strain in industrial work and occupational diseases such as tendinitis[23].

Localized fatigue often affects small muscles without causing general effects that lead to discontinuance of the work. One often finds in prolonged work that its intensity is chosen so as to produce a certain heart beat frequency. Overloading of small muscles and small muscle groups might in the long run cause chronic pain and other signs of deterioration. Myoelectric tests for muscle fatigue are thus necessary complements to the methods commonly used in work physiology.

The application of myoelectric power spectrum analysis to respiratory physiology is quite recent[19, 68]. Grassino and Bellemare[18] have studied the influence of force and duty cycle – measured as differential diaphragmatic pressure and inspiration time in relation to breathing cycle duration – on the spectral content of the myoelectric signal; their results are in agreement with those from periodic loading of skeletal muscles mentioned earlier. They concluded that ventilation and duty cycle in loaded inspiration are linked to the metabolic state of the inspiratory muscle. There is also general agreement that myoelectric spectral analysis can reliably detect diaphragmatic fatigue prior to the time when the muscle fails as a pressure generator[19].

One interesting application of myoelectric spectral analysis in respiratory physiology concerns the study of REM sleep in newborns[49]. During REM sleep intercostal muscles relax causing the rib cage to be partly distorted. The diaphragm then must work harder to maintain the tidal volume and shows myoelectric signs of fatigue in proportion to the rib cage distortion. Some infants hypoventilate for a period of time before they increase the activity of their intercostal muscles while others make use of a fatigue-recovering apnea for 5–30 s[49]. Diaphragmatic fatigue was likewise found in newborns with cardiopulmonary diseases who were being weaned off the respirator. In adults, muscle fatigue also contributed to the difficulty they experienced during weaning from artificial ventilation[62].

Local muscle fatigue seems to be very common in respiratory failure. In a number of diseases affecting respiration, patients are obviously working with their respiratory muscles very close to the critical levels of force and duty cycle where fatigue becomes significant. It has thus been stated that muscle fatigue probably is the limiting factor in patients with CO_2 retention that prevents them from maintaining normal Pa,co_2[62]. In quadriplegic patients, it has also been shown that only a moderate increase in respiratory resistance will cause localized fatigue in the inspiratory muscles.

There are many other potential applications for fatigue detection with myoelectric spectral analysis. One is quantification of severeness of peripheral circulatory disturbances. In contrast to plethysmographic methods now used, EMG spectral methods have increased sensitivity when blood flow decreases. The myoelectric method is also a functional test of the muscle: blood flow as well as oxygen utilization and enzyme efficiency are integrated by measuring spectral change.

Conclusions

The authors have discussed some features of EMG spectral analysis and described the use of spectra in studies of localized muscle fatigue. They foresee an extensive use of EMG spectral analysis in routine clinical diagnosis. The theoretical models describing EMG volume conduction and signal summation suggest numerous ways to extract important information from myoelectric signals.

In particular, propagation velocity, the width of the innervation zone and motor unit size (the number of fibers) are parameters of fundamental clinical interest which can be quantified through the power spectrum.

With reference to fatigue a few fields have been indicated with growing interest for application of EMG spectral methods, such as ergonomics and respiratory physiology. Further applications in this respect are the study of differential diagnosis of fatigue syndromes including those of psychogenic origin and also to non-invasive measurements of reduced buffering capacity in certain metabolic disorders. Another application is in the monitoring of the extraordinary fatigue during underwater work.

Technically, the EMG power spectrum analysis has required somewhat complicated equipment. With the recent appearance of micro processors, computer-based myoelectric signal analysis will be included in daily diagnostic routines.

References

1 BARCROFT, H. and MILLEN, J. L. E. The blood flow through muscle during sustained contraction. *Journal of Physiology*, **97**, 17–31 (1939)

2 BASS, L. and MOORE, W. J. The role of protons in nerve conduction. *Progress in Biophysics and Molecular Biology*, **27**, 143–171 (1973)

3 BORG, G. and NOBLE, B. I. Perceived exertion. In *Exercise and Sport Sciences Reviews*, **2**, edited by J. Wilmore, 131–153. New York, Academic Press (1974)

4 BROMAN, H. An investigation on the influence of a sustained contraction on the succession of action potentials from a single motor unit. *Electromyography and Clinical Neurophysiology*, **17**, 341–358 (1977)

5 CARLSÖÖ, S. The static muscle load in different work positions: an electromyographic study. *Ergonomics*, **4**, 193 (1961)

6 CHAFFIN, D. B. Localized muscle fatigue – definition and measurement. *Journal of Occupational Medicine*, **15**, 346–354 (1973)

7 COLE, K. S. *Membranes, Ions and Impulses*. Berkeley and Los Angeles, University of California Press (1968)

8 DAWSON, M. J., GADIAN, D. G. and WILKIE, D. R. Contraction and recovery of living muscles studied by ^{31}P nuclear magnetic resonance. *Journal of Physiology*, **267**, 703–735 (1977)

9 DOWLING, M. H., FITCH, P. and WILLISON, R. G. A special purpose digital computer (Biomac 500) used in the analysis of the human electromyogram. *Electroencephalography and Clinical Neurophysiology*, **25**, 570–573 (1968)

10 EDWARDS, R. H. T., HILL, D. K. and McDONNELL, M. Myothermal and intramuscular pressure measurements during isometric contractions of the human quadriceps muscle. *Journal of Physiology*, **224**, 58P–59P (1972)

11 EDWARDS, R. H. T., HILL, D. K. and McDONNELL, M. Metabolic heat production and relaxation rate of electrically stimulated contractions of the quadriceps muscle in man. *Journal of Physiology*, **231**, 81P–83P (1973)

12 EDWARDS, R. H. T., HILL, D. K. and JONES, D. A. Heat production and chemical changes during isometric contractions of the human quadriceps muscle. *Journal of Physiology*, **251**, 303–315 (1975)

13 EDWARDS, R. H. T., McDONNELL, M. I. and HILL, D. K. A thermistor probe for myothermal measurements in man. *Journal of Applied Physiology*, **36**, 511–513 (1974)

14 ERICSON, B. E. and HAGBERG, M. EMG power spectra versus muscular contraction level. *Acta Neurologica Scandinavica*, Supplementum **73**, 163 (1979)

15 FEX, J. and KRAKAU, C. E. T. Some experiences with Walton's frequency analysis of the electromyogram. *Journal of Neurology, Neurosurgery and Psychiatry*, **20**, 178–184 (1957)

16 FRAUENDORF, H., GELBRICH, W., KRAMER, H. and REIMER, W. Einfluss von lokaler Erwärmung auf die elektrische und thermische Leitfähigkeit der Haut und das Oberflächen-EMG. *European Journal of Applied Physiology*, **33**, 339–346 (1974)

17 GERSTEN, J. W., CENKOVICH, F. S. and JONES, G. D. Harmonic analysis of normal and abnormal electromyograms. *American Journal of Physical Medicine*, **44**, 235–240 (1965)

18 GRASSINO, A. and BELLEMARE, F. Respiratory muscle fatigue and its effects on the breathing cycle. In *Central Nervous Control Mechanisms in Breathing*, edited by C. von Euler and H. Lagercrantz, Wenner-Gren Center International Symposium Series, **32**, 465–472 (1978)

19 GROSS, D., GRASSINO, A., ROSS, W. R. D. and MACKLEM, P. Electromyogram pattern of diaphragmatic fatique. *Journal of Applied Physiology*, **46**, 1–7 (1979)

20 HAGBERG, M. and JONSSON, B. The amplitude distribution of the myoelectric signal in an ergonomic study of the deltoid muscle. *Ergonomics*, **18**, 311–319 (1975)

21 HANSON, J. Effects of repetitive stimulation on membrane potentials and muscle contraction. In vitro studies of muscle fibres from frog, rat and man. *Thesis*, Karolinska Hospital, Stockholm (1974)

22 HAYES, K. J. Wave analysis of tissue noise and muscle action potentials. *Journal of Applied Physiology*, **15**, 749–752 (1960)

23 HERBERTS, P. and KADEFORS, R. A study of painful shoulder in welders. *Acta Orthopaedica Scandinavica*, **47**, 381–387 (1976)

24 HUMPHREYS, P. W. and LIND, A. R. The blood flow through active and inactive muscles of the forearm during sustained hand-grip contractions. *Journal of Physiology*, **166**, 120–135 (1963)

25 KADEFORS, R., KAISER, E. and PETERSÉN, I. Dynamic spectrum analysis of myo-potentials with special reference to muscle fatigue. *Electromyography*, **8**, 39–74 (1968)

26 KADEFORS, R. and PETERSÉN, I. Industrial work and localized muscle fatigue. In *Symposia – Sixth International Congress of Electromyography* (Stockholm, Sweden, 1979), edited by A. Persson, Department of Clinical Neurophysiology, Huddinge Hospital, Sweden. 188–194 (1979)

27 KAISER, E., KADEFORS, R., MAGNUSSON, R. and PETERSÉN, I. Myoelectric signals for prosthesis control. *Medicinsk Teknik-Medicoteknik*, **1**, 14–42 (1968)

28 KAISER, E. and PETERSÉN, I. Frequency analysis of action potentials during tetanic contraction. *Electroencephalography and Clinical Neurophysiology*, **14**, 955 (1962)

29 KOGI, K. and HAKAMADA, T. Slowing of surface electromyogram and muscle strength in muscle fatigue. *Report of the Institute for Science of Labour*, **60**, 27–41 (1962)

30 KOMI, P. V. and VIITASALO, J. H. T. Signal characteristics of EMG at different levels of muscular tension. *Acta Physiologica Scandinavica*, **96**, 267–276 (1976)

31 KONDO, S. Anthropological study on human posture and locomotion mainly from the viewpoint of electromyography. *Journal of the Faculty of Science, University of Tokyo*, Series **V–II–2**, 189–260 (1960)

32 KOPEC, J. and HAUSMANOVA-PETRUSEWICZ, I. Application of harmonic analysis to the electromyogram's evaluation. *Acta Physiologica Polonica*, **XVII**, 597–608 (1966)

33 KWATNY, E., THOMAS, D. H. and KWATNY, H. G. An application of signal processing techniques to the study of myoelectric signals. *IEEE Transactions on Biomedical Engineering*, **BME–17**, 303–312 (1970)

34 LARSSON, L.-E. Frequency analysis of the EMG in neuromuscular disorders. *Electroencephalography and Clinical Neurophysiology*, **24**, 89 (1968)

35 LARSSON, L.-E., ERLANDSSON, P. and LUNDBERG, M. Erfarenheter av neurofysiologisk followup på patienter med regelbunden dialysbe-

handling. *Medicinsk Riksstämma, Stockholm,* (26–30 November) Stockholm, Swedish Medical Association (1969) In Swedish.

36 LINDSTRÖM, L. Filtering properties of EMG-electrodes. In *Proceedings of the 1st Nordic Meeting on Medical and Biological Engineering*, (Otaniemi, Finland), 134–136. Helsinki, Finnish Society for Medical and Biological Engineering (1970)

37 LINDSTRÖM, L. On the frequency spectrum of EMG signals. *Thesis*, Research Laboratories for Medical Electronics, Goteborg (1970)

38 LINDSTRÖM, L. Fatigue changes in the myoelectric signal during periodic muscle work. *Bulletin Européen de Physiopathologie Respiratoire*, **15**, 107–114 (1979)

39 LINDSTRÖM, L., BROMAN, H., MAGNUSSON, R. and PETERSÉN, I. On the interrelation of two methods of EMG analysis. *Electroencephalography and Clinical Neurophysiology*, **7**, 801 (1973)

40 LINDSTRÖM, L. and HELLSING, G. Masseter muscle fatigue objectively quantified by analysis of myoelectric signals. *Archives of Oral Biology* (in press)

41 LINDSTRÖM, L., KADEFORS, R. and PETERSÉN, I. An electromyographic index for localized muscle fatigue. *Journal of Applied Physiology*, **43**, 750–754 (1977)

42 LINDSTRÖM, L. and MAGNUSSON, R. I. Interpretation of myoelectric power spectra: A model and its applications. *Proceedings of the Institute of Electrical and Electronics Engineers*, **65**, 653–662 (1977)

43 LINDSTRÖM, L., MAGNUSSON, R. and PETERSÉN, I. Muscular fatigue and action potential conduction velocity changes studied with frequency analysis of EMG signals. *Electromyography*, **10**, 341–356 (1970)

44 LINDSTRÖM, L., MAGNUSSON, R. and PETERSÉN, I. Muscle load influence on myo-electric signal characteristics. *Scandinavian Journal of Rehabilitation Medicine*, Supplement 3, 127–148 (1974)

45 LLOYD, A. J. Surface electromyography during sustained isometric contractions. *Journal of Applied Physiology*, **30**, 713–719 (1971)

46 LYNN, P. A. Direct on-line estimation of muscle fiber conduction velocity by surface electromyography. *IEEE Transactions on Biomedical Engineering*, **BME–26**, 564–571 (1979)

47 MAGNUSSON, R. and PETERSÉN, I. Vocational electromyography. In *Proceedings of the Second Nordic Meeting on Medical and Biological Engineering*, 174–176. Oslo, Norwegian Society for Medical and Biological Engineering (1971)

48 MORTIMER, J. T., MAGNUSSON, R. and PETERSÉN, I. Conduction velocity in ischemic muscle: effect on EMG frequency spectrum. *American Journal of Physiology*, **219**, 1324–1329 (1971)

49 MULLER, N., GULSTON, G., CADE, D., WHITTON, J., FROESE, A. B., BRYAN, M. H. and BRYAN, A. C. Diaphragmatic muscle fatigue in the newborn. *Journal of Applied Physiology*, **46**, 688–695 (1979)

50 NAKAMARU, Y. and SCHWARTZ, A. The influence of hydrogen ion concentration on calcium binding and release by skeletal muscle sarcoplasmic reticulum. *Journal of General Physiology*, **59**, 22–32 (1972)

51 NIGHTINGALE, A. The analysis of muscle potentials by means of a Muirhead-Pametrada wave analyser. *Muirhead Technique*, **11**, 27–32 (1957)

52 NIGHTINGALE, A. 'Background noise' in electromyography. *Physics in Medicine and Biology*, **3**, 325–338 (1958/59)

53 NILSSON, B. and INGVAR, D. H. Intramuscular pressure and contractile strength related to muscle blood flow in man. *Scandinavian Journal of Clinical and Laboratory Investigation*, Supplement **93**, 31–38 (1966)

54 ÖRTENGREN, R. Electromygographic evaluation of localized muscle fatigue during static and dynamic loading. In *Symposia – Sixth International Congress of Electromyography* (Stockholm, Sweden, 1979), edited by A. Persson, Department of Clinical Neurophysiology, Huddinge Hospital, Sweden. 172–176 (1979)

55 PETERSÉN, I., HERBERTS, P., KADEFORS, R., PERSSON, I., RAGNARSSON, K. and TENGROTH, B. The measurement, evaluation and importance of electromyography and electroencephalography in arduous industrial work. In *Society, Stress and Disease – Working Life*, edited by L. Levi, Oxford, University Press (in press)

56 PETERSÉN, I. and KADEFORS, R. An electromyographic study of training technique in welding. In *Proceedings of the 19th International Congress of Electroencephalography and Clinical Neurophysiology*, Amsterdam (1977)

57 PETERSÉN, I. and MAGNUSSON, R. Vocational electromyography: methodology of muscle fatigue studies. *Digest of the Ninth International Conference on Medical and Biological Engineering*, 163. Melbourne (1971)

58 PETROFSKY, J. S. Frequency and amplitude analysis of the EMG during exercise on the bicycle ergometer. *European Journal of Applied Physiology*, **41**, 1–15 (1979)

59 RICE, S. O. Mathematical analysis of random noise. *Bell System Technical Journal*, **23/24** 1–162 (1944–45)

60 RICHARDSON, A. T. *St. Thomas' Hospital Reports*, Ser. 2, **7**, 164 (1951). Quoted by Walton (reference 74)

61 ROHMERT, W. Ermittlung von Erholungspausen für statische Arbeit des Menschen. *Internationale Zeitschrift für Angewandte Physiologie, Einschliesslich Arbeitsphysiologie*, **18**, 123–164 (1960)

62 ROUSSOS, C. Respiratory muscle fatigue in the hypercapnic patient. *Bulletin Européen de Physiopathologie Respiratoire*, **15**, 117–123 (1977)

63 SABBAHI, M. A., DeLUCA, C. J. and POWERS, W. R. Effect of ischemia, cooling and local anesthesia on the median frequency of the myoelectric signals. In *Fourth Congress of ISEK* (Boston, USA) Chairman: C. DeLuca, Children's Hospital Medical Center, Boston, USA. 94–95 (1979)

64 SATO, M. Some problems in the quantitative evaluation of muscle fatigue by frequency analysis of the electromyogram. *Journal of the Anthropological Society of Japan*, **73**, 20–27 (1965)

65 SATO, M., HAYAMI, A. and SATO, H. Differential fatiguability between one- and two-joint muscles. *Journal of the Anthropological Society of Japan*, **73**, 14–22 (1965)

66 SCHERRER, J. and MONOD, H. Le travail musculaire local et la fatigue chez l'homme. *Journal de Physiologie (Paris)*, **52**, 419–501 (1960)

67 SCHWEITZER, T. W., FITZGERALD, J. W., BOWDEN, J. A. and LYNNE-DAVIS, P. Spectral analysis of human inspiratory diaphragmatic EMGs. *Journal of Applied Physiology*, **46**, 152–165 (1979)

68 SCOTT, R. N. Myo-electric energy spectra. *Medical and Biological Engineering*, **5**, 303–305 (1967)

69 SHIGIYA, R., ITOH, K., SUHARA, K., SAMESHIMA, M. and SUZUKI, H. Spectral analysis of surface electromyogram. *Electroencephalography and Clinical Neurophysiology*, **34**, 799–800 (1973)

70 STÅLBERG, E. Propagation velocity in human muscle fibres in situ. *Acta Physiologica Scandinavica*, **70**, Supplementum 287 (1966)

71 SYLVEST, D. and HVID, N. Pressure measurements in human striated muscles during contraction. *Acta Rheumatolgica Scandinavica*, **5**, 216–222 (1959)

72 TASAKI, I., SINGER, I. and TAKENAKA, T. Effects of internal and external ionic environment on excitability of squid giant axon. *Journal of General Physiology*, **48**, 1095–1123 (1967)

73 TERAKAWA, S., NAGANO, M. and WATANABE, A. Intracellular pH and plateau duration of internally perfused squid giant axons. *Japanese Journal of Physiology*, **28**, 847–862 (1978)

74 WALTON, J. N. The electromyogram in myopathy: Analysis with the audio-frequency spectrometer. *Journal of Neurology, Neurosurgery and Psychiatry*, **15**, 219–226 (1952)

5
Electrophysiological tests of neuromuscular transmission
Erik Stalberg and Donald B. Sanders

Although it is not a common disease, myasthenia gravis (MG) has received much attention in recent years. One reason for this interest has been a major breakthrough in understanding the pathogenetic mechanisms. The defect of neuromuscular transmission in MG seems to be due mainly to an immunologically induced blockade and reduction of acetylcholine receptors on the muscle end-plate[1, 19]. The condition has been induced in animals by immunization with nicotinic receptor protein from, for example, the electric fish *Torpedo marmorata*[23, 34, 37]. Autoantibodies have been recognized in animals and in patients with MG, and their binding to the receptor has been demonstrated[18]. What triggers the autoimmune response is still unknown. Whether there are other abnormalities of the motor unit is also unknown. In addition, primary or secondary presynaptic defects have not been excluded, and an abnormality of the contractile mechanism has been suggested because of the absence of the so-called staircase phenomenon, which is seen in normal muscle following electrical stimulation[39].

Another reason for the recent interest in MG is the ability to reduce the symptoms by medical treatment in various ways, sometimes to complete remission. For instance, immunosuppressive agents and treatment by plasmapheresis reduce myasthenic symptoms.

The myasthenic syndrome, Eaton-Lambert syndrome, a condition that is even more uncommon than MG, presents similar clinical symptoms[14]. The principal neuromuscular defect is reduced acetylcholine release, however, and there are none of the immunological features seen in MG. In the majority of the cases there is a concomitant malignancy, usually oat cell cancer of the lung.

Patients with Eaton-Lambert syndrome must be distinguished from those with MG for several reasons. First, the high probability of lung cancer in patients with Eaton-Lambert syndrome should lead to a search for it though muscle symptoms may precede the clinical appearance of the cancer by many years. Secondly, patients with Eaton-Lambert syndrome should be treated differently from those with MG.

It is important, then, to recognize as soon as possible either Eaton-Lambert syndrome or MG amont patients who show symptoms of muscular fatiguability. Effective electrophysiological testing procedures are particularly valuable in providing early confirmation of diagnoses and in following the patient.

In this chapter some methods used in clinical neurophysiology to test neuromuscular transmission are presented. Other diagnostic techniques, for example, estimation of antibodies against cholinergic receptors, will not be described in detail but will be mentioned in a brief comparison of different diagnostic methods.

Normal neuromuscular transmission

After a terminal arborization, the intramuscular motor nerve ends in a number of so-called axonal expansions or presynaptic terminals, each of which lies in apposition to a motor end-plate that is located midway between the ends of a muscle fibre. The nerve terminal contains vesicles, some of which are concentrated in sites close to the membrane. These vesicles contain acetylcholine. A synaptic space of about 50 nm (500 A) separates the nerve terminal from the folded postsynaptic membrane of the muscle fibre. Cholinergic receptors are concentrated on the tips of the folds and are in juxtaposition to special structures of the presynaptic membrane that probably represent the sites of acetylcholine release.

Acetylcholine is synthesized inside the terminal and stored in the vesicles. During rest there is a slow spontaneous release of acetylcholine, some of which appears as packages, or quanta (corresponding to the content of a single vesicle), which are discharged into the synaptic gap. After discharge, the wall of the empty vesicle is incorporated into the presynaptic membrane. New vesicles are formed by invagination of the membrane. They are initially empty but become filled with acetylcholine in the terminal. A nerve impulse causes simultaneous release of many vesicles in the following way: depolarization of the

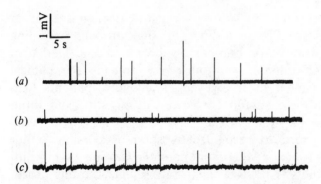

Figure 5.1 Miniature end-plate potentials recorded in
intercostal muscle fibres from a normal subject (*a*), a
patient with myasthenia gravis (*b*), and a patient with
Eaton-Lambert syndrome (*c*). The amplitude of the
spontaneously occurring MEPPs is reduced in (*b*) and
very small MEPPs may be hidden in the baseline,
producing an apparent reduction in frequency as well.
In (*c*), the amplitude and frequency of MEPPs is not
different from control recordings

nerve terminal membrane initiates a voltage-dependent calcium influx
into the nerve terminal which causes the vesicles to approach the
membrane and rupture into the synaptic space. Acetylcholine crosses
the synaptic space and binds to the receptors. The interaction produces local depolarization of the end-plate membrane, and when this
depolarization exceeds a certain threshold value a muscle action
potential is generated. Acetylcholine is then hydrolyzed by cholinesterase, and the resulting choline is resorbed into the terminal,
probably via specific channels.

These events can be monitored by means of intracellular microelectrodes in the end-plate area of muscle fibres. The spontaneous release
of quanta produces miniature end-plate potentials (MEPPs) with
amplitudes of 0.2–1.2 mV, well below the threshold necessary to
trigger an action potential, which requires a depolarization of 15–25
mV. MEPPs normally appear with a frequency of about 1 per 5 s
(*Figure 5.1*). After a nerve impulse the summated activity from many
quanta is seen as a larger depolarization called an end-plate potential
(EPP), which normally exceeds the firing threshold rapidly and
produces an action potential in the muscle fibre. From the MEPP
amplitude and frequency and the EPP amplitude, quantitative information is gained about neuromuscular transmission.

Electrodiagnostic tests

Progressive reduction or disappearance of visible muscle contraction during faradic stimulation in MG was described by Jolly[26] in 1895, who called this a 'myasthenic reaction.' The earliest reports of electromyographic abnormalities in MG were those of Lindsley[30] in 1935, who reported variability in the motor unit potential amplitude with consecutive discharges and of Harvey and Masland[21,22] in 1941, who in addition reported a decrementing muscle response with repetitive nerve stimulation. The first finding is still one of the major characteristics of conventional electromyography in MG but is usually not used for quantitative testing. The second observation has over the years become the basis of the most frequently used electrodiagnostic method in MG though it has undergone several modifications. The procedure whereby this test is performed in the authors' laboratories is described below.

Repetitive nerve stimulation

Surface electrodes are attached to the cleaned skin, one electrode over the motor end-plate zone, determined by recording compound muscle action potentials with a sharp negative take-off, and one electrode over an indifferent area. The stimulating electrode is placed proximally over the corresponding nerve.

As a standard procedure, stimulation frequency is started at 2 or 3 Hz, but never more than 5 Hz, and the negative amplitude of the first response is measured. Ten stimuli are given to define the pattern of any amplitude changes (decrement/increment) that are seen[33]. The change in amplitude between the first and fourth response is then calculated (*Figure 5.2*) The fifth response can also be used. If a computer is available the same calculations can be made for the area of the evoked compound muscle action potential. Discrepancies between changes in these two parameters usually indicate a technical artefact or so-called pseudofacilitation, which is due to synchronization of individual muscle fibre action potentials. This produces shortening of duration and an amplitude increase, but minimal or no change in the area. The amplitude is usually measured from film in other laboratories. It is recommended that the sweep speed used be fast enough for the waveform to be clearly discernible. Area measurements are too tedious to perform without a computer.

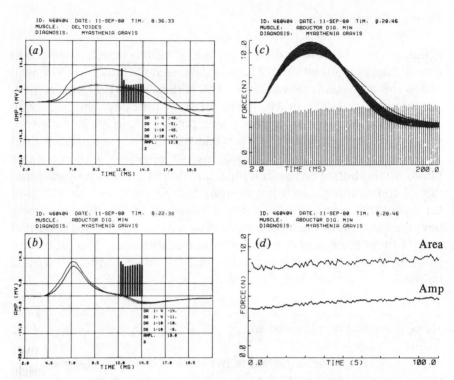

Figure 5.2 Computer printouts of recordings from a patient with myasthenia gravis. Surface recording of the muscle action potential after repetitive nerve stimulation (2 Hz) from (*a*) deltoid muscle, (*b*) ADM muscle. The decrement of amplitude and area are measured for the fourth and tenth response compared to the first. The amplitude changes are most pronounced in the deltoid muscle (decrement of the fourth response is 48 percent compared to 14 percent for the ADM muscle). In (*c*) and (*d*) the mechanical twitch amplitude and area of the ADM muscle are demonstrated. In this patient an increase is seen, so-called positive staircase, after an insignificant initial decrement, a normal finding

The patient is then asked to contract the muscle maximally for 20 s. The low frequency stimulation test is then repeated, first within 10 s after the end of the activation to demonstate facilitation (*Figure 5.3*) and then every minute or, later, every second minute for 10 min to study the post-activation exhaustion.

In cases of more pronounced MG an activation period of 20 s may be too long. In these cases the test will not show facilitation, only exhaustion. The activation time is then adjusted to an optimal duration. In cases of slight or moderate myasthenia, 20 s of activation may show facilitation but not give significant exhaustion. A longer period of muscle contraction is useful in such cases. For each patient the activation time is kept constant in follow-up investigations in order to obtain comparable results.

A more quantitative method of activation requires tetanic stimulation at 20–50 Hz for 10 s. This method is, in contrast to voluntary activation, somwhat painful and is not frequently used by the authors.

In some cases stimulation frequencies up to 10 Hz are useful. For example, when no decrement is found with 2 Hz, 10 Hz stimulation may reveal a decrement in children with MG. It is also useful, in addition to voluntary activation, to quantify the facilitation in Eaton-Lambert syndrome, when stimulation is continued for 10 s.

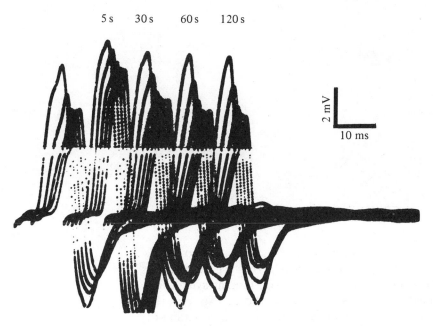

Figure 5.3 Repetitive nerve stimulation studies in the ADM of a patient with myasthenia gravis. The ulnar nerve was stimulated at 5 Hz before, and at indicated intervals after maximum voluntary contraction of the muscle for 30 s. Five seconds after the end of the voluntary contraction, the amplitude of the initial response was greater and the decrement was less, than they were originally ('facilitation'). After 60 s and 120 s the decrement was greater than originally (post-activation exhaustion)

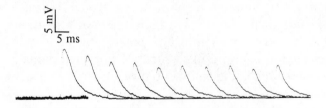

Figure 5.4 End-plate potentials (EPPs) recorded with
an intracellular microelectrode in an intercostal muscle
biopsy from a patient with myasthenia gravis, during
stimulation of the intramuscular nerve at 1 Hz. The
initial decrement ('rundown') has become maximal by
the fifth response; the variation in amplitude thereafter
results from normal fluctuations in the number of
acetylcholine quanta released from the nerve terminal

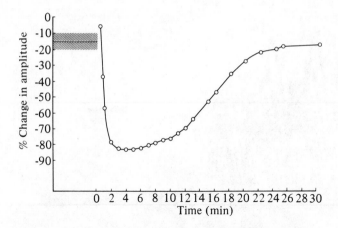

Figure 5.5 The decrement of muscle action potentials
recorded with surface electrodes on the gastrocnemius
muscle of a rabbit receiving a constant intravenous
infusion of *d*-tubocurarine. The vertical axis represents
the drop in amplitude of the fifth response to trains of
3 Hz stimuli applied to the sciatic nerve. At time 0, the
nerve was stimulated at 40 Hz for 10 s. The horizontal line
and shaded area represent the mean decrement ± 2 SD
recorded during a period of control observation prior to
activation with the high frequency stimulation. A brief
period of facilitation follows activation, and is followed by
a more prolonged period of 'post-activation exhaustion'

Background

Intracellular recordings from the myasthenic motor end-plate[17] show reduced amplitudes of MEPPs (*Figure 5.1*) and EPPs but a normal number of quanta in each EPP, i.e. normal quantal content. This is compatible with a postsynaptic defect.

The decrementing response seen in MG with repetitive nerve stimulation probably represents an unmasking of phenomena present in normal motor end-plates, but which is not detected because of the safety factor of neuromuscular transmission. *In vitro* recording of EPPs with an intracellular electrode in the partially blocked motor end-plate shows an initial decrement or 'rundown' in the EPP amplitude (*Figure 5.4*). There is also increased EPP amplitude during high frequency stimulation due to increased release of acetylcholine (facilitation) and reduced EPP amplitude ('exhaustion') thereafter. These variations in EPP amplitude do not produce any changes in strength or EMG measurements in normal muscle since all EPPs exceed the action potential threshold under the conditions described. The progressive weakness or excessive fatiguability that characterizes MG probably results from an unmasking of this 'normal' phenomenon of exhaustion following neuromuscular activation. The cause for this exhaustion is not known, but it is not specific to MG since it can also be seen after curarization (*Figure 5.5*).

In Eaton-Lambert syndrome (and in botulinum intoxication) there is also an initial decrement to repetitive nerve stimulation, but a much more pronounced facilitation is seen both after voluntary activation and during high frequency repetitive stimulation (*Figure 5.6*). In this condition the defect is due to impaired transmitter release. The decrement represents the unmasking of the normal rundown. The increase after activation is due to normally-present facilitation of acetylcholine release, which has an exaggerated effect in this disease in which release is impaired.

In normal muscle the electrical response from abductor digiti minimi and deltoid muscles shows the following characteristics: initial amplitude is more than 7 mV (normal values must be determined for each laboratory); decrement is less than 5 per cent; facilitation is less than 5 per cent; and there is no exhaustion.

In myasthenic muscle the amplitude of the initial muscle response is normal or reduced; decrement is more than 5 per cent and is more pronounced in proximal muscles; and facilitation is usually seen when the initial amplitude is reduced from normal. The amplitude usually increases by 10–50 per cent and/or there is less decrement. *Note*: the

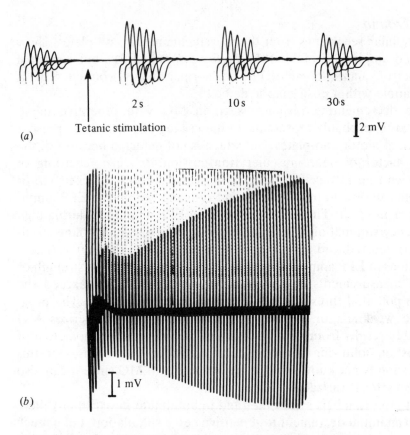

Figure 5.6 Surface recordings from the ADM muscle in a patient with Eaton-Lambert syndrome. (*a*) 5 Hz stimulation before and at indicated intervals after maximum voluntary muscle contraction for 20 s (arrow). The facilitation was 104 per cent. (*b*) 50 Hz stimulation for 1.5 s showing an initial decrement (partially obscured by baseline shift) and subsequent facilitation. The broken vertical lines are stimulus artefacts. (After Sanders *et al.*, *Journal of Neurology, Neurosurgery and Psychiatry*, **43**, 978–985, 1980)

test must be performed immediately after the end of activation, preferably within about 10 s. Post-activation exhaustion, i.e. reduced initial amplitude and/or increased decrement, may be seen after 2–5 min. In *Figure 5.7* it is seen between 1 and 3 min.

In Eaton-Lambert syndrome the amplitude of the initial response in the hand muscles is low, usually less than 2 mV; the decrement is similar to that in myasthenia; and facilitation back toward normal is

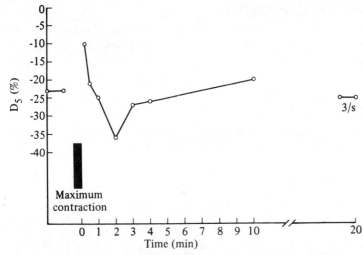

Figure 5.7 Amplitude decrement between the first and fifth responses (D_5) from ADM muscle in a patient with myasthenia gravis. Note the facilitation after 30 s of maximal voluntary activation and subsequent exhaustion

usually 200–300 per cent. Facilitation is also usually demonstrated during prolonged 10 Hz stimulation, which produces similar increases in amplitude. Post-activation exhaustion is also present, but may be difficult to demonstrate when the initial amplitude is very low.

Choice of muscle

The test can be performed in many muscles in the leg, arm or face. In many laboratories hand muscles are tested first because of the convenient recording and stimulation sites. Usually, however, the myasthenic abnormality is much easier to detect in proximal muscles, for example, biceps or deltoid[33]. A negative result in hand muscles should *always* be followed by tests in proximal muscles. In the authors' laboratories the deltoid muscle is always tested by stimulation at Erb's point or the biceps brachii by stimulation in the axilla. In patients with MG, decrement has been demonstrated in 38 per cent of the abductor digiti minimi muscles tested (202 patients) and in 64 per cent of the deltoid muscles tested (178 patients). In none of the patients have there been normal findings in deltoid or biceps when tests in the hand muscles were abnormal. It may be necessary to study facial muscles in patients with mainly ocular MG in order to demonstrate a decremental response.

Decrement enhancing methods

Exercise may unmask a mild neuromuscular abnormality and can be used as part of the diagnostic test. It should not be used for quantitative follow-up since it is impossible to standardize. *Increased muscle temperature* can be used to provoke abnormalities[25], since the decrement is greater after warming the muscle from resting values, which are usually below 30°C.

The increase in decrement with increased temperature varies among patients and muscles (*Figure 5.8*). Serial tests should be performed at

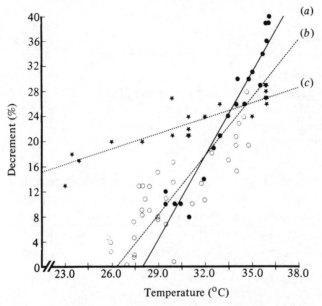

Figure 5.8 Effects of temperature on the decrement in 3 patients. (*a*) (●), and (*c*) (✻) from deltoid muscles, (*b*) (○) from ADM muscle

the same intramuscular temperature if comparisons are to be made among them. *Ischaemia* is used by some investigators[5, 10] by placing a blood-pressure cuff around the upper arm and performing repetitive nerve stimulation after three minutes. The authors' limited experience indicates that it is more useful to study an adequately warmed proximal muscle than to study an ischaemic distal muscle. In a few laboratories a small dose of *curare* is injected, usually as a regional test[20, 24], and its effect on neuromuscular transmission is studied.

Because this is a potentially hazardous test, it is not used in the authors' laboratories. Another way of testing neuromuscular transmission is to measure the mechanical twitch, which is technically more difficult than measuring the electrical responses. It should be said here that mechanical twitch measures the contractile characteristics of the muscle fibres as well as the neuromuscular transmission. With repetitive nerve stimulation the twitch amplitude typically decreases as previously described for the electrical response. Facilitation and post-activation exhaustion may also be seen with this technique.

Staircase phenomenon

When the nerve to a normal muscle is stimulated at 1–3 Hz, the mechanical twitch initially decreases by 10 per cent (negative staircase) but increases by 15–50 per cent with an average of 25 per cent after 3–5 min (positive staircase) (Figure 5.2). This phenomenon has been described in animal and human muscles[13, 39]. The positive staircase is characterized by increasing single twitch force, reduced contraction time and reduced relaxation time. It results from an intensification of the excitation–contraction process (active state). One hypothesis is that the muscle action potential releases an increased amount of calcium ions from the sarcoplasmic reticulum that enhances the twitch. The staircase is typically reduced in Duchenne dystrophy[11].

After curarization the mechanical twitch is reduced. In comparison to the electrical response, the mechanical responses initially decrease to the same extent but they show a slow increase to give a so-called relative staircase.

Slomic, Rosenfalck and Buchtal[39] reported the absence of the staircase phenomenon in MG. However, other investigators[12] found a positive staircase in 22 of 24 patients with MG after allowing for the simultaneous neuromuscular blockade.

The staircase phenomenon is difficult to interpret in MG because a decreasing number of fibres contributes to the mechanical twitch during continuous nerve stimulation.

Slomic, Rosenfalck and Buchtal[39] have reported cases of MG with no or minimal decrement with an abnormal staircase response, that is, absence of staircase. The value of the technique in the diagnosis of MG is still uncertain. It may have a role in further studies of contractile mechanisms in that disease.

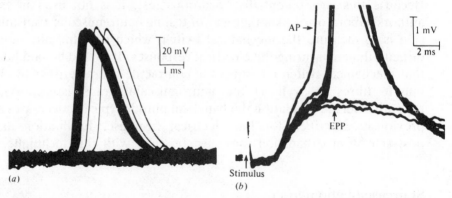

Figure 5.9(a) Intracellular recordings made at the end-plate in an intercostal muscle from a patient with myasthenia gravis during stimulation of the intramuscular nerve at 1 Hz. The variation and latency from stimulus (which occurred at a constant point just off the figure to the left) to response is the neuromuscular jitter. (*b*) Similar recordings made from curarized normal human intercostal muscle at a higher gain than in (*a*). The action potentials (AP) are truncated by the high gain used. Variations in latency from stimulus to AP result from variations in the time necessary for EPPs to reach threshold. When the threshold is not reached no action potential occurs (blocking) and the full EPP wave form can be seen

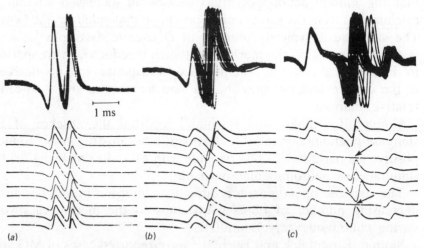

Figure 5.10 Single fibre recordings from the EDC muscle in a patient with MG. They show (*a*) normal jitter, (*b*) increased jitter, and (*c*) increased jitter with intermittent impulse blockings (arrows). (From Stalberg, Clinical electrophysiology in myasthenia gravis. *Journal of Neurology, Neurosurgery and Psychiatry*, **43**, 622–633 (1980), courtesy of the Editor and publisher)

Single fibre electromyography

By means of a selective EMG recording technique it is possible to study neuromuscular transmission quantitatively in individual motor end-plates *in situ*. This technique, called single fibre EMG (SFEMG), has been described in detail by Stålberg and Trontelj[43].

When action potentials are recorded from two muscle fibres in the same motor unit, the time interval between them varies during consecutive discharges, a phenomenon called *jitter*. Jitter is mainly due to variability in synaptic delay and is in the order of 10–50 µs expressed as the mean value of the consecutive time interval differences (MCD), in the normal muscle.

In cases of disturbed neuromuscular transmission, for example, after curare is administered, during ischaemia, during the early stages of re-innervation and in myasthenia gravis and Eaton-Lambert syndrome, the jitter is increased. With more pronounced disturbances, individual muscle impulses may be missing, that is, there is an intermittent or partial neuromuscular block. It is thus possible to detect slightly impaired neuromuscular function as increased jitter before any impulse blocking occurs, the latter phenomenon being necessary for clinical examinations and other tests to demonstrate abnormal neuromuscular transmission[15, 36, 44]. The synaptic events responsible for these phenomena can be demonstrated with intracellular recordings from the end-plate area of the muscle fibre (*Figure 5.9*).

The typical finding in a patient with myasthenia gravis is that some motor end-plates have normal jitter, others have increased jitter and still others show intermittent blocking (*Figure 5.10*). This spectrum of findings also occurs within a single motor unit. In order to quantify the results, 20 potential pairs are studied. The results are expressed as the frequency of potential pairs having normal jitter, increased jitter and increased jitter with blocking. The overall mean jitter for all fibres studied is also calculated.

The distribution of normal versus abnormal motor end-plates varies with the degree of clinical involvement (*Table 5.1*). Within the same patient, clinically involved muscles usually show more abnormalities than do muscles with normal strength. As a rule, jitter is abnormal in some fibres even in clinically normal muscles in the myasthenic patient, but no blockings are seen. For example, the extensor digitorum communis (EDC) muscle shows some abnormal motor end-plates in about 60 per cent of patients who have purely ocular myasthenia. A varying degree of electrophysiological abnormality is

Table 5.1 Single fibre findings* in the extensor digitorum communis muscle
in 141 patients with myasthenia gravis

Group (number)	Mean jitter, μs	% Normal fibre pairs	% Fibre pairs with blocking
Control (26)	27.6 ± 0.6 (22–33)	98 ± 0.5 (94–100)	0.5 ± 0.3 (0–6)
Remission (12)	35.9 ± 2.1 (25–52)	86 ± 3.5 (58–100)	2 ± 1.2 (0–12)
Ocular (19)	34.1 ± 1.7 (22–49)	84 ± 5.3 (0–100)	2.7 ± 1.3 (0–19)
Mild generalized without weak EDC (52)	45.1 ± 3.7 (22–199)	77 ± 2.9 (8–100)	9 ± 2.1 (0–77)
with weak EDC (22)	90.0 ± 5.8 (49–133)	24 ± 5.3 (0–71)	39 ± 6.1 (0–100)
Moderate and severe generalized (36)	121.6 ± 13.4 (36–276)	16 ± 4.5 (0–95)	60.0 ± 6.2 (0–100)

* Values given as group mean ± SEM (range). Patients in remission had been treated with prednisone and/or thymectomy. All other patients were studied at the time of initial diagnosis.

seen when patients are divided into clinical groups using the Osserman classification. Those with ocular myasthenia show the fewest abnormalities.

Jitter is affected by the same enhancing manoeuvres described for the decrement studies. Thus, in patients with MG, jitter increases with activity and with increasing temperature and decreases after edrophonium injection in patients who are not receiving cholinesterase inhibitors. The degree of blocking also decreases as the jitter value decreases towards normal. In patients treated with cholinesterase inhibitors, the jitter may increase in some motor end-plates after injection of edrophonium.

With certain criteria for abnormality (more than 2 abnormal recordings out of 20 or an average jitter among the 20 exceeding 34 μs), SFEMG has been positive in 95 per cent of 291 cases. It has been positive in 100 per cent of the cases when a weak muscle was tested. In ocular MG, 85 per cent of the patients have shown increased jitter in facial muscles and 59 per cent in the EDC muscle. Of 13 patients in clinical remission (no symptoms of MG or detectable weakness, receiving no cholinesterase inhibitors) four have shown normal SFEMG studies in EDC. In the others some abnormality has still been seen, usually with few fibres showing blocking.

In three patients with thymoma who had no symptoms of MG before the investigation, jitter was abnormal[36]. One of the patients later developed clinical evidence of MG. In another, abnormal neuromuscular transmission was confirmed by intercostal muscle biopsy.

In Eaton-Lambert syndrome the jitter is greatly increased and impulse blockings occur frequently. The main difference between jitter caused by Eaton-Lambert syndrome and that in MG is the effect of continuous activity. When the innervation frequency is increased, jitter increases in the typical case of MG but decreases in Eaton-Lambert syndrome. This response is expected considering what is known about the underlying abnormality of neuromuscular transmission in these two disorders.

Single fibre EMG is technically more complicated than decrement studies but gives information about the individual motor end-plate and is sensitive enough to detect abnormal neuromuscular transmission before impulse blockings occur. It should be re-stated that increased jitter is a sign of disturbed neuromuscular transmission and is not synonymous with a myasthenic defect (*see* p. 110).

Needle electromyography

The needle EMG (concentric or monopolar recording) is performed in patients suspected of having MG for two reasons. The first, and in the authors' opinion the most important, is to exclude other diseases that may resemble MG clinically or to find concomitant diseases, such as myositis or thyroid myopathy. The second reason is to make a positive diagnosis of MG.

As expected from the findings seen in SFEMG, when jitter is increased and impulse blocking is present, the motor unit action potential (MUP), which represents the temporal and spatial summation of action potentials from 5 to 15 muscle fibres, may show defective neuromuscular transmission as a shape variability at consecutive discharges (*Figure 5.11*). This is also the explanation for the variations in MUP amplitude that were described by Harvey and Masland[22] in 1941.

Another finding is a continuous change in the MUP, the amplitude and duration decreasing steadily during activity. The MUP may be normal at the beginning of a period of activity and return to normal after 10–30s of rest. The smallness of the MUP, caused by the neuromuscular block, has been misinterpreted as a sign of myopathy in MG. A superimposed myopathy is actually sometimes found and verified by biopsy. The clinically important question of whether

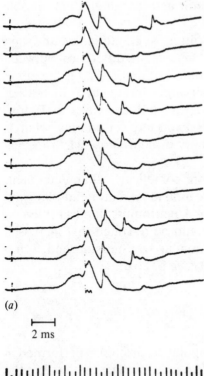

(a)

|———|
2 ms

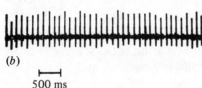

(b)

|———|
500 ms

Figure 5.11 Potentials recorded from a single motor unit with a concentric needle EMG electrode in a patient with MG during slight voluntary contraction. With a fast oscilloscope sweep speed (*a*), variations in the motor unit potential wave form can be seen. With a slower sweep speed (*b*), significant fluctuations in the motor unit potential amplitude can be appreciated

steroid myopathy is present in these patients may be very difficult to answer. The typical normalization of MUP after rest or edrophonium is not seen in motor units that are abnormal mainly due to myopathy, but it may be seen if the abnormality is due to a neuromuscular defect. Because these two conditions may co-exist, the differentiation is difficult.

Recently Boyd, Lawrence and Bratty[6] presented a technique to analyse variability of the motor unit potential. Using a concentric needle electrode they recorded the activity from one motor unit just outside its territory, as judged from the smooth, usually triphasic shape of the MUP. From the other studies[42] it is known that this MUP still represents only the part of the motor unit that is closest to the recording needle. Boyd, Lawrence and Bratty analyzed the shape variability of the action potential with consecutive discharges. In the myasthenic patient, this variability is greater than in normal muscle due to increased jitter and blocking among those fibres contributing to the recorded MUP. This analysis necessitates the use of a computer.

End-plate noise

When recording with concentric EMG needle electrodes in the end-plate zone of the muscle, it is every electromyographer's experience occasionally to record 'noise' of low amplitude, usually less than 50 μV. This is produced most likely by extracellularly recorded miniature end-plate potentials[46]. Their frequency is higher than seen *in vitro* with intracellular electrodes partly because more nerve endings are contributing to the signal and possibly also because the temperature in the muscle is higher than that usually used in the bath. In normal muscle end-plate noise amplitude is very dependent on the position of the recording electrode. The amplitude and frequency of this noise is said by some authors[31] to be decreased in MG corresponding to the decrease in MEPP amplitude seen in the *in vitro* studies. The problem, of course, is that a reduction of noise amplitude may also be due to positioning of the electrode. The absence of noise can probably not be used as a diagnostic criterion of MG since in the absence of noise there is no direct evidence that the recording is made in the immediate end-plate vicinity.

Stapedial reflex fatigue

The stapedius muscle acts to change the tension on the ear-drum, and its action can be inferred from measurements of the acoustic impedance of the tympanic membrane. Reflex contraction of this muscle is induced by sound presented to either ear; thus, stimulation of the stapedial reflex can be used to produce impedance changes that quantitatively reflect the tension of stapedial contraction (*Figure 5.12*).

Continuous sound stimulation produces sustained contraction of the stapedius; it has been shown that the reflex impedance progressively decreases in myasthenia gravis because of fatigue of this muscle[3, 45]. Technically, it is difficult to measure a steady impedance change for more than several seconds at a time. Sound stimulation, consisting of pulses of 200–500 ms duration separated by an equal duration 'off

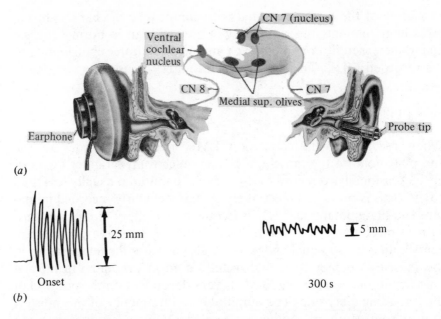

(a)

(b)

Figure 5.12 (a) Stapedial reflex recording system and reflex arc. The sound stimulus is presented to one ear via the earphone and tympanic membrane impedance is measured with a probe in the opposite ear canal. (b) Changes in the tympanic membrane impedance produced by pulsed sound stimuli in a patient with MG at the beginning and at the end of a 300 s period of stimulation. The drop in amplitude of impedance excursions can be at least partially reversed by the administration of edrophonium. (After Kramer *et al.*[28])

time', have been used to produce rapid changes in the acoustic impedance and the amplitude of these impedance excursions can be determined over prolonged periods[35]. When there is defective neuromuscular transmission in the stapedius muscle there is a decrementing pattern in these excursions (*Figure 5.12*), frequently reversed by edrophonium, similar to that seen in twitch tension and compound muscle action potential responses in other, more peripheral muscles.

Using pulsed sound stimulation, Kramer *et al.*[28] found an abnormal degree of stapedial reflex fatigue in 84 per cent of 89 myasthenic patients studied (*Table 5.2*). Those authors have also found abnormal stapedial reflex fatigue in other diseases of the motor unit, and the full range of diseases that can produce this abnormality has yet to be defined.

The technique for measuring stapedial reflex fatigue is painless and requires only minimal cooperation. Most of the equipment required is available in a well-equipped audiology laboratory. Since experience with the technique is still limited, it is advisable to establish local control values before using it in the clinical diagnosis of neuromuscular disorders.

Table 5.2 Stapedial reflex fatigue to pulsed sound stimulation in patients with myasthenia gravis

Class of disease (number of patients)	Percent abnormal studies (n)
Remission (6)	83(5)
Ocular (10)	90(9)
Mild generalized (54)	91(49)
Moderate or severe generalized (19)	63(12)

(From Kramer *et al.*[28], courtesy of the Editor and publishers, *Annals of Neurology*)

Oculography and tonometry

It is frequently difficult to confirm defective neuromuscular transmission in patients with myasthenia gravis whose weakness is limited to the extraocular muscles; thus, several techniques have been developed to demonstrate edrophonium responses in these muscles.

Ocular muscle EMG

Direct needle electromyography of ocular muscles may show a reduction in motor unit activity after sustained effort, with increased motor unit activity after administration of edrophonium[7]. This procedure is unpleasant and may not be tolerated by all patients. Quantitation of changes in motor unit activity is relatively crude and is usually subjective. This technique has not been tested in large disease and control populations and has limited clinical applicability.

Tonometry

Tonometric measurements of intraocular pressure demonstrate increases in pressure after edrophonium administration to patients with ocular myasthenia[27]. In a study of 22 patients with MG there was a significant tonometric response to edrophonium in all, but it was necessary to withhold cholinesterase inhibitors for two days prior to study[47]. False positive responses, however, were seen in nonmyasthenic disease controls. In another study of 17 patients with MG, tonometric responses were found in all patients except one whose ocular muscle weakness was fixed[8].

Oculography

Electronystagmography has been used to measure the amplitude of optokinetic nystagmus (OKN) excursions before and after administration of edrophonium. This procedure demonstrated significant increases in OKN amplitude after edrophonium in all 13 patients with MG reported in three studies[4, 32, 41] but in only 50 per cent of 12 patients reported in a fourth[8].

When infrared measurements of OKN deflections were used, an increase after edrophonium was seen in 100 per cent of 40 patients with MG, including eight without demonstrable ophthalmoparesis[40]. Increased amplitude and/or velocity of saccadic eye movements after edrophonium was found in 11 of 12 patients with MG, only three of whom had clinically apparent ocular muscle weakness[2].

Tests of ocular muscle function before and after the administration of edrophonium are probably quite sensitive in detecting the neuromuscular abnormality of MG, if local control values are established in normal and non-myasthenic disease populations.

Intercostal muscle biopsy

The physiological abnormalities characteristic of MG[17] and the Eaton-Lambert syndrome[16] can be demonstrated definitively in physiologically intact muscle biopsies, though this is much too complicated a technique to be used in routine clinical diagnosis.

The intercostal muscle is uniquely suited for these studies since the entire length of uncut fibres from an interspace can be obtained by removing periosteum with the muscle from the rib above and below. The biopsy can be performed laterally, near the anterior axillary line, or medially, near the costochondral junction. Since this procedure is usually performed at the time of thymectomy, the latter location avoids a separate incision and reduces postoperative discomfort.

Classical techniques for recording intracellular electrical events with glass microelectrodes allow the measurement of voltage changes at the muscle end-plate that reflect the amount of acetylcholine contained in each quantum released spontaneously from the nerve terminal, the responsiveness of the end-plate to each quantum and the number of quanta released by nerve stimulation. Single quanta of spontaneously released acetylcholine produce miniature end-plate potentials having normal amplitudes of approximately 1 mV. MEPPs are reduced in amplitude in MG[17] (*Figure 5.1*) as is the postsynaptic membrane's response to iontophoretically-applied acetylcholine[1]. In Eaton-Lambert syndrome, MEPP size is normal (*Figure 5.1*), but there is a reduction in the number of quanta released by nerve stimulation[16]. The fact that the neuromuscular defect is presynaptic in Eaton-Lambert syndrome and postsynaptic in myasthenia gravis explains many of the differences in the characteristic responses of each disease seen in decrement and jitter studies.

Other conditions with disturbed neuromuscular transmission

Neuromuscular transmission is also disturbed in conditions other than those having a primary effect on the motor end-plate, that is, myasthenia gravis, Eaton-Lambert syndrome, botulinum intoxication and some electrolyte disturbances. Transmission impairment is often seen with on-going re-innervation, such as after nerve trauma and in neuropathies, lower motor neuron disorders and polymyositis (*Figure 5.13*).

SFEMG recordings show increased jitter and partial blocking during re-innervation. In studies of muscle transplantation, it has been shown with SFEMG that impulse transmission is impaired during the first three to six months after initiation of re-innervation and is thereafter usually normal. The defect is thus most clearly seen during the phase of active re-innervation.

Edrophonium also improves transmission in these situations. In some recordings, a neurogenic block can be demonstrated during re-innervation. This type of transmission failure takes place peripherally in the intramuscular nerve tree, probably in the newly-formed nerve sprouts, and is also overcome by edrophonium. Thus, the administration of edrophonium will not distinguish between neurogenic and neuromuscular blocking.

Is disturbed neuromuscular transmission in these conditions also seen with tests other than SFEMG?

With repetitive nerve stimulation a decrement can be seen in some patients with polymyositis[38], and clinical fatiguability is often reported. A decrement of about 10 per cent, rarely more than 20 per cent, is sometimes found in patients with amyotrophic lateral sclerosis[9, 29, 38]. This decrement is usually progressive after the fifth response and without facilitation. In these patients the decrement may also be reversed or at least decreased after edrophonium[9].

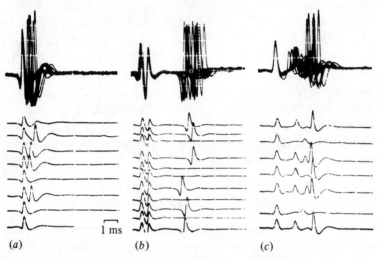

Figure 5.13 SFEMG recordings from EDC muscle in patients with myasthenia gravis (*a*), polymyositis (*a*) and amyotrophic lateral sclerosis (*c*). In each there is increased jitter and blocking. The fibre density was increased in the patients from whom (*b*) and (*c*) were recorded

Thus, decrement as such during repetitive nerve stimulation is not pathognomonic for a primary neuromuscular disease, such as myasthenia gravis, even when edrophonium has a positive effect. It is rather a sign of disturbed neuromuscular transmission.

In conventional EMG the neuromuscular defect is seen as variations in the shape of the MUP at consecutive discharges, sometimes with dropping-out of individual spike components. This is particularly true 1–3 months after nerve injury and in rapidly progressive lower motor neuron diseases, such as amyotrophic lateral sclerosis. The distinction between MG and other diseases where a decrement or increased jitter is present is usually easily made with other EMG techniques.

Comparison of techniques

A comparison of diagnostic tests is shown in *Table 5.3*. When all or several of these diagnostic techniques are available to the clinician, he has the luxury of deciding which are more valuable to him in the specific situation. Usually, however, it suffices to demonstrate that an abnormality exists in any one of these studies in order to confirm the clinical diagnosis. Much more critical is the situation that arises when one or more of the tests does not demonstrate the abnormality.

Table 5.3 A comparison of diagnostic tests for myasthenia gravis*

Group	SFEMG	Decrement: Abductor digiti minimi	Decrement: Biceps brachii, deltoid	Stapedius reflex decay	Anti-receptor antibodies
Ocular	85 (39)	4 (24)	19 (26)	90 (10)	76 (17)
Extensor digitorum communis	59 (39)				
Abnormal only in frontalis	32 (31)				
Mild generalized	96 (184)	31 (122)	68 (124)	91 (54)	76 (66)
Moderate or severe generalized	100 (68)	68 (56)	89 (28)	63 (19)	88 (19)
Remission	69 (13)	0 (5)	0 (5)	83 (6)	

* Percentage positive tests (n)

Decrement studies are most commonly available in the clinical EMG laboratory and offer the advantage of relative simplicity. Studies of the hand muscles are easily tolerated by most patients and offer few technical pitfalls. The hand must be warmed to at least 34°C before testing, and the decrement must be measured after exhaustion to obtain the maximum diagnostic yield. Even so, no more than 50 per cent of patients with MG will demonstrate an abnormality on this test. Decrement studies in proximal muscles will detect abnormalities in 65–70 per cent of all patients with MG, and up to 90 per cent of those with moderate or severe weakness. Studies of these muscles are more painful, however, especially if surface stimulation is used, and are more subject to artefactual changes that can hamper interpretation by the noncritical electromyographer. Decrement studies of facial muscles are frequently not tolerated by patients and are also prone to artefactual changes. SFEMG measurements require fairly elaborate equipment, extensive training and experience as well as patient cooperation. They have a very high diagnostic yield and can be especially valuable in demonstrating defective neuromuscular trans- mission in patients with the milder forms of MG and with purely ocular disease. The EDC should be tested first, since this will be abnormal in 95 per cent of patients with MG and no further examination is necessary. Most patients, including children older than seven years, can cooperate well enough for adequate study, although a distal tremor may make recording from the EDC muscle impossible..A more proximal muscle can usually then be studied successfully. Many find this test less uncomfortable than repetitive stimulation of the ulnar nerve for decrement studies. If SFEMG of the EDC is normal in a patient with ocular symptoms, then the frontalis should be tested and will be abnormal in over 80 per cent of such patients. If, on the other hand, weakness predominates proximally, then the deltoid or biceps should be investigated next.

Tests of intraocular tension, ocular movements or stapedial reflex fatigue are painless and require minimal patient cooperation, but the diagnostic specificity of these techniques has yet to be conclusively demonstrated. More widespread use of these tests will be necessary before their clinical applicability can be adequately assessed.

Titres of antibodies against nicotinic acetylcholine receptor are elevated in 78 per cent of patients with MG in the authors' experience, and demonstrate conclusively the immunologic abnormality. The advantages of this test are clear in confirming the diagnosis, though the level of antibodies does not correlate with clinical severity. It has yet to be shown that serial antibody determinations correlate with activity of the disease. Since antibody levels are elevated in only 76 per cent of patients with ocular MG, failure to demonstrate an elevation in such cases cannot be interpreted as excluding the disease. At the present time, accurate determinations of anti-receptor antibodies are not universally available. These tests should be regarded as com- plementing the physiological tests described.

In the authors' experience the diagnostic sensitivity of most of these tests is not affected by on-going treatment with cholinesterase inhibi- tors. Thus it is not usually necessary to withhold these drugs prior to testing. However, if quantitative comparisons of the physiologic abnormalities are to be made in the same patient over a period of time the tests should be performed with the same time-relationship to the previous drug adminstration.

Acknowledgements

Supported by the Swedish Research Council Grant No. 135 (ES).

References

1 ALBUQUERQUE, E. X., RASH, J. E., MAYER, R. F. and SATTERFIELD, J. R. An electrophysiological and morphological study of the neuromuscular junction in patients with myasthenia gravis. *Experimental Neurology*, **51**, 536–563 (1976)

2 BALOH, R. W. and KEESEY, J. C. Saccade fatigue and response to edrophonium for the diagnosis of myasthenia gravis. *Annals of the New York Academy of Sciences*, **274**, 631–641 (1976)

3 BLOM, S. and ZAKRISSON, J. E. The stapedius reflex in the diagnosis of myasthenia gravis. *Journal of the Neurological Sciences*, **21**, 71–76 (1974)

4 BLOMBERG, L. H. and PERSSON, T. A new test for myasthenia gravis. *Acta Neurologica Scandinavica*, **41**, Supplementum 13, 363–364 (1965)

5 BORENSTEIN, S. and DESMEDT, J. E. New diagnostic procedures in myathenia gravis. In *New Developments in Electromyography and Clinical Neurophysiology*, **1**, edited by J. E. Desmedt, 350–354. Basel, S. Karger (1973)

6 BOYD, D. C., LAWRENCE, P. D. and BRATTY, P. J. A. The effect of electromyographic jitter on single motor unit EMG potentials. *IEEE Transactions on Biomedical Engineering*, **BME–26**, (8), 471–478 (1979)

7 BREININ, G. M. Electromyography – a tool in ocular and neurological diagnosis. I. Myasthenia gravis. *Archives of Ophthalmology*, **57**, 161–175 (1957)

8 CAMPBELL, M. J., SIMPSON, E., CROMBIE, A. L. and WALTON, J. N. Ocular myasthenia: evaluation of Tensilon tonography and electronystagmography as diagnostic tests. *Journal of Neurology, Neurosurgery and Psychiatry*, **33**, 639–646 (1970)

9 DENYS, E. H. and NORRIS, F. H. Amyotrophic lateral sclerosis. Impairment of neuromuscular transmission. *Archives of Neurology*, **36**, 202–205 (1979)

10 DESMEDT, J. E. The neuromuscular disorder in myasthenia gravis. In *New Developments in Electromyography and Clinical Neurophysiology*, **1**, edited by J. E. Desmedt, 241–304. Basel, S. Karger (1973)

11 DESMEDT, J. E. and EMERYK, B. Disorder of muscle contraction processes in sex linked (Duchenne) muscular dystrophy, with correlative electromyographic study of myopathic involvement in small hand muscles. *American Journal of Medicine*, **45**, 853–873 (1968)

12 DESMEDT, J. E., EMERYK, B., HAINAUT, K., REINHOLD, H. and BORENSTEIN, S. Muscular dystrophy and myasthenia gravis. In *New Developments in Electromyography and Clinical Neurophysiology*, **1**, edited by J. E. Desmedt, 380–399. Basel, S. Karger (1973)

13 DESMEDT, J. E. and HAINAUT, K. Kinetics of myofilament activation in potentiated contraction. Staircase phenomenon in human skeletal muscle. *Nature (London)*, **217**, 529–532 (1968)

14 EATON, L. M. and LAMBERT, E. H. Electromyography and electric stimulation of nerves in diseases of motor unit: observations on the myasthenic syndrome associated with malignant tumors. *Journal of the American Medical Association*, **163**, 1117–1124 (1957)

15 EKSTEDT, J. and STÅLBERG, E. Myasthenia gravis. Diagnostic aspects by a new electrophysiological method. *Opuscula Medica*, **12**, 73–76, (1967)

16 ELMQVIST, D. and LAMBERT, E. H. Detailed analysis of neuromuscular transmission in a patient with the myasthenic syndrome sometimes associated with bronchogenic carcinoma. *Mayo Clinic Proceedings*, **43**, 689–713 (1968)

17 ELMQVIST, D., HOFMANN, W. W., KUGELBERG, J. and QUASTEL, D. M. J. An electrophysiological investigation of neuromuscular transmission in myasthenia gravis. *Journal of Physiology (London)*, **174**, 417–434 (1964)

18 ENGEL, A. G., LAMBERT, E. H. and HOWARD, F. M. Immune complexes (IgG and C3) at the motor end-plate in myasthenia gravis. Ultrastructural and light microscopic localization and electrophysiologic correlation. *Mayo Clinic Proceedings*, **52**, 267–280 (1977)

19 FAMBROUGH, D. M., DRACHMAN, D. B. and SATYAMURTI, S. Neuromuscular junction in myasthenia gravis: Decreased acetylcholine receptors, *Science*, **182**, 293–295 (1973)

20 FOLDES, F. F., KLONYMUS, M. W. and OSSERMAN, K. E. A new curare test for the diagnosis of myasthenia gravis. *Journal of the American Medical Association*, **203**, 113–127 (1968)

21 HARVEY, A. M. and MASLAND, R. L. A method for the study of neuromuscular transmission in human subjects. *Bulletin of the Johns Hopkins Hospital*, **68**, 81–93 (1941)

22 HARVEY, A. M. and MASLAND, R. L. The electromyogram in myasthenia gravis. *Bulletin of the Johns Hopkins Hospital*, **69**, 1–13 (1941)

23 HEILBRONN, E., MATTSSON, C., THORNELL, L., SJÖSTRÖM, M., STÅLBERG, E. HILTON-BROWN, P. and ELMQVIST, D., Experimental myasthenia gravis in rabbits: biochemical, immunological, electrophysiological, and morphological aspects. *Annals of the New York Academy of Sciences*, **274**, 337–353 (1976)

24 HOROWITZ, S. H. and SIVAK, M.The regional curare test and electrophysiologic diagnosis of myasthenia gravis: further studies. *Muscle and Nerve*, **1**, 432–434 (1978)

25 HUBBARD, J., JONES, S. F. and LANDAU, E. M. The effect of temperature change upon transmitter release, facilitation and post-tetanic potentiation. *Journal of Physiology (London)*, **216**, 591–609 (1971)

26 JOLLY, F. Über Myasthenia gravis pseudoparalytica. *Berliner Klinische Wochenschrift*, **32**, 1–7 (1895)

27 KORNBLEUTH, W., JAMPOLSKY, A., TAMLER, and ELWIN, M. Contraction of the oculorotary muscles and intraocular pressure. A tonographic and electromyographic study of the effects of edrophonium chloride (Tensilon) and succinylcholine (Anectine) on the intraocular pressure. *American Journal of Ophthalmology*, **49**, 1381–1387 (1960)

28 KRAMER, L. D., RUTH, R. A., JOHNS, M. E. and SANDERS, D. B. A comparison of stapedial reflex fatigue with repetitive stimulation and single fiber EMG in myasthenia gravis. *Annals of Neurology*, (in press)

29 LAMBERT, E. H. and MULDER, D. W. Electromyographic studies in amyotrophic lateral sclerosis. *Proceedings of Staff Meetings of the Mayo Clinic*, **32**, 441–446 (1957)

30 LINDSLEY, D. B. Electrical activity of human motor units during voluntary contraction. *American Journal of Physiology*, **114**, 90–99 (1935/36)

31 LOVELACE, R. E., OLARTE, M. R., ZABLOW, L. and PAI, J. Extracellular recording of miniature end-plate potentials in normals, myasthenia gravis and the experimental model. (Abstract) *Fifth International Congress of Electromyography* (Rochester, Minn. USA, Sept. 21–24, 1975). Omaha, NE, International Federation of Societies for Electroencephalography and Clinical Neurophysiology (1975)

32 METZ, H. S., SCOTT, A. B. and O'MEARA, D. M. Saccadic eye movements in myasthenia gravis. *Archives of Ophthalmology*, **88**, 9–11 (1972)

33 ÖZDEMIR, C. and YOUNG, R. R. The results to be expected from electrical testing in the diagnosis of myasthenia gravis. *Annals of the New York Academy of Sciences*, **274**, 203–222 (1976)

34 PATRICK, J. and LINDSTROM, J. Autoimmune response to acetylcholine receptor. *Science*, **180**, 871–872 (1973)

35 RUTH, R. A., JOHNS, M. E., KRAMER, L. D., SANDERS, D. B. and CANTRELL, R. W. Evaluation of the stapedius muscle in neuromuscular disorders.

Proceedings of the Fourth International Symposium on Acoustic Impedance Measurements, Lisbon (1980)

36 SANDERS, D. B., HOWARD, J. F. and JOHNS, T. R. Single fiber electromyography in myasthenia gravis. *Neurology (Minneapolis)*, **29**, 68–76 (1979)

37 SANDERS, D. B., SCHLEIFER, L. S., ELDEFRAWI, M. E., NORCROSS, N. L. and COBB, E. E. An immunologically-induced defect of neuromuscular transmission in rats and rabbits. *Annals of the New York Academy of Sciences*, **274**, 319–336 (1976)

38 SIMPSON, J. A. Disorders of neuromuscular transmission. *Proceedings of the Royal Society of Medicine*, **59**, 993–998 (1966)

39 SLOMIC, A., ROSENFALCK, A. and BUCHTHAL, F. Electrical and mechanical responses of normal and myasthenic muscle, with particular reference to the staircase phenomenon. *Brain Research*, **10**, 1–75 (1968)

40 SPECTOR, R. H. and DAROFF, R. B. Edrophonium infrared optokinetic nystagmography in the diagnosis of myasthenia gravis. *Annals of the New York Academy of Sciences*, **274**, 642–651 (1976)

41 STELLA, S. Optokinetic nystagmus in patients with ocular myasthenia. *Investigative Ophthalmology*, **6**, 668 (1967)

42 STÅLBERG, E. and ANTONI, L. Electrophysiological cross section of the motor unit. *Journal of Neurology, Neurosurgery and Psychiatry*. **43**, 469–474 (1980)

43 STÅLBERG, E. and TRONTELJ, J. *Single Fibre Electromyography*, 244 pp. Old Woking, Surrey, UK, Mirvalle Press (1979)

44 STÅLBERG, E., TRONTELJ, J. and SCHWARTZ, M. S. Single muscle fibre recording of the jitter phenomenon in patients with myasthenia gravis and in members of their families. *Annals of the New York Academy of Sciences*, **274**, 189–262 (1976)

45 WARREN, W. R., GUTMANN, L., CODY, R. C., FLOWERS, P. and SEGAL, A. T. Stapedial reflex decay in myasthenia gravis. *Archives of Neurology*, **34**, 496–497 (1977)

46 WIEDERHOLD, W. C. 'End-plate noise' in electromyography. *Neurology (Minneapolis)*, **20**, 214–224 (1970)

47 WRAY, S. H. and PAVAN-LANGSTON, D. A re-evaluation of edrophonium chloride (Tensilon) tonography in the diagnosis of myasthenia gravis. *Neurology (Minneapolis)*, **21**, 586–593 (1971)

6
Electrophysiological studies in peripheral neuropathy: early detection and monitoring

Bhagwan T. Shahani and Austin J. Sumner

Introduction

Estimation of conduction velocity in human motor and sensory nerves has been widely used for detection and documentation of peripheral nervous system pathology. However, conventional methods evaluate only the function of fastest conducting, and presumably largest diameter, axons in distal segments – proximal segments including anterior or posterior roots and intraspinal portions being excluded. Their diagnostic yield is therefore limited. Clinical neurophysiologists need techniques which can study function of motor and sensory axons with various conduction characteristics in their entirety from spinal cord or brain stem to their most distal segments. The purpose of the present review is to describe some of these newer techniques, especially late responses and collision techniques which, because of their precision, have proved useful in the early detection of subclinical peripheral neuropathies and in monitoring the response of patients' neuropathies to therapies or the passage of time. To assist in understanding changes noted in these electrophysiological studies, experimental work giving insights into the pathophysiology of a number of neuropathies encountered in the clinic is first reviewed.

Demyelinative versus axonal neuropathies

Anatomical features of a myelinated nerve fiber which are important to its conduction velocity are:

(1) diameter of the fiber;
(2) distance between nodes of Ranvier; and
(3) integrity of the myelin sheaths.

In peripheral nerve diseases with segmental demyelination, striking abnormalities in the velocity of nerve impulse propagation are observed. Maximum conduction velocities reduced by more than 40 percent from the mean normal value usually indicate the presence of segmental demyelination[29]. By contrast, axonal polyneuropathies (associated with alcoholism, uremia, multiple myeloma, carcinoma, diabetes, malnutrition, heavy metal intoxication and many toxic chemicals and drugs) are not associated with marked slowing of nerve conduction velocities. Early detection of these diseases may depend upon reduction of sensory (especially sural) or motor response amplitudes or abnormalities of late response studies rather than slowing of conduction velocity especially if the pathological process tends to spare larger diameter axons.

Physiological consequences of demyelination

Slowed conduction

Rapid advances in electrophysiological knowledge of peripheral neuropathy started with the observation that impulses can propagate at greatly reduced velocities in certain patients with peripheral nerve disease[34]. Ensuing experimental studies[39] of experimental diphtheritic and allergic polyneuritis showed this slowing could not be due to selective degeneration or functional elimination of the fastest fibers, to low temperature, or to nerve fiber regeneration. Segmental demyelination of Gombault[31] was noted especially in the regions adjacent to nodes of Ranvier and even relatively slight alterations of myelin sheaths were shown to greatly impair conduction velocity. More detailed observations on experimental diphtheritic neuritis by McDonald[55, 56] included recordings of slowed conduction in individual identified cutaneous or muscle afferents. These initial observations were subsequently confirmed in experimental allergic neuritis[14, 32] and with nerve compression[52] or local ligature[47].

Rasminsky and Sears[69] recorded from successive nodes of single undissected ventral root fibers in the rat. In fibers demyelinated by diphtheria toxin, slowing of conduction was shown to be due to increased internodal time; the magnitude of the change varies from segment to segment in keeping with the variety and distributions of pathological changes that occur with this type of lesion. It is now possible to record from a greater number of sites within each internode by using more closely spaced electrodes[6]. In some fibers, long after exposure to diphtheria toxin, continuous conduction of nerve impulses over lengths corresponding to approximately one internode has been observed. In a few, mean velocity in the segment with continuous conduction was in the range normal for unmyelinated fibers (1.1–2.3 m/s). Impulses can then resume saltatory conduction after a stretch of continuous conduction.

Continuous conduction has also been observed in dystrophic mice where there is a congenital defect in myelin formation in the mid-portion of the ventral root[68] and in regenerating nerve fibers[5]. Theoretically, continuous conduction is an important phenomenon because it could explain recovery in CNS demyelinative lesions where remyelination has not been seen[33, 57]. However, the frequency with which it appears and time course of its development are still to be determined. In the focal demyelinative lesion produced by intraneural injection of immune sera, electrophysiological demonstration of earliest recovery of conduction and the process of remyelination are closely correlated[74]. Recovery of conduction is not seen before some axons are invested with two to eight lamellae of myelin.

Conduction block

Although electrophysiological studies have emphasized slowing of conduction as an important physiological consequence of demyelination, conduction block is a much more serious consequence in terms of disturbed nervous system function. Conduction block was first inferred by Erb[25] from the observation that in certain patients with complete muscle paralysis due to peripheral nerve injury, contraction resulted from electrical stimulation below but not above the lesion. Direct compression of peripheral nerve by a tourniquet has provided a useful animal model in which to study this phenomenon[18, 27, 30, 52, 61, 62, 63] but conduction block independent of local trauma in a setting of a generalized peripheral nerve disease was first studied by McDonald[56] who showed that focal demyelination near the dorsal root ganglion produced by diphtheria toxin was associated with conduction block in that precise region.

Acute study

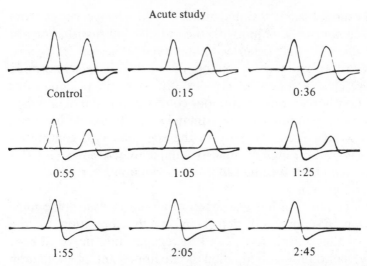

Figure 6.1 Motor responses recorded from a rat hind foot following supramaximal nerve stimulation at ankle (distal response) and sciatic notch (proximal response). From upper left, responses before and at various times after injection of 50μl EAE serum into sciatic nerve at mid-thigh. Conduction block of all motor axons is complete in 2 hours 45 min. (From Sumner *et al.*[91], courtesy of the Editor and publisher, *Neurology*)

More recently, acute conduction block has been produced by certain immune sera[73,76,77,91]. Peripheral demyelination can be produced with experimental allergic encephalomyelitis (EAE) or neuritis (EAN) serum or anti-galactocerebroside serum by an immunological effect which is antibody-dependent and complement-mediated[72,74]. Demyelinating activity associated with high galactocerebroside antibody titers is lost following absorption by galactocerebroside, indicating that antibodies against this component of myelin are responsible for electrophysiological and morphological effects. Direct injections of small volumes of active sera into rat sciatic nerve produce cytoplasmic alterations and vacuolation of Schwann cells, myelin splitting and vesiculation, macrophage phagocytosis of myelin and an associated acute inflammatory reaction. Within 30 min, conduction block in some motor axons can be detected by a decline in amplitude of the muscle response evoked by stimulation proximal to the injection site. Conduction block progresses over the next 2 to 4 hours (*Figure 6.1*) and is not associated with slowing of maximum conduction velocity until the block is well advanced, a surprising and unexpected observation.

Correlative studies indicate there are usually only subtle morphological changes in paranodal myelin at this time although over the next several hours active vesicular demyelination appears. Recovery from conduction block begins about the eighth day, initially with very slow velocity (estimated at 2–5 m/s) through the region in which some axons are thinly remyelinated. Subsequently, there is progressive recovery of conduction velocity which returns to control values over the next 25–35 days.

Unlike peripheral nerve where the perineurium normally forms a highly effective permeability barrier against demyelinating activity of active sera, a focal lesion can be produced in dorsal and ventral roots by the topical application of a drop of serum. This provides the opportunity to study single intact ventral root fibers up to the point of conduction block. Acute conduction block in single axons is preceded by progressive increase in conduction time within 10 min of serum application. Conduction times across short lengths of ventral root can increase by 400–700 µs prior to block which occurs within 60–90 min. The first fibers affected are invariably slowly conducting; faster conducting fibers show similar preblock changes which begin later with conduction block occurring 4–6 hours after exposure to serum. This selective early block of smaller diameter axons is not yet understood but may relate to reduced safety factors in these axons. Selective effects on slower conducting axons apparently explain relatively well-preserved maximum conduction velocities when populations of motor fibers are observed during acutely evolving conduction block.

In this experimental model, extensive morphological damage of the myelin sheath is not a prerequisite for acute conduction block; quite subtle morphological changes may be associated with complete failure of impulse propagation. Myelin that appears to be intact may possibly be 'short circuited' by communications between the peri-axonal space and extracellular fluid. The high series-impedance of normal myelin both prevents activation of any excitable channels in internodal axolemma and dwarfs the contribution of passive electrical properties of internodal membrane to total membrane impedance. With demyelination, however, this situation is completely altered and properties of an exposed internode will completely dominate behaviour of an entire axon. There is some evidence that internodal membrane may have different excitable properties from nodal membrane and these may alter as a consequence of demyelination[6, 12].

Some rabbits immunized repeatedly with bovine brain galactocerebroside develop a neuropathy characterized by flaccid paresis and hypoesthesia of all limbs 2–11 months after initial inoculation[75]. Serial studies of these animals show motor conduction velocities are usually normal at the time of onset of paresis. Within a week or two, markedly prolonged distal motor latencies and multifocal conduction block are seen in peripheral trunks. These abnormalities are strikingly similar to those found in human acquired demyelinative neuropathies such as Guillain-Barré syndrome and its relapsing and chronic variants. In these animals, perivascular demyelinative lesions associated with phagocytic mononuclear cells were prominent in spinal ganglia and roots, but were less frequent in distal nerves.

Physiological correlates of axonal neuropathies

Axonal neuropathies have been less intensively studied. Axonal degeneration, which is essentially similar to Wallerian degeneration, is believed to begin in the distal portion of axons and spread slowly proximally. The term 'dying-back' reaction is often used to describe this pattern of peripheral pathology[11]. The term 'distal axonopathy' has been introduced more recently because, in certain hexacarbon neuropathies, axonal degeneration did not seem to begin at the nerve terminals, but rather in a multifocal manner in the distal portion of axons. With continued intoxication, proximal spread of degeneration was multifocal, not seriate, with short lengths of axons undergoing simultaneous degenerative changes distal to nodal points at which giant axonal swellings had occurred[85].

A number of human neuropathies have been identified in which the most striking pathological change involves neurofilamentous aggregation within distal axons. These include giant axonal neuropathy of idiopathic childhood type and acquired neuropathies related to neurotoxic substances such as monomeric acrylamide, certain hexacarbons, and carbon disulfide[85]. Actin, tubulin, and the neurofilamentous polypeptide triplets (putative constituents of axonal filaments) comprise the bulk of proteins moving distally by slow axoplasmic transport. These filamentous structures account for more than 40 percent of total migratory protein synthesis in the neuronal perikaryon; a major part of the neuronal economy.

In distal axonopathies, degeneration concentrated in parts of the nerve fiber furthest from the perikaryon has led to the assumption that effects on the cell body itself result in failure to maintain integrity of most distal portions of the neuron. Many studies have attempted to demonstrate abnormalities in perikaryon synthesis or axoplasmic transport but no plausible explanation for this pathology has been forthcoming. Most distal axonopathies, e.g. acrylamide, triorthocresyl phosphate, and thiamine deficiency, show a clear fiber length suscepti- bility but in others (the neuropathy associated with acute intermittent porphyria) distal parts of fibers appear to degenerate irrespective of the length of axons[71].

Slowing of conduction velocity, not a prominent feature in axonal neuropathies, depends on three different mechanisms:

(1) loss of largest diameter axons;
(2) secondary changes in myelin sheaths; and
(3) axonal shrinkage.

Conduction in axonal neuropathies was first studied experimentally in guinea pigs with acute thallium poisoning[39]. In appropriate dosage, thallium produces an acute neuropathy with fall in amplitude of muscle response to nerve stimulation occurring every three or four days. Even when muscle responses are almost gone, conduction velocity is virtually unchanged. Thallium neuropathy is difficult to study because many animals either fail to develop neuropathy or die acutely. Experimental acrylamide neuropathy became widely adopted as the prototypical laboratory model for study of distal axonal neuropathy following the discovery that monomeric acrylamide ($CH_2CHCONH_2$) readily produces a pure axonal neuropathy in rats which otherwise remain in good health[28]. Their maximum motor conduction velocities fall progressively to approximately 80 percent of control values as the neuropathy advances in severity. When adminis- tration of acrylamide is stopped, animals recover from their neurolo- gical disabilities and conduction velocities return to normal. This is somewhat surprising because after mechanical division of the peripheral nerve, recovery of conduction velocity in regenerating fibers is incomplete[14]. In rats or baboons[38], investigators showed histological evidence of selective large diameter fiber loss and con- cluded that slowed conduction velocities resulted from selective axonal degeneration rather than slowing of conduction in individual axons.

This can be contrasted with experimental organophosphorus neuro- pathy which is not associated with conduction velocity slowing even when weakness is severe[35]. Fiber diameter histograms show that some large diameter fibers are spared in organophosphorus neuropathy even when there is severe generalized axonal loss whereas in acryla- mide neuropathy, the largest axons are always affected[49]. Recordings from single axons in this experimental neuropathy have confirmed large fiber susceptibility: (1) Ia and Ib afferent nerve fibers from primary muscle spindle and tendon organ endings in the cat become physiologically unresponsive at a time when most group 2 afferents from secondary spindle endings are functioning normally[90]; (2) A-α cutaneous afferent fibers from hair and touch receptors fail due to terminal degeneration at a time when most A-δ afferents from downy hair receptors are responding normally (*Figure 6.2*). Failure of axons

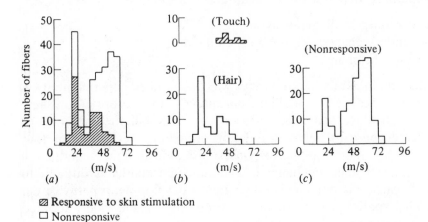

Figure 6.2 Histograms of velocities in sural cutaneous afferent fibers in cats with acrylamide neuropathy. (*a*) The solid line represents the conduction velocity distribution of the total population of units. In (*b*) and (*c*) the population has been subdivided into touch units or hair units, and nonresponsive units. The nonresponsive group is presumed to contain some non-receptor afferents (From Sumner[89], courtesy of the publishers, *Physiology and Pathobiology of Axons*)

to respond to physiological stimulation appears to be abrupt without evidence of progressive receptor dysfunction. This is consistent with morphological observations that earliest changes affect nodes of Ranvier a few internodes proximal to the receptor ending[78].

This hierarchy of vulnerability among different-sized sensory fibers did not apply to motor axons in the same peripheral nerve which were much less susceptible to neurotoxic actions of acrylamide than sensory fibers of similar size and length[89]. This difference may relate to total cell size; sensory axons, especially from lumbosacral root ganglion cells, have both large central and peripheral extensions, while anterior horn cells with their single peripheral axons have smaller cytoplasmic volumes. Central projections of primary sensory neurons taper to differing degrees with the largest diameter projections in cat dorsal columns subserving specialized Pacinian corpuscles in the footpad[8]. Schaumberg, Wisniewski and Spencer[78] showed these are the earliest nerve terminals to show morphological changes in acrylamide neuropathy. Although the earliest degenerative changes occur in terminal portions of dying-back axons, it can be shown (*Figure 6.3*) that

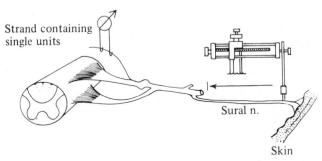

Strand containing single units

Sural n.

Skin

Figure 6.3 Stimulating and recording arrangement used in studies of dying-back axons. (From Sumner[88], courtesy of the publishers, *Physiology of Peripheral Nerve Disease*)

degeneration advances centripetally with continued intoxication. At any stage of disease, centripetal degeneration occurs earlier and to a greater extent in larger diameter axons than in smaller ones (*Figures 6.4 and 6.5*). With fairly acute acrylamide neuropathy, studied by these methods, conduction velocity appears to be uniform in proximal portions of dying-back axons without evidence of axonal tapering or shrinkage. In the most terminal few millimeters of a dying-back axon, the electrical threshold is much increased, sometimes associated with a short length of slowed conduction velocity which may be the consequence either of paranodal myelin changes in the giant axonal swellings which occur in this region or of short excitable regenerative sprouts[59, 88].

An important exception to the general rule that conduction velocities are not greatly reduced in axonal neuropathies is provided by the hexacarbon neuropathies caused by N-hexane and related industrial solvents. In a glue-sniffer who developed a severe N-hexane neuropathy[43], motor conduction velocities of 33.5 m/s in median nerve and 25 m/s were recorded in peroneal nerve. Sural nerve biopsy demonstrated prominent axonal degeneration but, in addition, many

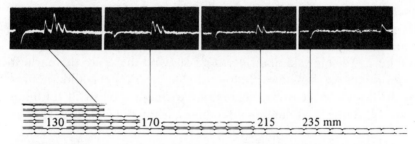

Figure 6.4 Recordings from an S1 dorsal root filament after supramaximal stimulation of sural nerve at 150, 170, 215 and 235 mm distance along the nerve, respectively. (From Sumner[88], courtesy of the publishers, *Physiology of Peripheral Nerve Disease*)

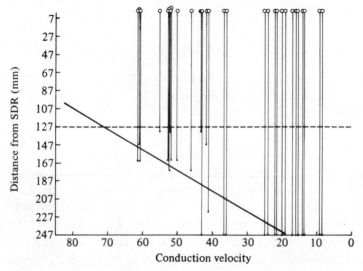

Figure 6.5 Relationship between axon size (conduction velocity) and the extent of centripetal degeneration in acrylamide neuropathy. SDR = dorsal root recording site. Distance refers to most distal excitable point. (From Sumner[88], courtesy of the publishers, *Physiology of Peripheral Nerve Disease*)

fibers contained giant axonal swellings associated with thinning of the overlying myelin and retraction of myelin sheaths in the paranodal region. These secondary changes in myelin probably explain the observed slowing of conduction velocity. Although axonal atrophy has frequently been advocated as a cause of slowed conduction velocity in axonal neuropathies, it has only recently been demonstrated in animals chronically intoxicated with β-iminodiproprionitrile (IDPN) which causes a reduction in axonal calibre and few other changes in peripheral nerve[87]. After 6 months, conduction velocities had fallen 12 percent and after 20 months as much as 40 percent proportional to the reduction in axonal diameter which occurred in the absence of significant demyelination or nerve fiber loss.

These animal studies demonstrate that early detection of axonal neuropathies depends upon development of newer electrophysiological techniques, especially those capable of measuring the distribution of conduction velocities in peripheral nerve[15, 19, 20, 81]. Another approach to early detection is to record from a cutaneous sensory nerve following mechanical stimulation of skin receptors and electrical stimulation of intracutaneous nerve terminals[9]. Such methods may detect early degenerative changes in sensory nerve terminals before abnormalities in conduction or amplitude are apparent in nerve trunks.

Clinical studies

Late responses

In recent years, many investigators have begun to use the monosynaptic H reflex (*Figure 6.6a*) and the F response, which is not a reflex, (*Figure 6.6b*) to evaluate function of the peripheral nervous system[2, 3, 4, 7, 13, 24, 40, 41, 42, 44, 46, 54, 64, 65, 66, 67, 70, 82, 84, 86, 94, 95]. The H reflex, an electrically elicited ankle jerk, was named after its discoverer Paul Hoffman[36] by Magladery and McDougal[51]; another 'late response', i.e. those with latencies greatly prolonged beyond the direct M response, with latency similar to the H reflex but requiring a stronger stimulus was called the F response by the same authors. F responses are produced by centrifugal discharges from individual motoneurons each of which is initiated by an antidromic volley artificially produced in its axon[17, 53, 58, 83, 86, 92]. Since their latencies are similar – F response latency being a few milliseconds longer in the same muscle – it may sometimes be difficult to ascertain exactly what percentage of a late response recorded with surface electrodes is made up of motor units active in an F response versus an H reflex. However, a clear distinction between these two responses must be made because they provide different types of information about the peripheral and central nervous systems[82, 83]. Whereas conduction only in an α-motor axon is tested by F response latency, H reflex latency gives information about activity in large afferent (Ia) as well as efferent fibers.

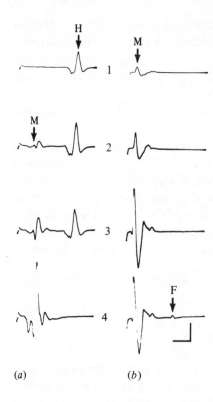

Figure 6.6 (a) H reflex (soleus). Increasing stimulus from trace 1 to 4. Note the appearance of H reflex in 1 before the M response clearly seen in 2, 3 and 4. *Calibration*: traces 1 and 2 vertical 500 μV, traces 3 and 4 vertical 1 mV. Horizontal 10 ms. (*b*) F response (abductor pollicis brevis). Increasing stimulus and calibration as for (*a*)

Some studies of late responses have attempted to measure conduction velocity in different segments of a peripheral nerve, including proximal segments and nerve roots. Because formulae used to convert minimal latencies of these two late responses to conduction velocities are based on several unproven assumptions, it is recommended that the clinical neurophysiologist, as a rule, restrict his studies to the measurement of minimal latencies of both responses[96]. Some of the problems which make it impossible to measure conduction velocity on the basis of F response studies are:

(1) exact distance from site of recording and stimulation to that motoneuron pool in the spinal cord which is responsible for the appropriate late response cannot be measured;
(2) precise time for central delay of H reflex and F response is unknown in human subjects; and
(3) the initial motor unit activated in a late response evoked by stimulation at different sites may be entirely different so that basic requirements for conduction velocity measurements are not fulfilled.

In contrast to the H reflex which can be easily recorded only from resting soleus muscle in adult subjects, F responses are found in almost every skeletal muscle, making them more versatile for evaluation of conduction in motor nerve fibers. Moreover, F responses are evoked every time tests of motor conduction velocity are performed. By changing the oscilloscope sweep speed to permit visualization of approximately 100 ms after the stimulus, one can record F responses whenever supramaximal stimuli for direct muscle responses are delivered. That response, out of 10 or 20 consecutive ones, which has minimal latency provides information regarding conduction in the fastest and presumably largest diameter α-motor axons activated in the F response.

As expected, there is a direct relationship between minimal latency of these two late responses and distance from points of stimulus and recording to the activated spinal motoneuron pool. In the clinical setting, minimal latencies of late responses should be correlated with height (*Figure 6.7*) and/or length of the appropriate extremity[13, 45, 46, 83]. The authors find it simpler and more accurate to record height than measure distance between various anatomical landmarks. Nomograms with minimal latency plotted for different heights provide accurate normative information regarding conduction in motor and/or group Ia afferent (in case of H reflex) nerve fibers. Interlimb differences for

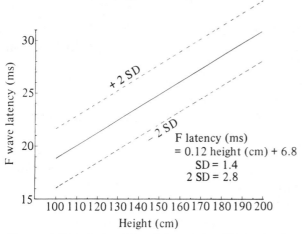

F latency (ms)
= 0.12 height (cm) + 6.8
SD = 1.4
2 SD = 2.8

Figure 6.7 Relationship of the minimal latency of the F response (abductor pollicis brevis) to height in normal subjects. (From Lachman, Shahani and Young[45], courtesy of the Editor and publisher, *Journal of Neurology, Neurosurgery and Psychiatry*)

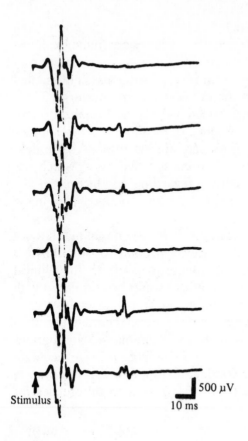

Stimulus

500 μV

10 ms

Figure 6.8 F response from the abductor digiti minimi muscle in a patient with Charcot-Marie-Tooth disease. Note the prolonged latency for the F response, 40 ms compared with 30 ms as upper normal limit

minimal latencies of responses described above are normally less than 2 ms.

Abnormalities of late responses have been demonstrated in neuropathies (*Figure 6.8*), both the primarily 'axonal' type as well as the segmental demyelinating types (*Table 6.1*)[45, 83]. In some neuropathies with specific disorders of large sensory fibers, such as pure pansensory neuropathy[3] and Friedreich's ataxia, H reflexes and tendon jerks are absent though F response latencies remain normal[45, 79]. In many metabolic-nutritional types, such as alcoholic and uremic neuropathies[1, 2, 22, 45, 46], prolongations of late response can be demonstrated in the same peripheral nerve distribution in which conventional methods of motor and sensory conduction may be normal. For example, Lefebvre-D'Amour *et al.*[46] performed conventional motor conduction velocity studies of median, ulnar, peroneal and tibial nerves and sensory conduction studies of ulnar and median nerves in 30 alcoholic subjects and a similar group of age-matched controls.

Table 6.1 Late responses in neuropathy

Type of neuropathy	Number examined	Abnormal late response; normal NCS*	Normal late response; abnormal NCS	Abnormal late response; abnormal NCS	Normal late response; normal NCS
Uremic	7	3	0	3	1
Diabetic	13	3	1	9	0
Alcoholic-nutritional	6	1	0	2	3
Porphyric	1	0	0	0	1
Diabetic and uremic	1	0	0	1	0
Charcot-Marie-Tooth chronic demyelinating neuropathy	10	0	0	10	0
Refsum's disease	1	0	0	1	0
Guillain-Barré syndrome	11	2	1	8	0
Total	50	9	2	34	5

* NCS: nerve conduction studies.
(From Lachman, Shahani and Young[45], courtesy of the Editor and publisher, *Journal of Neurology, Neurosurgery and Psychiatry*)

These results were compared with sural nerve and late response studies which included recording H reflexes from soleus as well as F responses from abductor pollicis brevis (median nerve), abductor digiti minimi (ulnar nerve), extensor digitorum brevis (peroneal nerve) and flexor hallucis brevis (tibial nerve). These two newer techniques improved the diagnostic yield in this patient population by 20 percent. Abnormal sural nerve or late responses were found in 93 percent of these patients (*Table 6.2*) although only 84 percent were symptomatic, thus indicating the importance of these studies in early detection of peripheral nerve disorders[45, 46, 83]. In a recent study, detailed electrophysiological investigations, including conventional

Table 6.2 Electrophysiological studies in 30 alcoholic subjects

	Percent
1 Abnormal motor or sensory (median or ulnar) study	73
1 Abnormal late response or sural conduction study	93
1 Abnormal study (motor, sensory or late response)	93

(From Lefebvre-D'Amour *et al.*[46], courtesy of the Editor and publisher, *Neurology*)

motor and sensory conduction as well as sural sensory conduction and F response studies were undertaken in 75 patients with diabetes mellitus (Stålberg, personal communication, 1980); the 'latency value' for F responses was measured as F latency minus distal latency in order to exclude abnormalities of conduction in distal segments. Parenthetically, it should be emphasized that the first motor unit activated in the M response may not be the same as that activated for the minimal-latency F response and therefore the 'latency value' may not be truly representative of conduction in any particular axon. Stalberg found evidence of neuropathy in 70 out of 75 patients and the most sensitive parameters for its detection were F response latencies in the tibial (81 percent) and peroneal nerves (76 percent) followed by sural sensory conduction which was abnormal in 72 percent (*Table 6.3*). Late response and sural conduction studies could detect abnormalities in 94 percent of diabetic patients, a figure similar to that (93 percent) found for alcoholic subjects[46]. Similar electrophysiological studies, along

Table 6.3 Electrophysiological studies in diabetes. Abnormal results in 70 patients with peripheral neuropathy

	Percent
F latency value – tibial nerve	81
F latency value – peroneal nerve	76
Sural conduction	72
F latency value – ulnar nerve	58
Peroneal MCV	52
Tibial MCV	49
F latency value – median	43
Median sensory – palmar	40
Ulnar MCV	33
Ulnar sensory – palmar	30
Ulnar digit V – sensory	27
Median MCV	24

MCV: motor conduction velocity
(From Stålberg, personal communication, 1980)

with detailed quantitative examinations of sensory function, have been used to assess and monitor function of peripheral nerves in patients with diabetic[16] and uremic[22] neuropathies; however, no mention was made of any particular physiological parameter being most sensitive for early detection of peripheral neuropathies.

On the other hand, in patients with neuropathies in which the primary pathology appears to be segmental demyelination, such as Guillain-Barré syndrome, prolongation of late response latencies may be the first quantifiable sign. Prolongation of late response latencies has been seen in patients with Guillain-Barré syndrome at a time when conventional measurements of motor and sensory conduction, including distal latencies, were normal and there was no increase in cerebrospinal fluid protein. In other patients with Guillain-Barré syndrome, one finds considerable prolongation of late response latencies with only minor changes in conduction in distal segments, thereby localizing most lesions to the proximal part of the nerve. In a recent report, serial electrophysiological studies were performed in patients with acute Guillain-Barré syndrome treated with plasma exchange[80]. Changes in shape, amplitude and configuration of compound muscle action potentials (CMAP), absent or asynchronous late responses and abnormalities of blink reflexes provided early and sensitive indications of peripheral and cranial nerve dysfunction. Clinical improvement was accompanied by early increase in amplitude of CMAP, reappearance of previously absent F responses and decrease in latency of both components of the blink reflex at a time when conventional motor conduction velocity studies showed little change. These studies highlight the importance of conduction block which, as mentioned earlier, is a far more significant consequence of segmental demyelination in its acute stages than slowing of conduction.

The usefulness of late response studies has been demonstrated not only in the evaluation of peripheral neuropathies but also in the assessment of entrapment neuropathies and root compression syndromes. Abnormal prolongation of minimal late response latencies in entrapment neuropathies is an important adjunct to routine motor and sensory nerve conduction studies. Appropriate abnormalities of late responses have been recorded in the carpal tunnel syndrome, ulnar compression syndrome, and surgically proven thoracic-outlet syndrome[23, 50, 81]. Similarly, studies of H reflex and F responses both recorded from soleus provide useful information in root compression syndromes affecting S1/S2 roots[7, 21, 26, 60, 93]. F responses in other muscles such as extensor digitorum brevis (L5/S1) provide further information regarding lesions of those roots[93]. Prolongation of H reflex latency is usually correlated with reduction in ankle jerk on the appropriate side. When the tendon jerk cannot be elicited it is usually not possible to record an H reflex. It must be emphasized that every patient with a root compression syndrome will not have prolonged minimal latency of late responses. However, whenever abnormal, studies of H reflex and F responses can be extremely useful in localizing lesions in patients with lumbo-sacral or cervical root disease.

Late responses in pediatric patients

H reflexes can be elicited in intrinsic hand muscles of the newborn and may be present up to the age of one year. In addition, F responses can also be recorded from almost every skeletal muscle. Since minimal latency recorded for late responses depends upon both conduction velocity and height, and maximum motor or sensory conduction velocity in the newborn is approximately half the adult value, minimum latencies for F response and H reflexes are longer (when compared with adult values) in relation to the height. That is, age is a more important factor in the interpretation of these studies than height at least up to two years.

Some advantages of late response studies in children are:

(1) a single site of stimulation produces responses which provide information regarding conduction in the entire nerve;
(2) there is no need to measure distance, which is often even more difficult to record accurately in a pediatric population. Short distance measurements tend to introduce larger errors in calculations of conduction velocity in children;
(3) the range of normal minimal latencies is relatively narrower than that for MCV; and
(4) late response studies improve the diagnostic yield of electrophysiological studies.

Newer F response parameters

In addition to recording minimal latency, one can measure minimal–maximal F latency differences, duration of F complexes, and maximal F amplitude estimated as percentage of maximal CMAP.

Some of these can be abnormal at a time when other studies of conduction, including minimal F latency, are within normal limits[80] because these newer F parameters provide information regarding conduction in different size α-motor axons. Each time an F response is evoked, it represents activation of a different motoneuron and axon with its specific conduction velocity. By measuring minimum and maximum latencies, one can determine the range of conduction velocities in different diameter axons. Increased duration of an F response complex may, on the other hand, either represent activity of different motor units or a re-innervated prolonged-duration single motor unit potential. Similarly, interpretations based on amplitude of an F response must be made with caution; increased amplitude may be due either to synchronization of different motor units activated in the F response, as in chronic spasticity, or to re-innervated large amplitude single motor units, as seen in neurogenic disorders[80].

Other methods for estimation of conduction velocity in different diameter motor and sensory fibers

By improving signal-to-noise ratio with special input circuits and electronic averaging, Buchthal, Rosenfalck and Behse[10] have recorded sensory potentials from different diameter axons of normal and diseased peripheral nerves. A sensory potential evoked by stimulation of digits and recorded at the wrist has, in addition to the main triphasic component recorded routinely, four or five small components of less than $0.5\,\mu V$ amplitude, each corresponding to groups of smaller diameter sensory nerve fibers. With this technique, the average minimum conduction velocity in myelinated nerve fibers is 15 m/s for sural and 16 m/s for ulnar and median nerves; components which conduct at less than 2 m/s originate in unmyelinated C fibers[10].

Hopf's 'collision technique'[37] has been used to measure minimum as well as maximum conduction velocity of motor axons[48, 81]. A graphic display of disorders in motor axons of intermediate and slow conduction velocity can be produced from data obtained by this technique[19] (*Figure 6.9*). Supramaximal stimulation is delivered at two sites over one nerve; proximal stimulation, e.g. axillary, is paired with a preceding distal stimulus, e.g. at the wrist, at known variable intervals. CMAP produced by proximal stimulation grow with increasing interstimulus intervals as antidromic impulses from distal stimulation pass the proximal stimulus site, first in the fastest and then in increasingly

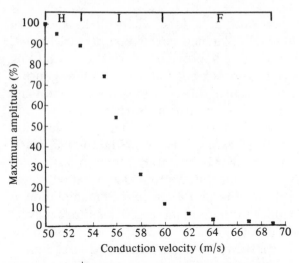

Figure 6.9 Amplitude of the CMAP plotted
against conduction velocity at different interstimulus intervals in a normal subject. The 'head'
(H), intermediate zone (I) and 'foot' (F) of the
sigmoid curve give information regarding conduction in slow, medium-sized and fast conducting
α-motor axons respectively. Details in the text.

slower axons – impulses in them are then no longer blocked by
collision with impulses from the distal stimulus. In normal subjects,
plots of amplitude of CMAP versus conduction velocity at each
interstimulus interval form a smooth sigmoid curve as in *Figure 6.9*.
The 'foot' of this curve represents activity in largest diameter fastest
conducting axons, the intermediate steep part represents medium-
sized axons and the 'head' represents smallest diameter, slowest
conducting motor axons. Thus one can document involvement of
larger diameter motor axons in patients with entrapment
neuropathies[48, 81] whereas abnormalities of the mid-portion of this
curve, suggesting dysfunction in fibers of intermediate conduction
velocity, are seen in patients with metabolic-nutritional
neuropathies[19]. Using these collision techniques, the conduction
velocity of different diameter sensory fibers has also been estimated[20].
When amplitude of compound sensory nerve action potentials
(CSNAPs) is plotted against conduction velocity, the 'sensory' curve
has the same appearance as the foot of the 'motor' curve. In contrast
to *in vitro* sensory nerve conduction studies, where A-α, A-δ and C

peaks are distinctly seen, CSNAPs recorded routinely in most EMG laboratories represent activity only in largest diameter A-α fibers.

Using conventional electrophysiological studies, it has only been possible to correlate clinical signs and symptoms of peripheral nerve dysfunction with abnormalities of conduction in the largest motor and sensory fibers. In most metabolic-nutritional neuropathies, it was only possible to show abnormalities when results from populations of patients were contrasted with those from large numbers of normal subjects; when individual patients were studied, values for maximal motor and sensory conduction were often found to be within normal limits, even in patients who had obvious clinical features of polyneuropathy. With newer techniques described above, early detection of a peripheral neuropathy is now possible even in an asymptomatic individual patient whose clinical course can then be monitored by performance of serial physiological studies. Effects of therapy or the passage of time can therefore be quantitated. F responses can be used to provide more accurate studies of largest motor fibers, with many fewer false negatives. Combined with collision techniques, they can also quantitate conduction in smaller diameter fibers.

References

1 ACKIL, A. A., SHAHANI, B. T. and YOUNG, R. R. Usefulness of late response and sural conduction studies in patients with chronic renal failure. *Electroencephalography and Clinical Neurophysiology*, **49,** 20P (1980)

2 ACKIL, A. A., SHAHANI, B. T. and YOUNG, R. R. Sural conduction studies and late responses in children undergoing hemodialysis. *Archives of Physical Medicine and Rehabilitation*, **59,** 562 (1978)

3 ADAMS, R. D., SHAHANI, B. T. and YOUNG, R. R. A severe pansensory familial neuropathy. *Transactions of the American Neurological Association*, **98,** 67–69 (1973)

4 ALBIZZATI, M. G., BASSI, S., PASSERINI, D. and CRESPI, V. F-wave velocity in motor neurone disease. *Acta Neurologica Scandinavica*, **54,** 269–277 (1976)

5 BOSTOCK, H., FEASBY, T. E. and SEARS, T. A. Continuous conduction in regenerating myelinated nerve fibres. *Journal of Physiology*, **269,** 88P (1977)

6 BOSTOCK, H. and SEARS, T. A. The internodal axon membrane: electrical excitability and continuous conduction in segmental demyelination. *Journal of Physiology*, **280**, 273–301 (1978)

7 BRADDOM, R. I. and JOHNSON, E. W. Standardization of H-reflex and diagnostic use in S–1 radiculopathy. *Archives of Physical Medicine and Rehabilitation*, **55**, 161–166 (1974)

8 BROWN, A. G. Cutaneous afferent fiber collaterals in the dorsal column of the cat. *Experimental Brain Research*, **5**, 293–305 (1968)

9 BUCHTHAL, F. Action potentials in the sural nerve evoked by tactile stimuli. *Mayo Clinic Proceedings*, **55**, 223–230 (1980)

10 BUCHTHAL, F., ROSENFALCK, A. and BEHSE, F. Sensory potentials of normal and diseased nerves. In *Peripheral Neuropathy*, edited by P. J. Dyck, P. K. Thomas and E. H. Lambert, 442–464. Philadelphia, W. B. Saunders, (1975)

11 CAVANAUGH, J. B. The significance of the 'dying-back' process in experimental and human neurological disease. *International Review of Experimental Pathology*, **3**, 219–267 (1964)

12 CHIU, S. Y. and RICHIE, J. M. Potassium channels on nodal and internodal axonal membrane of mammalian myelinated fibres. *Nature*, **284**, 170–171 (1980)

13 CONRAD, B., ASCHOFF, J. C. and FISCHLER, M. Der diagnostische Wert der F-Wellen latenz. *Journal der Neurologie*, **210**, 151–159 (1975)

14 CRAGG, G. C. and THOMAS, P. K. The conduction velocity of regenerated peripheral nerve fibers. *Journal of Physiology*, **171**, 164–175 (1964)

15 CUMMING, K. L., PERKEL, D. H. and DORFMAN, L. J. Nerve fiber conduction velocity distributions. I. Estimation based on the single fiber and compound action potentials. *Electroencephalography and Clinical Neurophysiology*, **46**, 647–658 (1979)

16 DAUBE, J. R., SERVICE, F. J. and DYCK, P. J. Acute effects on nerve conduction of strict control of blood sugar with an artificial pancreas. *Muscle and Nerve*, **3**, 437 (1980)

17 DAWSON, G. D. and MERTON, P. A. Recurrent discharges from motoneurones. *Procès de Congrés International de Physiologie* (Bruxelles), 221–222. Brussels, St. Catherine Press (1956)

18 DENNY-BROWN, D. and BRENNER, C. Paralysis of nerve induced by direct pressure and by tourniquet. *Archives of Neurology and Psychiatry* (*Chicago*), **51**, 1–26 (1944)

19 DOMINGUE, J., SHAHANI, B. T. and YOUNG, R. R. *In vivo* documentation of dysfunction in alpha motor axons of different diameter. *Annals of Neurology*, **8**, 126 (1980)

20 DOMINGUE, J., SHAHANI, B. T. and YOUNG, R. R. Conduction velocity in different diameter ulnar sensory and motor nerve fibers. *Muscle and Nerve*, **3**, 437 (1980)

21 DRESCHLER, B., LASTOUKA, M. and KALVODOVA, E. Electrophysiological study of patients with herniated intervertebral disc. *Electromyography*, **6**, 187–204 (1966)

22 DYCK, P. J., JOHNSON, W. J., LAMBERT, E. H., O'BRIEN, P. C., DAUBE, J. R. and UVIATT, K. F. Comparison of symptoms, chemistry and nerve function to assess adequacy of hemodialysis. *Neurology*, **29**, 1361–1368 (1979)

23 EGLOFF-BAER, S., SHAHANI, B. T. and YOUNG, R. R. Usefulness of late responses in diagnosis of entrapment neuropathies. *Electroencephalography and Clinical Neurophysiology*, **45**, 16P (1978)

24 EISEN, A., SCHOMER, D. and MELMED, C. The application of F-wave measurements in the differentiation of proximal and distal upper limb entrapments. *Neurology (Minneapolis)*, **27**, 662–668 (1977)

25 ERB, W. Diseases of the peripheral cerebrospinal nerves. In *Cyclopaedia of the Practice of Medicine*, XI, edited by H. von Ziemmsen. London, Samson Low, Marston, Searle and Rivington (1876)

26 FISHER, M. A., SHIVDE, A. J., TEIXERA, C. and GRAINER, L. S. Clinical and electrophysiological appraisal of the significance of radicular injury in back pain. *Journal of Neurology, Neurosurgery and Psychiatry*, **41**, 301–306 (1978)

27 FOWLER, T. J., DANTA, G. and GILLIATT, R. W. Recovery of nerve conduction after a pneumatic tourniquet: observations on the hind limb of a baboon. *Journal of Neurology, Neurosurgery and Psychiatry*, **35**, 638–647 (1972)

28 FULLERTON, P. M. and BARNES, J. M. Peripheral neuropathy in rats produced by acrylamide. *British Journal of Industrial Medicine*, **23**, 210–221 (1966)

29 GILLIATT, R. W. Applied electrophysiology in nerve and muscle disease. *Proceedings of the Royal Society of Medicine*, **59**, 989–992 (1966)

30 GILLIATT, R. W., McDONALD, W. I. and RUDGE, P. The site of conduction block in peripheral nerves compressed by a pneumatic tourniquet. *Journal of Physiology*, **238**, 31P (1974)

31 GOMBAULT, A. Contribution à l'étude anatomique de la nevrite parenchymateuse subaigue et chronique – nevrite segmentaire periaxile. *Archive d'Neurologie (Paris)* **1**, 11 (1880)

32 HALL, J. I. Studies on demyelinated peripheral nerves in guinea pigs with experimental allergic neuritis. A histological and electrophy-

siological study. II. Electrophysiological observations. *Brain*, **90**, 313–332 (1967)

33 HALLIDAY, A. M. and McDONALD, W. I. Pathophysiology of demyelinating disease. *British Medical Bulletin*, **33**, 21–27 (1977)

34 HENRIKSON, J. D. Conduction velocity of motor nerves in normal subjects and patients with neuromuscular disorders. *MS Thesis*, University of Minnesota (1956)

35 HERN, J. E. C. Tri-ortho cresyl phosphate neuropathy in the baboon. In *New Developments in Electromyography and Clinical Neurophysiology*, **2**, edited by J. E. Desmedt, 181–187. Basel, S. Karger, (1973)

36 HOFFMAN, P. Über die Beziehungen der Sehnenreflexe zur Willkurlichen Bewegung und zum Tonus. *Zeitschrift für Biologie (Munich)*, **68**, 351–370 (1918)

37 HOPF, H. C. Untersuchungen über die Unterschiede in der Leitgeschwindigkeit motorischer Nervenfassern beim Menschen, *Deutsche Zeitschrift für Nervenheilkunde*, **183**, 579–588 (1962)

38 HOPKINS, A. P. and GILLIATT, R. W. Motor and sensory nerve conduction velocity in the baboon: normal values and changes during acrylamide neuropathy. *Journal of Neurology, Neurosurgery and Psychiatry*, **34**, 415–426 (1971)

39 KAESER, H. E. and LAMBERT, E. H. Nerve function studies in experimental polyneuritis. *Electroencephalography and Clinical Neurophysiology*, **22**, 29 (1962)

40 KIMURA, J. F-wave velocity in the central segment of the median and ulnar nerves. A study in normal subjects and in patients with Charcot-Marie-Tooth Disease. *Neurology*, **24**, 539–546 (1974)

41 KIMURA, J. and BUTZER, J. F. F-wave conduction velocity in Guillain-Barré syndrome. *Archives of Neurology*, **32**, 524–529 (1975)

42 KING, D. and ASHBY, P. Conduction velocity in the proximal segments of a motor nerve in the Guillain-Barré syndrome. *Journal of Neurology, Neurosurgery and Psychiatry*, **39**, 583–544 (1976)

43 KOROBKIN, R., ASBURY, A. K., SUMNER, A. J. and NIELSON, S. L. Glue-sniffing neuropathy. *Archives of Neurology*, **32**, 158–162 (1975)

44 LACHMAN, T., SHAHANI, B. T. and YOUNG, R. R. Late responses as diagnostic aids in Landry-Guillain-Barré syndrome. *Electroencephalography and Clinical Neurophysiology*, **43**, 147 (1977)

45 LACHMAN, T., SHAHANI, B. T. and YOUNG, R. R. Late responses as aids to diagnosis in peripheral neuropathy. *Journal of Neurology, Neurosurgery and Psychiatry*, **43**, 156–162 (1980)

46 LEFEBVRE-D'AMOUR, M., SHAHANI, B. T., YOUNG, R. R. and BIRD, K. T. The importance of studying sural nerve conduction and late responses in the evaluation of alcoholic subjects. *Neurology*, **29**, 1600–1609 (1979)

47 LEHMAN, H. J. and ULE, G. Electrophysiological findings and structural changes in circumscript inflammation of peripheral nerves. *Progress in Brain Research*, **6**, 169 (1964)

48 LEIFER, L. J., MEYER, M. A., MORF, M. and PETRIG, B. Nerve bundle conduction velocity distribution measurements and transfer function. *Proceedings of the Institute of Electrical and Electronics Engineers*, **65**, 747–755 (1977)

49 LeQUESNE, P. M. Neurophysiological investigation of subclinical and minimal toxic neuropathies. *Muscle and Nerve*, **1**, 392 (1978)

50 MACCABEE, P. J., SHAHANI, B. T. and YOUNG, R. R. Usefulness of double simultaneous recording (DSR) and F response studies in the diagnosis of carpal tunnel syndrome (CTS). *Electroencephalography and Clinical Neurophysiology*, **49**, 18P (1980)

51 MAGLADERY, J. W. and McDOUGAL, D. B. Electrophysiological studies of nerve and reflex activity in normal man. I. Identification of certain reflexes in the electromyogram and the conduction velocity of peripheral nerve fibres. *Bulletin of Johns Hopkins Hospital*, **86**, 265–290 (1950)

52 MAYER, R. F. and DENNY-BROWN, D. Conduction velocity in peripheral nerve during experimental demyelination of the cat. *Neurology*, **14**, 714–726 (1964)

53 MAYER, R. F. and FELDMAN, R. G. Observations on the nature of the F-wave in man. *Neurology*, **17**, 147–156 (1967)

54 MAYER, R. F. and MAWDSLEY, C. Studies in man and cat of the significance of the H reflex. *Journal of Neurology, Neurosurgery and Psychiatry*, **28**, 201–209 (1965)

55 McDONALD, W. I. Conduction in muscle afferent fibers during experimental demyelination in cat nerve. *Acta Neuropathologica (Berlin)*, **1**, 425 (1962)

56 McDONALD, W. I. The effects of experimental demyelination on conduction in peripheral nerves: A histological and electrophysiological study: I. Clinical and histological observations. *Brain*, **86**, 501–524 (1963)

57 McDONALD, W. I. Remyelination in relation to clinical lesions of the central nervous system. *British Medical Bulletin*, **30**, 186–189 (1974)

58 McLEOD, J. G. and WRAY, S. H. An experimental study of the F-wave in the baboon. *Journal of Neurology, Neurosurgery and Psychiatry*, **29**, 196–200 (1966)

59 MORGAN-HUGHES, J. SINCLAIR, S. and DURSTON, J. H. H. The pattern of peripheral nerve regeneration induced by crush in rats with severe acrylamide neuropathy. *Brain,* **97,** 235–250 (1974)

60 NOTERMANS, S. L. H. and VINGERHOETS, H. M. The importance of the Hoffman reflex in the diagnosis of lumbar root lesions. *Clinical Neurology and Neurophysiology*, **1,** 54–65 (1974)

61 OCHOA, J., DANTA, G., FOWLER, T. J. and GILLIATT, R. W. Nature of the nerve lesion caused by a pneumatic tourniquet. *Nature,* **233,** 265 –266 (1971)

62 OCHOA, J., FOWLER, T. J. and GILLIATT, R. W. Anatomical changes in peripheral nerves compressed by a pneumatic tourniquet. *Journal of Anatomy*, **113,** 433–455 (1972)

63 OCHOA, J., FOWLER, T. J. and GILLIATT, R. W. Changes produced by a pneumatic tourniquet. In *New Developments in Electromyography and Clinical Neurophysiology*, **2,** edited by J. E. Desmedt, 174–180. Basel, S. Karger, (1973)

64 PANAYIOTOPOULOS, C. P. F-wave conduction velocity in the proximal segment of the deep peroneal nerve: Charcot-Marie-Tooth Disease and dystrophica myotonica. *Muscle and Nerve*, **1,** 37–44 (1978)

65 PANAYIOTOPOULOS, C. P., SCARPALEZOS, S. and NASTAS, P. E. F-wave studies in the deep peroneal nerve. Part 1. Control subjects. *Journal of Neurological Science*, **31,** 319–329 (1977)

66 PANAYIOTOPOULOS, C. P. and SCARPALEZOS, S. F-wave studies in the deep peroneal nerve. Part 2. 1, chronic renal failure; 2, limb-girdle muscular dystrophy. *Journal of Neurological Science*, **31,** 331–341 (1977)

67 PANAYIOTOPOULOS, C. P., SCARPALEZOS, S., and NASTAS, P. E. Sensory (Ia) and F-wave conduction velocity in the proximal segment of the tibial nerve. *Muscle and Nerve*, **1,** 181–189 (1978)

68 RASMINSKY, M., KEARNEY, R. E., AGUAYO, A. J. and BRAY, G. M. Conduction of nervous impulses in spinal roots and peripheral nerves of dystrophic mice, *Brain Research*, **143,** 71–85 (1978)

69 RASMINSKY, M. and SEARS, T. A. Internodal conduction in undissected demyelinated nerve fibers. *Journal of Physiology*, **227,** 323–350 (1972)

70 RENSHAW, B. Influence of discharge of motoneurones upon excitation of neighboring motoneurones. *Journal of Neurophysiology*, **4,** 167 –183 (1941)

71 RIDLEY, A. Porphyric neuropathy. In *Peripheral Neuropathy*, edited by P. J. Dyck, P. K. Thomas and E. H. Lambert, 942–956. Philadelphia, W. B. Saunders (1975)

72 SAIDA, K., SAIDA, T., BROWN, M. J. and SILBERBERG, D. H. *In vivo* demyelination induced by intraneural injection of anti-galactocerebroside serum. A morphologic study. *American Journal of Pathology*, **95,** 99–110 (1979)

73 SAIDA, K., SAIDA, T., BROWN, M. J., SILBERBERG, D. H. and ASBURY, A. K. Antiserum-mediated demyelination in vivo. A sequential study using intraneural injection of experimental allergic neuritis serum. *Laboratory Investigation*, **39,** 449–462 (1978)

74 SAIDA, K., SUMNER, A. J., SAIDA, T., BROWN, M. J. and SILBERBERG, D. H. Antiserum-mediated demyelination: relationship between re-myelination and functional recovery. *Annals of Neurology*, **8,** 12–24 (1980)

75 SAIDA, T., SAIDA, K., BROWN, M. J. and SILBERBERG, D. H. Peripheral nerve demyelination induced by intraneural injection of ex-perimental allergic encephalomyelitis serum. *Journal of Neuro-pathology and Experimental Neurology*, **38,** 498–518 (1979)

76 SAIDA, T., SAIDA. K., DORFMAN, S. H., SILBERBERG, D. H., SUMNER, A. J., MANNING, M. C., LISAK, R. P. and BROWN, M. J. Experimental allergic neuritis induced by sensitization with galactocerebroside. *Science*, **204,** 1103–1106 (1979)

77 SAIDA, T., SAIDA, K., SILBERBERG, D. H. and BROWN, M. J. Transfer of demyelination by intraneural injection of experimental allergic neuritis serum. *Nature*, **272,** 639–641 (1978)

78 SCHAUMBERG, H. H., WISNIEWSKI, H. M. and SPENCER, P. S. Ultrastructu-ral studies of the dying back process. I. Peripheral nerve terminal and axon degeneration in systemic acrylamide intoxication. *Journal of Neuropathology and Experimental Neurology*, **33,** 260 (1974)

79 SHAHANI, B. T. Flexor reflex nerve afferents in man. *Journal of Neurology, Neurosurgery and Psychiatry*, **33,** 792–800 (1970)

80 SHAHANI, B. T., POTTS, F. and DOMINIGUE, J. N. F-response studies in peripheral neuropathies. *Neurology*, **30,** 409 (1980)

81 SHAHANI, B. T., POTTS, F., JUGUILON, A. and YOUNG, R. R. Maximal–minimal motor nerve conduction and F-response studies in normal subjects and patients with ulnar compression neuropathies. *Muscle and Nerve*, **3,** 182 (1979)

82 SHAHANI, B. T. and YOUNG R. R. Effect of vibration on the F-response. In *The Motor System: Neurophysiology and Muscle Mechanisms*, edited by M. Shahani, 185–195. Amsterdam, Elsevier (1976)

83 SHAHANI, B. T. and YOUNG, R. R. Studies of reflex activity from a clinical viewpoint. In *Electrodiagnosis in Clinical Neurology*, edited

by M. J. Aminoff, 290–304. New York, Churchill Livingstone (1980)

84 SHAHANI, B. T., YOUNG, R. R. and LACHMAN, T. Late responses as aids to diagnosis in peripheral neuropathy. *Journal of Postgraduate Medicine*, **21,** 7 (1975)

85 SPENCER, P. S. and SCHAUMBERG, H. H. (Editors). *Experimental and Clinical Neurotoxicology*, Baltimore, Williams and Wilkins (1980)

86 STÅLBERG, E. and TRONTELJ, J. *Single Fibre Electromyography*. Old Woking, Surrey, UK, Mirvalle Press (1979)

87 STANLEY, E. F., LONG, R. R., GRIFFIN, J. W. and PRICE, D. L. Experimental axonal atrophy reduces nerve conduction velocity. *Neurology*, **30,** 370 (1980)

88 SUMNER, A. J. Axonal neuropathies. In *Physiology of Peripheral Nerve Disease*, edited by A. J. Sumner. Philadelphia, W. B. Saunders (1980)

89 SUMNER, A. J. The physiology of dying back neuropathies. In *Physiology and Pathobiology of Axons*, edited by S. G. Waxman, 349–359. New York, Raven Press (1978)

90 SUMNER, A. J. and ASBURY, A. K. Physiological studies of the dying-back phenomenon. I. Effects of acrylamide on muscle stretch afferents. *Brain*, **98,** 91–100 (1975)

91 SUMNER, A. J., SAIDA, K., SAIDA, T., BROWN, M. J., SILBERBERG, D. H., ASBURY, A. K. Acute conduction block produced by intraneural injection of EAE serum: A correlative electrophysiological and morphological study. *Neurology*, **29,** 581 (1979)

92 THORN, J. Central responses to electrical activation of the peripheral nerves supplying the intrinsic hand muscles. *Journal of Neurology, Neurosurgery and Psychiatry*, **28,** 482–495 (1965)

93 TONZOLA, R., ACKIL, A., SHAHANI, B. T. and YOUNG, R. R., Usefulness of electrophysiological studies in the diagnosis of lumbosacral root disease, *Electroencephalography and Clinical Neurophysiology*, **49,** 17 (1980)

94 WAGER, E. E., JR. and BUERGER, A. A. H-reflex latency and sensory conduction in normal and diabetic subjects. *Archives of Physical Medicine and Rehabilitation*, **55,** 126–219 (1974)

95 WAGER, E. E., JR. and BUERGER, A. A. A linear relationship between the H-reflex latency and sensory conduction velocity in neuropathy. *Neurology*, **24,** 711–715 (1974)

96 YOUNG, R. R. and SHAHANI, B. T. Clinical value and limitations of F-wave determination. *Muscle and Nerve*, **1,** 248–250 (1978)

7

New aspects of sympathetic function in man

B. Gunnar Wallin

Introduction

From a practical viewpoint, autonomic symptoms are rarely dominant features of neurological diseases and for most neurologists and clinical neurophysiologists, the autonomic nervous system is still *terra incognita*. On the one hand, when major autonomic symptoms do occur, they often fall within the realm of, for example, cardiologists or urologists and the neurologist may not have prime responsibility for diagnostic and therapeutic measures. On the other hand, autonomic neural functions are difficult to study. Most commonly, conclusions about autonomic drive have been drawn somewhat indirectly from various effector organ activities, e.g. heart rate, blood flow, blood pressure and sweat production. Unfortunately such data are difficult to interpret, both because effector organs react slowly to variations in autonomic neural drive and because they also react to hormonal and local chemical stimuli. Nevertheless, such recordings have been used to develop a battery of clinical tests which have proved useful for the detection of dysfunction in different autonomic regions. For a description of these tests the reader is referred to a recent text[21] and to a review[45] dealing with disorders of the autonomic nervous system.

Owing to difficulties in interpreting recordings of autonomic effector organ activities in neural terms, our understanding of neurophysiological mechanisms underlying various autonomic reflexes is still very incomplete. It was therefore a considerable methodological advance when the microneurographic technique of percutaneous introduction *in vivo* of a tungsten microelectrode into nerves within human limbs, was found to be useful for recording sympathetic action potentials in peripheral nerves of awake, unanaesthetized human

145

subjects[18, 36]. It then became possible to get direct information about sympathetic neural outflow to skin and muscle in man both at rest and during various manoeuvres. Visceral sympathetic activity (and parasympathetic activity) is still inaccessible but data obtained with the new technique has nevertheless provided new insights into specific sympathetic reflex mechanisms and also new data which modify the current concept of the term 'sympathetic tone'. This chapter will summarize these results. Consequently, rather than describing new tests for diagnoses of autonomic disorders, it will present new physiological data which hopefully afford better understanding of the usefulness and limitations of those autonomic tests already in clinical use.

Technique

Nerve recordings utilize tungsten microelectrodes with a tip diameter of a few microns. The recording electrode is inserted manually, through intact skin, into an underlying nerve with a reference electrode placed subcutaneously 1–2 cm away. Usually, multi-unit recordings are obtained but a few single unit recordings have been reported[20]. Most recordings have been made from the peroneal nerve at the fibular head but sometimes median, radial, tibial, sural or posterior antebrachial cutaneous nerves are used. In general, mixed nerves are impaled as far distally as possible in order to obtain recordings from relatively 'pure' muscle or skin nerve fascicles. In some experiments, blood pressure was recorded in the brachial artery; in others, electrical resistance of skin and a finger or toe plethysmogram (photoelectric) were monitored. Usually nerve recordings cause only minimal discomfort. Detailed descriptions of the technique as well as evidence for the sympathetic nature of the recorded impulses have been given previously[4, 12, 33, 36]. Ganglionic blocking agents such as trimetaphan (Arfonad), when given intravenously, reversibly depress or eliminate the recorded activity.

Anatomical background

The large majority of postganglionic sympathetic fibres to skin and muscles in the extremities run in peripheral nerves, each of which is composed of a varying number of fascicles. Fascicles are most numerous distally where each contains fibres connected only to skin or only to muscles, but they become confluent and in the proximal part of an extremity all fascicles are composed of a mixture of skin and muscle fibres. For example, there are 20–35 fascicles in the median nerve at the wrist but only 3–13 fascicles proximally in the upper arm[32]. Unmyelinated C fibres, both somatic afferent and sympathetic efferent, are not diffusely distributed in the fascicles but lie clustered within groups of Schwann cells[2, 17]. This agrees with the author's experience from microelectrode recordings where sympathetic activity can be recorded only from certain intrafascicular sites.

The segmental sudomotor innervation of skin was mapped by Richter and Woodruff[29] who measured resistance changes in skin denervated by lumbar or sacral sympathectomies. Recently Normell[24] made similar mappings of vasomotor innervation of skin by recording vasomotor-induced changes in skin temperature in paraplegic patients. In Normell's study, loss of thermoregulatory sweating was also measured with a simple and elegant method which permitted direct comparison between skin areas deprived of vasomotor and sudomotor function. He showed differences between areas of sudomotor and vasomotor loss, sometimes corresponding to several somatosensory dermatomes, in about 50 per cent of 57 paraplegic patients. This strongly suggests an anatomical dissociation of vasomotor and sudomotor efferent pathways.

Functional organization of sympathetic outflow

Traditionally, sympathetic reactions were thought to be slow and protracted and to occur in parallel in different parts of the body[10]. This view of a diffusely acting system led to the term 'sympathetic tone' to describe a presumed global level of activity in sympathetic nerves – clinically, subjects are often classified as having 'high' or 'low sympathetic tone'. Unfortunately this concept is too simplistic. When recordings are made selectively from sympathetic nerves supplying well-defined effector organs, there are clear differences between the activity in one nerve and that in another as would be expected with differentiated regional control of sympathetic outflow. For example, when comparing sympathetic activity recorded in nerve fascicles innervating skin or muscles, temporal patterns of activity are different even at rest. Muscle sympathetic activity (MSA) is characterized by fairly regular pulse-synchronous bursts of impulses, often occurring in short sequences separated by periods of neural silence[12]. Skin sympathetic activity (SSA), on the other hand, consists of more irregular

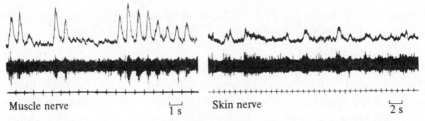

Muscle nerve   1 s   Skin nerve   2 s

Figure 7.1 Typical patterns of multi-unit sympathetic activity at rest in human muscle and nerve fascicles. Traces from above: mean voltage neurograms (time constant 0.1 s); original neurograms; ECG. (From Wallin, Delius and Hagbarth[38], courtesy of the publishers, *Central Rhythmic and Regulation*)

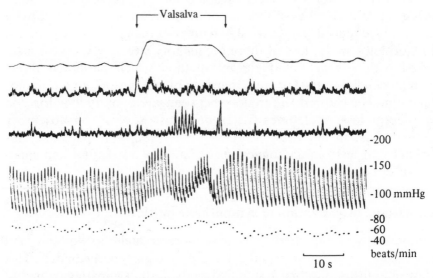

Figure 7.2 Effects of the Valsalva manoeuvre on SSA (second trace) and MSA (third trace) recorded simultaneously from left and right peroneal nerves. Upper trace: respiratory movements (inspiration upwards); fourth trace: blood pressure; bottom trace: instantaneous heart rate. (From Wallin, Delius and Hagbarth[38], courtesy of the publishers, *Central Rhythmic and Regulation*)

bursts of impulses, varying in strength and duration, and without relationship to the pulse[19]. Examples of the two types of activity are shown in *Figure 7.1*. In addition, various manoeuvres affect these activities differently. Body cooling leads to a clear increase of SSA without much change in MSA[13, 14] and in contrast, the Valsalva manoeuvre (*Figure 7.2*) always causes an increase in MSA but no consistent change in SSA[13, 14]. Arousal stimuli or stimuli with emotional effects, which lead to an increase of SSA, may sometimes even cause a decrease in MSA, i.e. the responses may be opposite in direction[13, 14, 37]. *Table 7.1* summarizes effects of different manoeuvres on SSA and MSA. In contrast to this evidence for differences between

Table 7.1 Comparison of effects of various manoeuvres on sympathetic activity in skin and muscle nerves

Manoeuvres	SSA		MSA	References
	Vasoconstrictor	Sudomotor		
Cooling	+	−	0	4, 13, 14
Warming	−	+	0	4, 5, 13, 14, 25
Arousal	+	+	0,−	4, 5, 12, 19, 37
Emotional stress	+	+	0,±	4, 5, 13, 14, 37
Deep breath	+	+	0,−	12, 19
Hyperventilation	+		−	13, 14
Smoking	+		−	13, 14
Muscle work	+,0		±,0	13, 14, 37
Orthostatic stress	0		+	8, 13
Raising the legs	0		−	13
Valsalva	0,+		+	13, 14, 37
Stim arterial baroreceptors	0		−	3, 41
Stim low pressure receptors			−	35
General anaesthesia	−			40

The signs +, − and 0 indicate increase, decrease and no change of activity, respectively. From hyperventilation and onwards the effects on SSA refer to a mixture of sudomotor and vasoconstrictor impulses.

sympathetic outflows to skin and muscle, there is remarkable parallelism between the two neurograms when MSA is recorded simultaneously in different nerves in recumbent subjects. Virtually every burst of sympathetic impulses can be identified in muscle nerves from both upper and lower extremities and even the strength of individual bursts varies in parallel[33]. In a corresponding way, double recordings of SSA from skin nerves innervating the palm of the hands and the feet reveal a similar close parallelism between both neurograms[5]. These findings show there are different populations of sympathetic neurons, each of which is subjected to its own homogenous supraspinal drive which may be different from that of other populations. Consequently there is no common 'sympathetic tone'; if the term is to be retained, it should be used only when considering the sympathetic drive in specified nerves supplying well-defined effector organs.

Sympathetic outflow to skin

The two most important autonomic effector organs in human skin, blood vessels and sweat glands, are innervated by separate sets of sympathetic fibres. The conduction velocity is 1.0–1.4 m/s in sudomotor and approximately 0.7 m/s in vasoconstrictor fibres[15]. In nerves supplying the palm of the hands and the feet, sudomotor and vasoconstrictor impulses can be recorded from the same intrafascicular site, suggesting that the fibres are intermingled[4, 19]. At rest at normal room temperature (22–24°C), some spontaneous bursts are followed by both transient changes in skin resistance and plethysmographic signs of vasoconstriction indicating that each burst contains a mixture of vasoconstrictor and sudomotor impulses (*Figure 7.3a*). Other bursts, such as in *Figure 7.3c*, contain only vasoconstrictor impulses (i.e. they are followed by transient vasoconstrictions but not by skin resistance changes) whereas pure sudomotor bursts are unusual at normal room temperature (*Figure 7.3d*). The sympathetic impulses in skin nerves are not grouped with the pulse rhythm, they show no

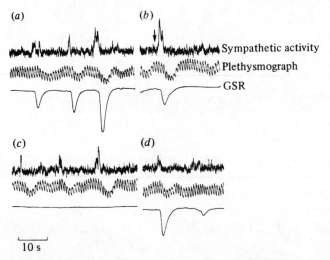

Figure 7.3 Spontaneous (*a, c, d*) and evoked (*b*) bursts of skin sympathetic activity in median nerve (upper traces) with accompanying finger plethysmographic (center traces) and palmar electrodermal (lower traces) responses. Room temperature 22–24°C. The arrow in (*b*) indicates the electrical skin stimulus on the contra-lateral arm. (From Bini *et al.*[4], courtesy of the Editor and publisher, *Journal of Physiology*.)

correlation with spontaneous fluctuations of blood pressure[19] (cf. *Figure 7.1* and *Figure 7.2*) and are not affected in a reproducible way by electrical stimulation of carotid sinus nerves[42]. These findings suggest that arterial baroreflex modulation of skin sympathetic activity is weak or absent. There is a loose coupling between the occurrence of sympathetic bursts and the respiratory rhythm and a sudden deep inspiration will regularly evoke a strong burst of impulses. On the other hand, these discharges are not inhibited during apnoea[19].

Previous recordings of cutaneous effector-organ responses have shown that spontaneous electrodermal and plethysmographic activity occurs in parallel in hands and feet[6, 9, 31] and a similar parallelism in the underlying sympathetic discharges has now been demonstrated[5, 37]. This parallelism does not apply to all skin areas, however, and during exposure to different temperatures there are differences in sympathetic drives between, for example, the median nerve innervating the palm of the hand and the dorsal cutaneous nerve of the forearm[5].

Thermoregulatory effects

The skin is important for thermoregulation and an efficient way of influencing the strength of skin sympathetic activity is to change environmental temperature. *Figure 7.4* illustrates changes of sympathetic activity in the median nerve during changes in ambient

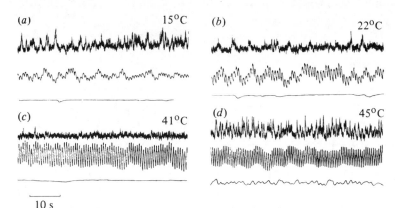

Figure 7.4 Thermoregulatory changes in sympathetic activity recorded in median nerve innervating the palm of the hand. Traces as in *Figure 7.3*. (*a–c*) Decreasing vasoconstrictor activity with rising temperature (from 15 to 45°C). (*d*) Strong sudomotor activity at 45°C. (From Bini *et al.*[4], courtesy of the Editor and publisher, *Journal of Physiology*.)

temperature. At 15°C strong sympathetic bursts occurred at high rates. They were associated with plethysmographic signs of skin vasoconstriction and absence of electrodermal activity within the neural innervation zone, indicating that in this situation neural activity consisted of only vasoconstrictor impulses (*Figure 7.4a*). As ambient temperature was increased, vasoconstrictor activity was reduced and at 35–40°C, usually there was neural silence with no signs of vasoconstriction or electrodermal activity (*Figure 7.4b* and *7.4c*). A further rise in temperature led to reappearance of sympathetic bursts at the same time as the subject started sweating and irregular fluctuations appeared in the skin resistance record, i.e. now the bursts were composed entirely of sudomotor impulses. (*Figure 7.4d*). When sweating first began each sudomotor burst was followed by a distinct electrodermal response and in this situation there was a linear relationship between mean-voltage amplitudes of sudomotor bursts and amplitudes of corresponding changes in skin resistance[4]. When sweating was more pronounced, successive electrodermal responses merged and a similar quantitative correlation could not be made.

These results show that by changing environmental temperature one can obtain selective activation of either the sudomotor or the vasoconstrictor neural system with suppression of spontaneous activity in the other system. These changes in central excitatory drives on the two systems were also reflected in different sudomotor and vasoconstrictor responsiveness to arousal stimuli at different ambient temperatures (*see below*).

The effects of mental stimuli

In agreement with the fact that stimuli with emotional effects may change skin colour and moisture, such stimuli, pleasant or unpleasant, regularly caused an increase of skin sympathetic activity[14, 19]. Any unexpected stimulus, such as a sudden sound, a sudden touch or a sudden pain stimulus anywhere on the skin surface, regularly evoke a a single burst of impulses which occurred after a latency of 0.5–1)s, depending on the recording site and the subject's height. (*Figure 7.3b*). This latency was shorter in proximal than in distal recording sites and short subjects had shorter latencies than tall subjects. The differences are due mainly to differences in conduction time in postganglionic sympathetic C fibres and reflex latencies can be used as an indirect measure of sympathetic conduction velocity[15]. In contrast to thermoregulatory reflexes, which cause opposite responses in sudo- and vasomotor fibres, arousal reflexes usually involve simultaneous activation of sudomotor and vasoconstrictor fibres, i.e. sympathetic bursts were followed both by plethysmographic and electrodermal responses (*Figure 7.3b*). This simultaneous activation constitutes the basis for 'cold sweat'. The strength of neural and effector organ responses varied considerably and habituation often occurred[19]. As mentioned above, responsiveness of the two fibre systems to arousal stimuli was dependent on room temperature[4]. In a cool environment with ongoing spontaneous vasoconstrictor activity in the nerve and no spontaneous variations of skin resistance, weak arousal stimuli could evoke sympathetic bursts followed by clear plethysmographic but no electrodermal responses. On the other hand, when vasoconstrictor tone was reduced by moderate warming many bursts triggered by weak arousal stimuli seemed to be composed exclusively of sudomotor impulses. These findings show that in recordings of electrodermal activity, results may be influenced by the subject's thermoregulatory state. They also illustrate that the final effect of a manoeuvre on sympathetic outflow is determined by interaction between different reflexes which are integrated in central sympathetic structures.

Emotional excitement, brought on by a stressed conversation or a sudden request to solve an arithmetical problem, usually leads to an increase of skin sympathetic activity which is more long-lasting than that caused by arousal stimuli[14]. Such an increase may occasionally last for several minutes after the end of the stimulus[25]. In simultaneous recordings from nerves supplying the palm of the hand and the foot, neural responses to emotional stimuli are virtually identical but differences have been observed between nerves innervating the dorsal side of the forearm and the palm of the hand[5]. It is a common finding that at the beginning of an experiment, 'spontaneous' sympathetic activity to the skin is intense, and then gradually subsides as the subject gets used to the situation. Changes in wakefulness also cause marked changes in strength of neural activity and, for example, loss of consciousness with general anaesthesia virtually abolished spontaneous skin sympathetic activity[40].

Clinical suggestions

Though microneurographic recordings are too time-consuming for routine diagnostic purposes cutaneous sympathetic reflexes are easy to demonstrate with the aid of a photoelectric plethysmograph and/or a device for recording changes in skin resistance. If such recordings reveal clear variations of pulse amplitude and/or skin resistance, either spontaneously or in response to arousal stimuli, the reflex arc is qualitatively intact. Since sympathetic outflow to hands and feet occurs in parallel, simultaneous monitoring from two digits or extremities may be of value for demonstrating localized lesions. Absence of skin wrinkling on prolonged immersion of hands or feet in water provides another simple test of cutaneous sympathetic function which occasionally may be useful for demonstrating localized lesions[7, 27]. When recording effector organ responses from the palm of the hand or sole of the foot, absence of plethysmographic or skin resistance responses usually indicates an interrupted reflex arc. The sitution is more complex when recording from other skin areas. For example, the excitability level of sudomotor neurons supplying forearm skin seems to be more dependent on thermal factors than neurone supplying glabrous skin. In a warm environment, arousal stimuli usually give rise to clear-cut changes in resistance of forearm skin, but if the subject is cold responses may be difficult or impossible to elicit[4]. This agrees with Carmichael *et al.*[11], who found that when a subject was vasodilated and the skin warm, skin resistance responses could be recorded from most skin areas. In contrast, the author was not able to record arousal-induced transient changes of pulse amplitude in the plethysmogram from forearm skin although mean pulse amplitudes decreased with decreasing ambient temperature. The reason is not clear but may be due to insufficient plethysmograph sensitivity.

Absolute values for changes in skin resistance and pulse amplitudes in the plethysmogram depend not only on the strength of sympathetic discharges but also on local factors such as skin colour and thickness so that quantitative comparisons of effector organ responses between individuals cannot be made. Semi-quantitative estimates are, however, feasible. In a study of patients with polyneuropathy[16], skin resistance responses to arousal stimuli weresionall defined as weak if, using standardized amplifier settings, the responses never exceeded a certain voltage. Similarly, pulse plethysmographic responses were considered weak if the amplitude reduction was less than 25 per cent of the pre-stimulus amplitude. Using these criteria, a significant correlation was found between weak responses and symptoms of autonomic impairment such as dryness of hands and feet, orthostatism, impotence and bladder dysfunction. In addition, in microelectrode recordings no sympathetic recording sites were found in skin nerves in 67 per cent of extremities with one or both cutaneous effector organ responses weak or absent; when effector organ responses were normal, there were no failures.

Sympathetic outflow to muscles

Relationship to blood pressure

As mentioned above, bursts of sympathetic impulses recorded in muscle nerves are synchronous with the pulse and usually occur intermittently in short sequences. As *Figure 7.5* illustrates, they are

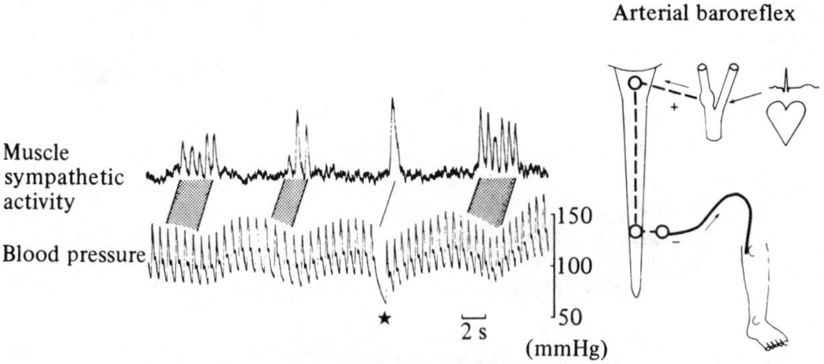

Figure 7.5 The relationship between spontaneous fluctuations of blood pressure and muscle nerve sympathetic activity (*left*). The baroreflex modulation (*right*) accounts for the pulse synchrony of nerve activity and the inverse relationship to blood pressure fluctuations. The star symbol indicates diastolic blood pressure fall due to sudden AV block. Shading indicates corresponding sequences of bursts and heartbeats. (From Wallin, Sundlöf and Lindblad[44], courtesy of the publishers, *Baroreceptors and Hypertension*.)

most frequent during spontaneous transient reductions in blood pressure and disappear when blood pressure goes up[12, 34, 37]. These findings agree with the notion that the bursts are composed of vasoconstrictor impulses controlled by arterial baroreflexes. A fall in pressure is sensed by the baroreceptors and counteracted by increasing vasoconstriction. According to this view, bursts correspond to diastolic blood pressure reductions whereas pauses between successive bursts correspond to systolic inhibitions. Several findings support this interpretation.

In cardiac arrhythmias with pronounced variations of blood pressure, a close correlation was observed between pressure variations and occurrence of bursts[38]. As shown in *Figure 7.5*, atrioventricular block, with a sudden fall in diastolic blood pressure during a single heart beat (marked by a star in the figure), is regularly followed by a strong sympathetic burst. The latency between the pressure fall and the burst is approximately 1.3 s which corresponds to the delay in the baroreflex arc. The delay was similar when sympathetic bursts were inhibited by electrical stimulation of carotid sinus nerves[42]. As with sympathetic reflexes in skin nerves, the delay is related to the subject's height and

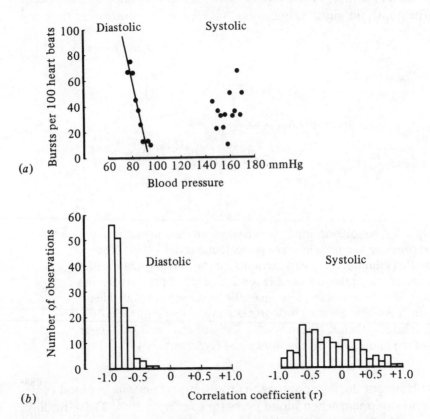

(a)

(b)

Figure 7.6 Occurrence of sympathetic bursts in relation to diastolic and systolic blood pressure. (*a*) Example of relationship during 3 min rest period from normotensive subject. Correlation coefficients for linear regression −0.95 (diastolic) and +0.21(systolic). (*b*) Distribution of correlation coefficients for 156 rest periods from 16 normotensive subjects. (From Sundlöf and Wallin[34], courtesy of the Editor and publisher, *Journal of Physiology*.)

can be used as an indirect measure of sympathetic conduction velocity[15]. By compensating for the reflex delay one can decide which heart beat a burst corresponds to and thereby analyze which blood pressure parameters determine the out-flow of sympathetic activity. As illustrated in *Figure 7.6*, the occurrence of bursts correlated intimately with diastolic blood pressure but showed no systematic relationship to systolic blood pressure. The finding is logical; the arterial baroreflex is inhibitory and since systolic inhibitions were always complete one expects activity to be determined by diastolic pressure variations.

Strength of activity is also dependent on the direction of an ongoing blood pressure change[34]. In *Figure 7.5* the shaded areas indicate which heart beats the bursts correspond to and it is quite clear that for a given blood pressure level, more bursts occur during falling than during rising pressure. This directional dependence may be due to arterial baroreceptor firing being stronger during increasing than during decreasing pressure[1]. In contrast to this intimate relationship between *dynamic variations* of diastolic blood pressure and MSA, there was no correlation if subjects were compared with regard to their *mean levels* of diastolic blood pressure and sympathetic activity. This suggests that sympathetic outflow to muscles is important for *buffering temporary changes of blood pressure but has little influence on long term blood pressure levels*[34]. Confirmation of this hypothesis came from a study of patients with essential hypertension which gave no evidence that the increased blood pressure level was due to an abnormally high traffic of sympathetic impulses in muscle nerves[41].

Other evidence strengthens the idea that MSA is primarily sensitive to *variations* in blood pressure. When carotid baroreceptors were stimulated by application of subatmospheric pressure in a collar around the neck (neck suction), dynamic stimuli were quite effective in influencing the activity whereas continuous neck suction only had minor and inconsistent effects[3]. This explains why previous investigators found only small changes of forearm blood flow during continuous neck suction. The result may in part be due to counterregulation from aortic and other extracarotid blood pressure receptors which do not sense the suction stimulus. Since the suction stimulus induces a maintained reduction of blood pressure the data nevertheless suggest that carotid sinus control of other effector organs than skeletal muscle is more static in nature or less attenuated by impulses from extracarotid baroreceptors.

Apart from arterial baroreceptors so-called 'low pressure receptors' also influence sympathetic outflow to muscles. These receptors, which are volume receptors primarily located in the heart and vessels entering the heart, are stimulated by changes in central blood volume. When blood is pooled in the legs by applying subatmospheric pressure around the lower body, there is an increase of MSA which cannot be explained as an arterial baroreceptor effect[35]. Interestingly enough, this increase in sympathetic activity did not wear off during 3 min and perhaps therefore, low pressure receptors exert a more static influence on MSA than arterial baroreceptors.

Relationship to heart rate

If mean *levels* of heart rate and MSA are compared amongst recumbent subjects at rest, subjects with low heart rates tend to have more sympathetic activity than subjects with high heart rates. In an unselected group of subjects with a wide age range, this correlation was low[43] but it was fairly high in a more homogenous group with a narrower age range[3]. These findings suggest that in recumbent subjects a low level of resting MSA in some way is balanced by a high heart rate and vice versa. There is also evidence that baroreceptor-induced *changes* of heart rate and MSA vary with pre-existing tone in cardiac and muscle autonomic nerves[3]. Thus, subjects with low incidence of sympathetic bursts while recumbent exhibited greater increases in sympathetic activity, and smaller changes of heart rate, on transition to sitting or standing than subjects with many bursts while lying[8]. In agreement with these two sets of findings there was also an inverse linear relationship between heart rate while lying and the change in heart rate induced by a standardized orthostatic test[23].

Relationship to plasma noradrenaline

In a study of normal variability of MSA in the recumbent posture Sundlöf and Wallin[33] found that mean burst incidence ranged from less than 10 to more than 90 bursts per 100 beats. There was a tendency for increasing values with increasing age. For each individual the value was remarkably constant, not only during the experiment, but also when recordings were repeated with intervals of many months; it was concluded that different subjects have different levels of 'sympathetic

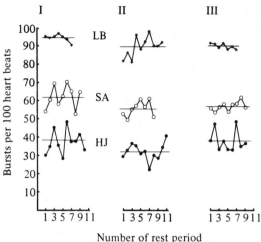

Figure 7.7 Quantitative analyses of repeated recordings of MSA in three different subjects (LB, SA, HJ) at rest. Each point represents the number of bursts per 100 heart beats determined from a rest period of approximately 3 min duration. The thin horizontal lines represent the mean value for each experiment. Recording I in subject SA was made in the right median nerve, all the others were made in either of the peroneal nerves. (From Sundlöf and Wallin[33], courtesy of the Editor and publisher, *Journal of Physiology*.)

tone' in their muscle nerves. This is illustrated in *Figure 7.7* which shows the results of repeated recordings of MSA in three different subjects. Similar results have been obtained for plasma noradrenaline, i.e. in a given subject, plasma concentrations of noradrenaline are reproducible from day to day but there are wide interindividual differences and concentrations tend to increase with increasing age[22, 28, 30]. Recently a link between these two sets of observations was obtained when a linear correlation ($r = 0.65$, $P < 0.01$, $n = 20$) was found between plasma concentrations of noradrenaline in forearm venous blood and the incidence of sympathetic bursts in muscle nerves in normotensive subjects at rest[43]. Since sympathetic outflow differs in different sympathetic nerves, such a correlation may seem surprising. The most probable explanation is that muscles, comprising about 40 per cent of total weight, contain such a large number of adrenergic terminals that overflow of transmitter from these becomes the major determinant of the plasma concentration of noradrenaline.

As mentioned above there is no correlation between mean levels of MSA and blood pressure. If the plasma concentration of noradrenaline is determined by the level of MSA it becomes understandable why most investigations have not been able to demonstrate a relationship between resting levels of noradrenaline and blood pressure in normotensive subjects. For the same reason one must also question to what extent determinations of noradrenaline at rest give useful information about hypertensive mechanisms.

The effect of various manoeuvres

In contrast to skin sympathetic activity, the outflow of sympathetic impulses to muscles is stable and not easily affected by minor disturbances such as arousal stimuli which do not themselves affect blood pressure. Any manoeuvre or situation associated with a change in blood pressure, however, *is* likely to produce a change of MSA. Low diastolic blood pressure induced by an extrasystole or an AV block is regularly followed by a strong sympathetic burst (*Figure 7.5*). A Valsalva manoeuvre (*Figure 7.2*), which causes a transient fall in blood pressure is the most reliable method for causing a short lasting increase of MSA[13, 37]. Emotional stress elicited by a request to solve an arithmetic problem usually leads to a blood pressure increase which sometimes is associated with a decrease of MSA[13]. These are examples in which changes of nerve activity can be regarded as secondary to blood pressure changes, i.e. they may be elicited from arterial baroreceptors. On the other hand, emotional stress may sometimes lead to an increase of MSA at the same time as blood pressure goes up[37] and similar effects have been observed during muscle work[13]. Since, in these latter examples, a modulating effect of the arterial baroreflex was still noticable, influence from other regulatory mechanisms must have been superimposed to produce parallel effects upon blood pressure and sympathetic activity. Increased MSA induced by reductions of central blood volume is an example of such an influence[35]. Changes in posture from lying to sitting to standing induce progressive increases of MSA which presumably are due to unloading of both arterial and central volume receptors[7]. Another type of influence comes from the respiratory rhythm which may also modulate MSA in the absence of respiratory-induced blood pressure fluctuations (Wallin, unpublished observations).

Clinical suggestions

There are several difficulties when one tries to evaluate sympathetic outflow to muscles from blood flow measurements in man. Apart from specific technical problems, available methods are too slow and/or measurements are taken intermittently. This is a serious drawback when examining arterial baroreflex effects. As discussed above, muscle sympathetic activity operates in a highly dynamic fashion responding to blood pressure variations from one heart beat to the next. Even if corresponding variations of vascular resistance are smoothed out and slowed they will rarely show up in blood flow measurements. More long-lasting and complex baroreceptor stimuli such as those induced by (static) neck suction are not suitable since they cause only minor changes in sympathetic activity and blood flow. Because of these difficulties, it is preferable to use reflexes elicited from 'low pressure receptors', for example by lower body negative pressure, when testing sympathetic control of muscle blood vessels. Such stimuli give rise to more long-lasting changes in sympathetic activity and corresponding changes of vascular resistance are easy to demonstrate. The Valsalva manoeuvre is an example of a simple test causing muscular vasoconstriction (presumably due to combined stimulation of high and low pressure receptors) which can be detected by blood flow measurements.

At present there is no satisfactory method to estimate interindividual differences in the level of muscle sympathetic activity from measurements of effector organ activities. However, at rest in the recumbent position both the level of plasma noradrenaline and the heart rate are related to the level of sympathetic activity and even if scatter is considerable, these parameters will at least give a semiquantitative estimate of neural activity.

Pathophysiological studies

Polyneuropathy

In polyneuropathy some patients have symptoms of autonomic impairment suggesting that sympathetic mechanisms are affected by the disease. Recently sympathetic activity was studied in a group of patients with polyneuropathies of different aetiology[16]. Sympathetic activity could be recorded in most patients and the pattern of activity was normal regardless of whether the patient had 'autonomic symptoms' or not. Furthermore sympathetic conduction velocity, estimated from sympathetic reflex latencies, was normal irrespective of the degree of slowing in motor conduction velocity – minimal MCV was 12 m/s in a patient with Charcot-Marie-Tooth disease. Patients with symptoms of autonomic impairment such as orthostatism, impotence, bladder dysfunction, and dryness of hands and feet, often had impaired cutaneous sympathetic effector organ responses (electrodermal or plethysmographic) to arousal stimuli. In many of these cases, especially those with diabetic polyneuropathy, it was not possile to find any sympathetic activity at all in the microelectrode recordings from the nerve. These findings suggest: (1) in polyneuropathy conduction velocities of postganglionic sympathetic C fibres are normal as long as the fibres conduct. This may indicate that the disease does not change C fibre membrane properties and axon diameters in a major way before conduction block occurs. (2) Degeneration of sympathetic fibres may be especially common with diabetic neuropathy.

Syncope

On two occasions, in conjunction with different manoeuvres, sympathetic activity was recorded by the author during so called 'vasovagal syncope'. In both subjects, sympathetic impulse traffic had been elevated for some time when heart rate began to fall and all sympathetic bursts disappeared. In one case, the syncope, which occurred while standing, terminated the recording[8] but the other subject (unpublished) was recumbent and recovery could be monitored. For approximately 1 min there were only occasional sympatheic bursts and during this period blood pressure was approximately 80/40 mmHg with heart rate around 60 beats/min. During the following 5 min there was a continuous slow rise of blood pressure, heart rate and sympathetic activity towards normal levels. These findings confirm the supposition that vasovagal syncope is associated with peripheral sympathetic silence in the face of an unchanged or increased vagal influence on the heart, but give no clue to the mechanisms triggering the attack.

Essential hypertension

Pathologically high activity in the sympathetic nervous system is often considered an important factor in the pathogenesis of essential hypertension but circulatory studies have failed to produce conclusive evidence supporting this hypothesis. Microelectrode recordings of sympathetic outflows at rest and during various manoeuvres revealed no *qualitative* differences either in MSA or SSA between normotensive and hypertensive subjects[35]. This suggests that the sympathetic activity recorded in hypertensive subjects is made up of impulses from fibre populations similar to those in normotensive subjects and that the outflow of these impulses is controlled by similar mechanisms in the two groups. A *quantitative* comparison of MSA between hypertensive and normotensive subjects[39] also did not provide evidence for an increased level of sympathetic activity in the hypertensive subjects. In the hypertensive subjects higher blood pressures were needed to inhibit the pulse-synchronous sympathetic bursts than in the normotensive controls, indicating an elevated working range of the arterial baroreflex. This was interpreted, however, as a secondary effect of the hypertension caused by the well-known resetting of the arterial baroreceptors[26]. *To summarize* the results from sympathetic recordings in hypertension, sympathetic outflow to the muscles does not appear to be involved in the pathogenetic process. There are no qualitative changes in skin sympathetic activity but a quantitative comparison still remains to be made.

Concluding remarks

Sympathetic nerve recordings in man offer several important advantages. The results give direct information about sympathetic mechanisms which often cannot be obtained from studies of sympathetic effector organ responses. In comparison with nerve recordings in animal studies it is a considerable advantage to be able to record from subjects who are awake, have not undergone anaesthesia and surgery and who can cooperate with the experimenter so that both emotional and mental reactions can be investigated. The method is safe and associated with only minor discomfort. To judge from present experience it will probably not be much used for routine diagnostic purposes but it seems well suited for physiological, pathophysiological and pharmacological studies. Future investigations of this kind will no doubt promote better understanding of autonomic involvement in various disease processes.

Acknowledgements

Supported by the Swedish Medical Research Council Grant No. B 80–14X–03546–09B.

References

1 ANGELL-JAMES, J. E. Characteristics of single aortic and right subclavian baroreceptor fibre activity in rabbits with chronic renal hypertension. *Circulation Research*, **32**, 149–161 (1973)

2 AGUAYO, A. J., BRAY, G. M., TERRY, L. C. and SWEEZEY, E. Three dimensional analysis of unmyelinated fibres in normal and pathologic autonomic nerves. *Journal of Neuropathology and Experimental Neurology*, **35**, 136–151 (1976)

3 BÅTH, E., LINDBLAD, L.-E. and WALLIN, B. G. Effects of dynamic and static neck suction on muscle nerve sympathetic activity, heart rate and blood pressure in man. *Journal of Physiology*, **311**, 551–564 (1981)

4 BINI, G., HAGBARTH, K.-E., HYNNINEN, P. and WALLIN, B. G. Thermoregulatory and rhythm-generating mechanisms governing the sudomotor and vasoconstrictor outflow in human cutaneous nerves. *Journal of Physiology*, **306**, 537–552 (1980)

5 BINI, G., HAGBARTH, K.-E., HYNNINEN, P. and WALLIN, B. G. Regional similarities and differences in thermoregulatory vaso- and sudomotor tone. *Journal of Physiology*, **306**, 553–565 (1980)

6 BLOCH, V. Le controle de l'activité electrodermal. *Journal de Physiologie*, **57**, supplement 13, 1–132 (1965)

7 BRAHAM, J. SADEH, M. and SAROVA-PINHAS, I. Skin wrinkling on immersion of hands. *Archives of Neurology*, **36**, 113–114 (1979)

8 BURKE, D., SUNDLÖF, G. and WALLIN, B. G. Postural effects on muscle nerve sympathetic activity in man. *Journal of Physiology*, **272**, 399–414 (1977)

9 BURTON, A. C. The range and variability of the blood flow in the human fingers and the vasomotor regulation of body temperature. *American Journal of Physiology*, **127**, 437–453 (1939)

10 CANNON, W. B. *Bodily Changes in Pain, Hunger, Fear and Rage*. New York, Appleton (1915)

11 CARMICHAEL, E. A., HONEYMAN, W. M., KOLB, L. C. and STEWART, W. K. Peripheral conduction rate in the sympathetic nervous system of man. *Journal of Physiology*, **99**, 338–343 (1941)

12 DELIUS, W., HAGBARTH, K.-E., HONGELL, A. and WALLIN, B. G. General characteristics of sympathetic activity in human muscle nerves. *Acta Physiologica Scandinavica*, **84**, 65–81 (1972)

13 DELIUS, W., HAGBARTH, K.-E., HONGELL, A. and WALLIN, B. G. Manoeuvres affecting sympathetic outflow in human muscle nerves. *Acta Physiologica Scandinavica*, **84**, 82–94 (1972)

14 DELIUS, W., HAGBARTH, K.-E., HONGELL, A. and WALLIN, B. G. Manoeuvres affecting sympathetic outflow in human skin nerves. *Acta Physiologica Scandinavica*, **84**, 177–186 (1972)

15 FAGIUS, J. and WALLIN, B. G. Sympathetic reflex latencies and conduction velocities in normal man. *Journal of the Neurological Sciences*, **47**, 433–448 (1980)

16 FAGIUS, J. and WALLIN, B. G. Sympathetic reflex latencies and conduction velocities in patients with polyneuropathy. *Journal of the Neurological Sciences*, **47**, 449–461 (1980)

17 GASSER, H. S. Properties of dorsal root unmedullated fibres on the two sides of the ganglion. *Journal of General Physiology*, **38**, 709–728 (1955)

18 HAGBARTH, K.-E., VALLBO, Å. B. Pulse and respiratory grouping of sympathetic impulses in human muscle nerves. *Acta Physiologica Scandinavica*, **74**, 96–108 (1968)

19 HAGBARTH, K.-E., HALLIN, R. G., HONGELL, A., TOREBJÖRK, H. E. and WALLIN, B. G. General characteristics of sympathetic activity in human skin nerves. *Acta Physiologica Scandinavica*, **84**, 164–176 (1972)

20 HALLIN, R. G. and TOREBJÖRK, H. E. Single unit sympathetic activity in human skin nerves during rest and various manoeuvres. *Acta Physiologica Scandinavica*, **92**, 303–317 (1974)

21 JOHNSON, R. H. and SPALDING, J. M. K. *Disorders of the Autonomic Nervous System*. Oxford, Blackwell Scientific Publications (1974)

22 LAKE, C. R., ZIEGLER, M. G. and KOPIN, I. J. Use of plasma norepinephrine for evaluation of sympathetic neuronal function in man. *Life Sciences*, **22**, 1315–1326 (1976).

23 LINDBLAD, L.-E., ATTERHÖG, J. H. and WALLIN, B. G. Sympathetic activity in muscle nerves – a factor influencing the postural heart rate increase? *Acta Physiologica Scandinavica* (in press)

24 NORMELL, L. A. Distribution of impaired cutaneous vasomotor and sudomotor function in paraplegic man. *Scandinavian Journal of Clinical and Laboratory Investigation*, **33**, supplement 138, 25–41 (1974)

25 NORMELL, L. A. and WALLIN, B. G. Sympathetic skin nerve activity and skin temperature changes in man. *Acta Physiologica Scandinavica*, **91**, 417–426 (1974)

26 McCUBBIN, J. W., GREEN, J. H. and PAGE, J. H. Baroreceptor function in chronic renal hypertension. *Circulation Research*, **4**, 205–210 (1956)

27 O'RIAIN, S. New and simple test of nerve function in hand. *British Medical Journal*, **3**, 615–616 (1973)

28 PEDERSEN, E. G. and CHRISTENSEN, N. J. Catecholamines in plasma and urine in patients with essential hypertension determined by double-isotope derivation techniques. *Acta Medica Scandinavica*, **198**, 373–377 (1975)

29 RICHTER, C. P. and WOODRUFF, B. G. Lumbar sympathetic dermatomes in man determined by the electrical skin resistance method. *Journal of Neurophysiology*, **8**, 323–338 (1945)

30 SEVER, P. S., BIRCH, M., OSIKOWSKA, B. and TUNBRIDGE, R. D. G. Plasma noradrenaline in essential hypertension. *Lancet*, **1**, 1078–1081, (1977)

31 SOUREK, K. *The Nervous Control of Skin Potentials in Man.* Prague, Czechoslovak Academy of Science (1965)

32 SUNDERLAND, S. The intraneural topography of the radial, median and ulnar nerves. *Brain*, **68**, 243–299 (1945)

33 SUNDLÖF, G. and WALLIN, B. G. The variability of muscle nerve sympathetic activity in resting recumbent man. *Journal of Physiology*, **272**, 383–397 (1977)

34 SUNDLÖF, G. and WALLIN, B. G. Human muscle nerve sympathetic activity at rest. Relationship to blood pressure and age. *Journal of Physiology*, **274**, 621–637 (1978)

35 SUNDLÖF, G. and WALLIN, B. G. Effect of lower body negative pressure on human muscle nerve sympathetic activity. *Journal of Physiology*, **278**, 525–532 (1978)

36 VALLBO, Å. B., HAGBARTH, K.-E., TOREBJÖRK, H. E. and WALLIN, B. G. Somatosensory, proprioceptive and sympathetic activity in human peripheral nerves. *Physiological Review*, **59**, 919–957 (1979)

37 WALLIN, B. G., DELIUS, W. and HAGBARTH, K.-E. Comparison of sympathetic nerve activity in normotensive and hypertensive subjects. *Circulation Research*, **33**, 9–21 (1973)

8 WALLIN, B. G., DELIUS, W. and HAGBARTH, K.-E. Regional control of sympathetic outflow in human skin and muscle nerves. In *Central Rhythmic and Regulation*, edited by W. Umbach and H. P. Koepchen, 190–195. Stuttgart, Hippokrates Verlag (1974)

9 WALLIN, B. G., DELIUS, W. and SUNDLÖF, G. Human muscle nerve sympthetic activity in cardiac arrhythmias. *Scandinavian Journal of Clinical and Laboratory Investigation*, **34**, 293–300 (1974)

0 WALLIN, B. G. and KÖNIG, U. Changes of skin nerve sympathetic activity during induction of general anaesthesia with thiopentone in man. *Brain Research*, **103**, 157–160 (1976)

1 WALLIN, B. G. and SUNDLÖF, G. A quantitative study of muscle nerve sympathetic activity in resting normotensive and hypertensive subjects. *Hypertension*, **1**, 67–77, (1979)

2 WALLIN, B. G., SUNDLÖF, G. and DELIUS, W. The effect of carotid sinus nerve stimulation on muscle and skin nerve sympathetic activity in man. *Pflügers Archiv*, **358**, 101–110 (1975)

3 WALLIN, B. G., SUNDLÖF, G., ERIKSSON, B.-M., DOMINIAK, P., GROBECKER, H. and LINDBLAD, L.-E. Plasma noradrenaline correlates to sympathetic muscle nerve activity in normotensive man. *Acta Physiologica Scandinavica*, **111**, 69–73 (1981)

4 WALLIN, B. G., SUNDLÖF, G. and LINDBLAD, L.-E. Baroreflex mechanisms controlling sympathetic outflow to the muscles in man. In *Baroreceptors and Hypertension*, edited by P. Sleight, 101–107. Oxford, University Press (1980)

5 YOUNG, R. R., ASBURY, A. L., CORBETT, J. L. and ADAMS, R. D. Pure pandysautonomia with recovery-description and discussion of diagnostic criteria. *Brain*, **98**, 613–636 (1975)

8
Quantitative testing of sensibility including pain
Ulf Lindblom

Introduction

Somatosensory dysfunction, due to a lesion of a sensory nerve or tract, is at least as common as motor disturbances in clinical neurology, but has not attracted the same interest for exact diagnosis. Conventional sensibility tests, although useful for screening examinations, are neither quantitative nor selective with regard to different modalities of sensation. Thus, testing with tubes of hot and cold water, or thermal disks, only reveals the presence or absence of warm and cold sensation and discrimination at the particular temperatures used, and co-activation of mechanoreceptors always occurs when the test probes are applied on the skin. Von Frey hairs are a semi-quantitative way of testing tactile sensibility, but the rate of application, which is the most important stimulus parameter for activation of the receptors, is not controlled. Furthermore, hairs of a few grams or more will produce noxious stimulation by exciting nociceptive endings in addition to touch and pressure receptors[22, 36, 73].

There were two developments during the last decade which enabled quantitative assessment of sensibility disturbances. The first development was the appearance of graded and modality-specific stimulation techniques. The second development was the elaboration of some psychophysical methods which were simpler than the old ones and more easily applicable in the clinic. It has thus become possible to define sensory disturbances in terms of changes of perception threshold, or of psychophysical magnitude functions, for different modes of stimulation. The most common sensory disturbance is hypoesthesia with augmented thresholds and reduced suprathreshold responses, but there may also be hyperphenomena which can be demonstrated as subnormal thresholds or exaggerated magnitude functions. It is also possible to quantify abnormalities of temporal and spatial summation, and of adaptation. Furthermore, there are special types of sensory disturbances, which are common in neuralgia when, for example, a cold stimulus feels warm and a tactile stimulus produces pain (allodynia[59]). At present, such qualitative abnormalities can only be partially quantified.

There was a third development which makes sensibility measurements especially meaningful today. This is the consolidation of knowledge of sensory nerve physiology, based on experiments in animals, especially subhuman primates, and largely confirmed in conscious man by means of percutaneous microneurography[75]. There is now general agreement that the largest afferent fibres from the skin mediate touch and vibration, small myelinated fibres mediate pricking pain and cold sensation, and unmyelinated fibres, warmth and aching pain. It is therefore possible to deduce, from the profile of the sensory impairment, information about the underlying nerve lesion with regard to the type and extent of injury or dysfunction of various fibre groups. Furthermore, since different disease agents may affect the fibre spectrum differentially, knowledge of the lesion pattern may give hints as to the etiology.

Modality-specific sensibility tests may thus provide information from all types of afferent fibres, not only the largest ones, and are more physiological than conduction velocity and action potential height in the sense that they are aimed directly at the sensory function of the system. The main drawback with sensibility tests is that they measure subjective responses and are therefore less objective. Furthermore, they do not show whether the lesion is peripheral or central, which has to be evaluated on the basis of the clinical syndrome and other tests. Nevertheless it is reasonable to assume that sensibility measurements will become an important complement to conventional clinical and electrophysiological examinations. Compared with conventional clinical evaluation, precise sensory tests are generally superior, as can be expected, quantitatively and qualitatively[10]. Furthermore, it is conceivable that sensibility measurements may become helpful in the differential diagnosis between peripheral and central disturbances, and between central dysfunctions of various kinds. This might be an especially valuable application in patients with chronic pain, where today there is considerable uncertainty regarding the role of peripheral and central pathogenetic mechanisms.

The most common cause of somatosensory dysfunction is probably a lesion of a peripheral nerve or sensory root in association with of some kind of mechanical injury, such as entrapment. Irritative phenomena, pain and paresthesiae, are usually early clinical manifestations in these cases. In toxic and metabolic neuropathies, subclinical sensory deficits are often the first sign of injury, while the symptoms come later. In the central nervous system, common causes of sensory disturbances are cerebrovascular lesions and focal demyelination in the spinal cord due to multiple sclerosis.

Mechanosensation

General

Touch, pressure and vibration are three dimensions of mechanosensation which are usually not well differentiated. Transient deformation of the skin is the adequate stimulus for the dynamically sensitive, rapidly adapting receptors which, on good grounds, are believed to mediate touch. Constant pressure can only be signalled by slowly adapting receptors situated in or beneath the skin. Pacinian corpuscles are very sensitive mechanoreceptors and are capable of transmitting high frequency sustained vibration, but they do not respond to constant pressure or slow deformation, as was thought when they were first discovered. There is no recognized clinical counterpart to this physiological differentiation of three types of mechanoceptive apparatus and sensation. All three receptor types are innervated by large myelinated fibres. Agents which affect the nerves rather than receptor structures cannot be expected to produce a differential disturbance within these mechanosenses. The observation that Pacinian endings are affected early in acrylamide poisoning[70] forecasts, however, the possibility of such a differentiation. It has also been found that an externally applied local anesthetic may produce hypoesthesia for one type of touch (von Frey hairs) but not another (mechanical pulses), which suggests that superficial touch may be mediated by different receptor populations[30].

Touch

There are several exact methods for determination of tactile thresholds[8, 11, 49, 50, 78] which are excellent for research purposes, and which have been used to establish specific and important physiological pathophysiological correlations. It has thus been confirmed that loss of tactile or vibratory sensation correlates with damage of the largest sensory fibres from the skin[9]. It has been demonstrated that the perceptual threshold approaches the physiological threshold of the rapidly adapting intracutaneous mechanoreceptors in the finger pads[39]. In other areas the psychophysical threshold is higher indicating that more spatial summation is required to produce a sensation. The exactness of mechanical pulse stimulation has also been utilized to re-examine the tactile sensitivity of different sexes, sides and sites and on different occasions in normal and blind subjects[53].

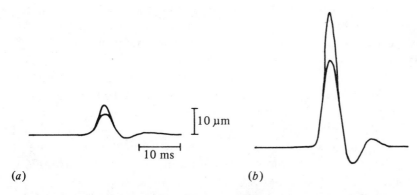

(*a*)   (*b*)

Figure 8.1 Tactile thresholds, determined with short mechanical pulses according to the method of limits, on the index fingers of a patient with sutured median nerve. Oscillographic records of threshold pulses from normal side, (*a*) and injured side, (*b*). Upper pulse contour indicates the lowest amplitude of the ascending stimulus series which was felt, and lower contour the highest pulse of the descending series which was not felt. (From Lindblom[50], courtesy of the publishers, *Progress in Brain Research*)

Figure 8.1 illustrates threshold determination with a short mechanical pulse in a patient with a median nerve lesion, several years after suture. Subjectively, the pulses are felt as taps on the skin. The double contours of the pulses in *Figure 8.1* which were recorded on an oscilloscope, represent the essence of threshold determination according to the methods of limits[23]. The upper pulse contour indicates the amplitude at which the pulse was first perceived when the stimulus was increased stepwise from zero (ascending series, 'yes' response). The lower contour indicates the highest amplitude which was not felt when the stimulus was decreased from a slightly supra-threshold value (descending series, 'no' response). The threshold, which is the mean of the 'yes' and 'no' responses, was 9 µm on the normal side (*Figure 8.1a*) and 42 µm on the injured side (*Figure 8.16*).

The method of limits is convenient and easy to use in patients who are, as a rule, inexperienced in sensory testing. From a scientific point of view, signal detection methods[23], which include null stimuli, are desirable and, for example, the forced choice procedure may be adapted to clinical use. The method of limits includes elements of signal detection testing, as clearly, subthreshold stimuli will alternate with near-threshold and suprathreshold stimuli during the ascending and descending series. It is not thought that there would be major differences in the results of various methods due to criterion or motivational factors if the subjects are properly prepared and instructed.

With pulses of various suprathreshold amplitudes, stimulus-response functions for touch can be determined by direct magnitude estimation[15, 29, 35, 41, 46]. Alterations of these functions have been described in patients with sutured median nerves[15] and peripheral neuralgia[57]. The form of the mechanical pulse, for instance, the rate of rise, is also relevant for the touch sensation, but this has so far not found any clinical application.

With single mechanical pulses it is easy to measure the latency of the sensation which may give valuable information. Although the reaction time includes the delay of the subject's response to the sensory event, it is as short as 0.2–0.3 s on stimulation with suprathreshold pulses. This is because the tactile impulses are conducted in the fastest afferent fibres from the skin, and because virtually no temporal summation is needed. Reaction time measurements may be used to analyze the afferent pathways[16, 18, 57, 79], and have the advantage of being a functional index that refers to the actual sensation. Exact conduction times can, of course, only be obtained by means of evoked potential techniques.

With these methods, normal and abnormal functions of passive touch can be studied in great detail, but the procedures may be too time-consuming for more or less routine clinical investigations. The stimulators are costly and may be difficult to adapt to various skin regions. Therefore, the classical von Frey hairs still hold their place in the quantitation of tactile sensibility, in spite of their many limitations, some of which were mentioned in the introduction. When the threshold for touch is normal or close to normal, the hairs primarily stimulate the rapidly adapting cutaneous receptors and there is a gross correlation between bending force and indentation depth relative to the sensation magnitude[40]. The use of a set of hairs or nylon threads with logarithmically-spaced bending pressures, e.g. 0.1–100 mN, is recommended. Sets can be made from nylon threads of different diameters and lengths, and are also commercially available. The perception threshold is titrated by finding the hair that is felt in about half of the applications, 5 times out of 10 for instance. A more precise assessment of the sensitivity can be obtained by means of a two-alternative, forced-choice paradigm[71].

For screening of tactile discrimination, figure writing is suitable and may be quantified as the minimum height of a correctly interpreted figure written on the skin with a blunt pencil. This height is normally 0.5 cm on the finger pads, and 4 cm on the dorsal surface of the foot. Figure writing is a combined test for spatial and temporal discrimination, while the two-point limen and localization tests measure the capacity of spatial resolution, unless they are modified to include movement on the skin[6].

The conventional test for stereognosis, when patients are asked to identify objects with their hands, is a test of active touch, in contrast to all the above-mentioned tests that pertain to passive touch. A simple test of active touch, which may give a numerical value, is Moberg's picking-up test[63]. There are also other methods for more precise analysis[44]. It is not possible to compare any measures of active touch with those of passive touch; there is a profound difference in the bias of the central nervous system. Not only will the volitional command signals condition the parietal lobe in active touch, but the movement *per se* will activate and produce a considerable background activity in the primary afferents[37].

Pressure

Sustained pressure is easier to measure than rate and depth of skin indentation, but the sensation of pressure is subject to pronounced adaptation and other influences, for instance thermal interference, which makes it difficult and impractical to work with. Pressure is primarily used as a noxious stimulus to study pain sensitivity (*see below*).

Vibration

Vibration is the type of mechanical stimulus which can be produced most easily in a uniform, measurable fashion. It has been used extensively by psychologists and also in clinical neurology ever since it was recognized, at around the turn of the century, that loss of vibratory sensation was common in patients with spinal cord lesions. To quantify the impairment, the perception threshold is nowadays measured by means of electromagnetic devices, a process known as vibrametry. Systemic lesions like polyneuropathy and myelopathy are the commonest indications for vibrametry. It is used to exclude or confirm an impairment which has been suspected on screening with the tuning fork, or to follow the course of a disease and evaluate therapeutic effects by repeated measurements. When the lesion is confined to a single nerve, vibrametry is less reliable because of stimulus spread to areas innervated by neighbouring intact nerves. Vibrametry may tentatively be used in cerebral lesions, but the exact relation between impaired vibration sense and the type of cerebral lesion has not yet been established. The old notion that subcortical lesions are more apt to affect the vibration sense[14] should be re-examined with modern methods of localizing cerebral lesions, such as computerized tomography. Vibrametry may also be used to map tissue viability and the extent of burns or traumatic lesions.

Most vibrators produce a continuous sinusoidal vibration of a standard frequency, for example, 100 or 120 Hz. Studies with different frequencies have not revealed any clinically relevant profiles[25], but it is conceivable that they may exist. The perception of low frequency vibration and 'flutter' is mediated by intracutaneous receptors rather than Pacinian corpuscles[47, 54, 61, 72]. The high frequency thresholds increase with age which can be explained by structural changes of the Pacinian corpuscles[76]. A similar impairment might be expected in the early stages of acrylamide intoxication which, as has already been mentioned, primarily affects these endings[70].

Clinical vibrametry is usually performed with a hand-held vibrator and a rather large probe, which is applied on the skin at a certain, undefined, pressure. To reduce the variability and enable comparison between different investigators and occasions, it is necessary to use a standardized technique. Due to differences in tissue damping, which are illustrated in *Figure 8.2*, and other technical variables, the actual vibrator movement is a better measure than the applied voltage[26]. It is also possible to use a pressure indicator to standardize the application

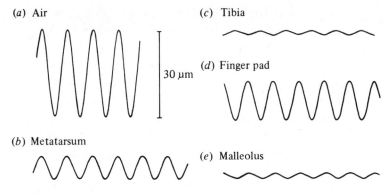

(a) Air

(c) Tibia

30 µm

(d) Finger pad

(b) Metatarsum

(e) Malleolus

Figure 8.2 The vibration amplitude of a 100 Hz sine wave, recorded by means of an accelerometer, when the applied voltage
was held constant and the vibrator was moving freely (a), or
applied at various body sites (b–e). (From Goldberg and
Lindblom[26], courtesy of the Editor and publisher, *Journal of
Neurology, Neurosurgery and Psychiatry*)

pressure, and to select certain stimulus points for which reference
values are available[26].

Clinical vibrametry has been limited to threshold determinations.
Magnitude functions, temporo-spatial integration and other aspects of
vibratory sensation do not seem to have been explored in patients. The
vibration threshold may be recorded as the perception threshold
(VPT), which is the amplitude at which vibration is first felt when the
stimulus is increased from zero. The disappearance threshold (VDT) is
the somewhat lower amplitude at which the vibration disappears on
subsequently decreasing the stimulus strength. VDT is less distinct
than VPT, especially in some patients with neuropathy. As with single
mechanical pulses, and according to the method of limits, the
threshold (VT) is preferably given as the average of VPT and VDT. In
certain situations it may be sufficient to record VPT, the variance of
which is not greater than that of VT[26].

The sensitivity of vibrametry as an index of neuropathy is rather
high. In a retrospective analysis of workers exposed to jet fuel, the
vibration threshold was the only sign of peripheral nerve lesion which
was significantly abnormal[52]. It is well known that the vibration
thresholds are increased early in diabetes and various metabolic and
toxic conditions associated with neuropathy. As well as its diagnostic
value, vibrametry may be used as an index of therapeutic effects, e.g.

in uremia[2, 4, 12, 67]. The sensitivity can be compared with that of conduction velocity (CV) determinations[28, 31, 68] (*see also* Chapter 6). In the author's experience, reduced sensory conduction velocity is frequently, but not always, encountered earlier than increased VT as a sign of subclinical neuropathy. The exact relationship between the two methods, and their relevance as disease indicators, has not yet been established. Apparently, they complement each other. For neuropathies of a very slow time course, CV studies are probably superior, while vibrametry appears as a more dynamic index of peripheral nerve

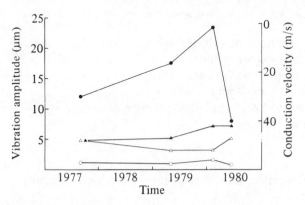

Figure 8.3 Vibrametry in patient with uremia and slight polyneuropathy. Thresholds in μm at second metacarpal bone (○), and first metatarsal bone (●). The thresholds increased to definitely abnormal levels in January 1980, and were normalized 4 months later. Conduction velocities (△, distal SCV of median nerve; ▲, MCV of peroneal nerve) varied insignificantly within normal limits. No action potentials were obtained from the sural nerve on any occasion

dysfunction. This is illustrated in *Figure 8.3* which shows vibration thresholds and conduction velocities in a female patient, born 1911, with uremia due to polycystic kidneys. On admission in 1977, and at the second neurological examination in 1979, there were no unequivocal signs of neuropathy. Hemodialysis was started in 1979. At the third neurological examination, in January 1980, there was a paresis of the dorsiflexors of the great toes and the vibration thresholds were definitely abnormal, both in the hands and feet. Four months later, the vibration thresholds were normalized without significant changes of other neurological parameters. The distal sensory conduction velocity of the median nerve, and the peroneal motor conduction velocity were within normal limits throughout the observation period. No action potentials could be recorded from the sural nerve on any occasion. Vibrametry may thus reflect deteriorations and improvements in the disease more closely than the conduction velocity (but *see* pp. 131–133). The vibration threshold may display a transient improvement on the day after dialysis[12], and during short-term treatment of diabetic neuropathy[13]. Vibrametry may also be used to study the effects of dorsal column stimulation[55] or neurolysis[77].

In normal subjects, the variance of closely repeated threshold determinations is small[26], but in patients with increased vibration thresholds, repeated successive measurements, or measurement at nearby sites, sometimes yield unexpected differences. This is probably an expression of the nerve fibre dysfunction and critical shifts in the number of excited afferents at the particular stimulus site. Non-sensory events, such as criterion shifts, do not appear to be important for the observed variations in mechanoceptive thresholds.

The results of vibrametry should always be evaluated together with the clinical picture. An isolated augmented vibration threshold may not have any actual clinical relevance, and has to be judged with the same caution as the finding of reduced conduction velocity[24]. As with exact tactile stimulation, a standardized vibrametry technique of the type described requires specialized, although less costly, equipment. In certain cases, even the inexpensive tuning fork may provide clinically useful qualitative data[7].

Temperature sensation

The sense of cold or warmth is physiologically distinct from the mechanosenses[44, 48, 65]. The initiation time in the receptors and the afferent conduction time are much longer. The delay of perception is also longer because of the dependency on temporal and spatial summation. There is a neutral zone at about 30–36°C where no sensation occurs at constant temperatures, due to complete adaptation. The threshold sensation of both warm and cool are dependent on the baseline temperature and the rate of change. All these characteristics have to be taken into account when stimulation procedures are designed. The lack of a suitable apparatus for specific measurement of temperature sensitivity in patients instigated the development of the Marstock method[21], which is based on the Peltier principle[43], previously used for adaptation and threshold studies[45]. The stimulator,

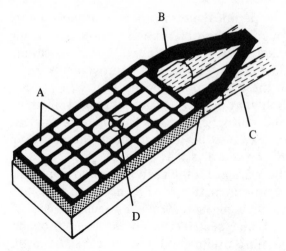

Figure 8.4 The Marstock stimulator for temperature stimulation. A, Peltier elements; B, current cable; C, water tube; D, thermocouple. (From Fruhstorfer *et al.*[21] courtesy of the Editor and publisher, *Journal of Neurology, Neurosurgery and Psychiatry*)

which is shown in *Figure 8.4* consists of series-coupled Peltier elements which will warm or cool the skin depending upon the direction of the applied current. The stimulator has to be in good contact with the skin surface and attached with surgical tape without pressure or strain to avoid interference with the circulation of the skin and co-activation of mechanoreceptors. The size of the stimulator, 25×50 mm (1250 mm^2) makes is applicable in most regions, but in sensitive or curved skin areas, such as face and the fingers, a smaller probe is preferred. In the thermode, water of 30°C is circulated to produce a constant baseline temperature in the neutral range, and to eliminate heat. A thermocouple is fixed to the center of the thermode, the signal of which is amplified and after calibration, potentiometrically recorded to display the interface temperature between the probe and skin surfaces in the centre of the stimulated area. The subject is instructed to press a switch as soon as clear cool or warmth is perceived. This will reverse the current to the stimulator, and thus the temperature change. The resulting zig-zag curve is illustrated in *Figure 8.5* (*left*). The interrupted line through the upward peaks represents the warm threshold, and the downward peaks the cold threshold. Since the corresponding values

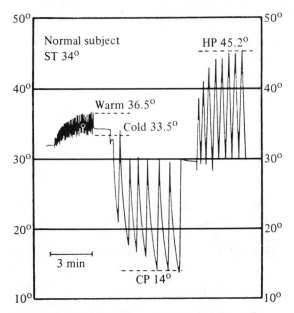

Figure 8.5 Typical Marstock record from the right thenar region of a normal subject. When determining thermal pain thresholds the current was reversed at indifferent temperatures by the operator. ST, skin temperature; CP, cold pain threshold; HP, heat pain threshold. (From Fruhstorfer *et al.*[21], courtesy of the Editor and publisher, *Journal of Neurology, Neurosurgery and Psychiatry*)

include delay of perception and the reaction time of the subject to pressing the button, they do not represent the absolute thresholds. This is especially important when patients with nerve lesions are tested. The sensation delay may then be prolonged by as much as three times[33].

Defective warm or cold sensation will appear as a broadening of the curve as is illustrated in *Figure 8.6* in record (*c*) from the right foot. The abnormal difference limen of warm and cold indicates dysfunction or loss of unmyelinated, or small myelinated fibres, or both, and can be taken as a measure of thermal hypoesthesia, which is the commonest finding in patients with peripheral nerve lesions or polyneuropathies[19,21]. It is not uncommon, however, to find lowered thresholds indicating thermal hyperesthesia[51], which may be of either peripheral or central origin.

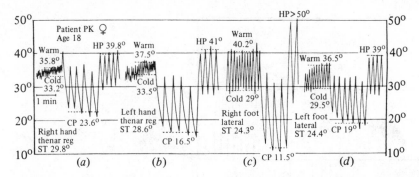

Figure 8.6 Marstock records from both hands (*a*, *b*) and feet (*c*, *d*) of a patient with peripheral neuropathy. On the right foot (record *c*) the warm–cold difference limen was abnormally wide and the heat pain threshold was not reached (HP > 50°C; the current was reversed at 50°C by the operator to avoid burning). Hyperalgesia is indicated by low heat pain thresholds on both hands and left foot (HP normally about 45°C, cf. *Figure 8.5*)

Warm and cold perception thresholds display considerable intra-individual fluctuations depending upon the state of adaptation at the time of the examination, and on shifts in the subject's criterion. It is evident that such shifts will occur more often with thermal sensations than with the more distinct mechanoceptive perceptions. Threshold changes from time to time should therefore be carefully evaluated and reference measurements made in an unaffected skin region which would reveal alterations of the subject's internal standard. With these reservations, the Marstock method seems to meet a need for quantitation of thermal sensitivity in the clinic. Besides the stimulator, the equipment consists of commercially available components.

A Peltier device may also be used for thermal pulse stimulation[33], but the maximum rate of rise is limited. There are other methods which are more suitable for this type of stimulation in reaction time and evoked potential studies [1, 5, 16, 17, 20]. The more sophisticated laser and focused ultrasound techniques have the most exact temporal and spatial characteristics[48, 62, 64, 74].

Pain

Measurement of spontaneous pain is usually made with verbal rating scales which vary from the simplest four step scale, i.e. none/slight/

moderate/severe, to elaborate questionnaires. Both verbal rating scales and analogue scales have their definite limitations but can be fitted to scientific as well as clinical needs. In the clinic, a combination of visual analogue scaling and pain drawing is becoming increasingly popular. Pain drawing can be used to obtain information about qualitative and affective aspects of the pain in addition to its spatial distribution. It is not within the scope of this presentation to describe these methods in detail and the reader is referred to a recent review[27].

Some methods of induced pain are discussed here which are suitable for measuring altered pain sensitivity in patients (hypo- or hyperalgesia). Usually, only stimuli which are potentially noxious, i.e. produce pain before tissue damage, should be used in the clinic, both for methodological and for obvious ethical reasons. A stimulus which causes tissue damage or alters the excitability cannot be repeated and is therefore unsuitable.

Pain sensitivity of the skin can be tested by a variety of noxious stimuli but only mechanical or thermal stimuli are practical. The old qualitative pin-prick test for pain of the A-δ type ('first pain') may be applied with a graded pressure and thus quantified, but the method gives very variable results and is therefore not much used. Stimuli with some areal distribution yield better uniformity and reproducibility. The author uses forceps with a flat surface of 20 mm² which can be applied in all regions where a fold of skin can be gripped (*Figure 8.7*).

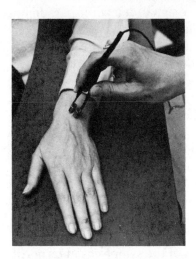
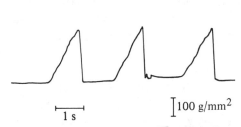

Figure 8.7 Forceps algometer and oscilloscopic recordings of strain gauge signal indicating pinch pressure at pain threshold in carpal hairy skin of normal subject. Three successive stimulations

The signal from a strain gauge in the shaft of the forceps is amplified and displayed on an oscilloscope to guide the examiner to apply the pressure at a certain constant speed. The subject is asked to report the appearance of pain and the pressure is immediately released. The corresponding amplitude, which is calibrated in g/mm^2, is taken as an estimate of the mechanical pain threshold. The average of at least three measurements from different adjacent skin folds is recorded for each site and occasion. Reference values are always collected from homologous skin outside the pain area, if possible contralaterally. There are several sources of variation with this technique. The innervation density may be different in adjacent skin folds, the subject may change the criterion for pain report and both the subject's and the examiner's reaction times are included. The method is, however, very easy and quick and with proper controls it is surprisingly reproducible and may be used to study therapeutic effects and pain mechanisms[3, 55, 58]. Perpendicularly-applied pressure algometers have been used in several studies and designs through the years[34, 38, 42, 60]. These instruments primarily measure the pain sensitivity of subcutaneous tissues. They are suitable for monitoring pressure hyperalgesia of musculoskeletal disorders and probably deserve a wider clinical use.

The most well-known technique for thermal pain stimulation, the radiant heat method of Hardy, Wolff and Goodell[34], has recently been further improved[66]. This, and similar methods, are useful experimentally and have been applied in a signal detection paradigm, which is necessary in studies on the pain sensitivity of different ages and populations where criterion differences should be avoided. The cold pressure test is less exact and limited to hands and feet but can be used up to the tolerance level without causing damage. For clinical routine or experimental investigations, the Marstock is suitable since it is quick and repeatable, and can be applied in almost any desired skin area. *Figure 8.5* illustrates cold and heat pain threshold determination with this method. The heat pain threshold (HP) is normally about 45°C, somewhat less in the face, and somewhat higher on part of the trunk and legs. In the patient with polyneuropathy in *Figure 8.6*, HP was increased in the right foot (>50°C, hypoalgesia) and decreased in the left foot (39°C, hyperalgesia). In patients with neuralgia, who complain of abnormal temperature sensitivity, the Marstock method enables documentation and quantification of the symptoms in terms of altered thermal and thermal pain thresholds[57]. Comparison with controls from records of homologous normal skin ensures that the patient is not generally hypo- or hypersensitive.

There are several other methods of measuring pain sensitivity and producing experimental pain[69], such as electrical stimulation, the tourniquet test, or injection of chemicals or hypertonic solutions, each of which may be the method of choice in a particular investigation. The greatest variable by far in the assessment of pain thresholds and tolerance levels is the subjects' response bias which varies between stoic and sensitive individuals who report at high or low stimulus intensities, respectively. There are also intra-individual variations depending upon expectation, anxiety, and reassurance. The best possible control of these factors will reduce the variability and strengthen the results.

The value of sensibility measurements may be summarized.

(1) Quantitative sensory tests are a useful complement to conventional clinical evaluation of sensory disturbances. They may also be complementary to electrodiagnostic procedures in the diagnosis of peripheral nerve disorders.

(2) A precise description of a lesion or dysfunction of a sensory nerve or tract can be achieved by combining the various tests for touch, vibration, temperature and pain. It is often possible to outline a characteristic sensibility profile.

(3) The course of a particular disease, and therapeutic effects, may be assessed by repeated measurements in the same patient.

(4) Some sensory tests are suitable for screening of neurotoxic effects on peripheral nerves.

(5) In neuralgia and other types of neurological pain conditions, sensibility measurements with analysis of the accompanying hyperalgesia may elucidate the pain mechanisms[51].

(6) The interference with the somatosensory functions produced by electrical stimulation of the CNS can be studied qualitatively and quantitatively[3, 55, 56].

(7) Some of the stimulation techniques may be used in evoked potential and reaction time studies, or combined with microneurography[32, 41], to analyze peripheral or central mechanisms of sensory disturbances including pain.

Acknowledgements

This work was supported by the Swedish Medical Research Council (Project number B80–14X–04256–06). Berit Lindblom, Gillis Agneflo, Bo Johansson and the late Sigge Ottosson are gratefully acknowledged for their skilful and dedicated technical assistance.

References

1 BECK, P. W., HANDWERKER, H. O. and ZIMMERMANN, M. Nervous outflow from the cat's foot during noxious radiant heat stimulation. *Brain Research*, **67**, 373–386 (1974)

2 BERGSTRÖM, J., LINDBLOM, U. and NOREE, L. O. Preservation of peripheral nerve function in severe uremia during treatment with low protein, high calorie diet and surplus of essential amino acids. *Acta Neurologica Scandinavica*, **51**, 99–109 (1975)

3 BOETHIUS, J., LINDBLOM, U., MEYERSON, B. A. and WIDÉN, L. Effects of multifocal brain stimulation on pain and somatosensory functions. In *Sensory Functions of the Skin in Primates*, **27**, edited by Y. Zotterman, 531–548. Oxford, Pergamon Press (1976)

4 DANIEL, C. R. III, BOWER, J. D., PEARSON, J. E. and HOLBERT, R. D. Vibrometry and uremic peripheral neuropathy. *Southern Medical Journal*, **70**, 1311–1316 (1977)

5 DARIAN-SMITH, I., JOHNSON, K. O. and DYKES, R. 'Cold' fiber population innervating palmar and digital skin of the monkey: responses to cooling pulses. *Journal of Neurophysiology*, **26**, 325–346 (1973)

6 DELLON, A. L. The moving two-point discrimination test: clinical evaluation of the quickly adapting fiber/receptor system. *Journal of Hand Surgery*, **3**, 474–481 (1978)

7 DELLON, A. L. Clinical use of vibratory stimuli to evaluate peripheral nerve injury and compression neuropathy. *Plastic and Reconstructive Surgery*, **65**, 466–476 (1980)

8 DYCK, P. J. Quantitation of cutaneous sensation in man. In *Peripheral Neuropathy*, edited by P. J. Dyck, P. K. Thomas and E. H. Lambert, 465–479. Philadelphia, W. B. Saunders (1975)

9 DYCK, P. J., LAMBERT, E. H. and NICHOLS, P. C. Quantitative measurement of sensation related to compound action potential and number and sizes of myelinated and unmyelinated fibers of sural nerve in health, Friedreich's ataxia, hereditary sensory neuropathy, and tabes dorsalis. In *Handbook of Electroencephalography and Clinical Neurophysiology*, **9**, edited by A. Rémond, 83. Amsterdam, Elsevier (1971)

10 DYCK, P. J., O'BRIEN, P. C., BUSHEK, W., OVIATT, K. F., SCHILLING, K. and STEVENS, J. C. Clinical vs quantitative evaluation of cutaneous sensation. *Archives of Neurology*, **33**, 651–655 (1976)

11 DYCK, P. J., ZIMMERMAN, I. R., O'BRIEN, P. C., NESS, A., CASKEY, P. E., KARNES, J. and BUSHEK, W. Introduction of automated systems to evaluate touch-pressure, vibration, and thermal cutaneous sensation in man. *Annals of Neurology*, **4**, 502–510 (1978)

12 EDWARDS, A. E., KOPPLE, J. D. and KORNFELD, C. M. Vibrotactile threshold in patients undergoing maintenance hemodialysis. *Archives of Internal Medicine*, **132**, 706–708 (1973)

13 FAGIUS, J. and JAMESON, S. Treatment of diabetic polyneuropathy with an aldose reductase inhibitor – a clinical and neurophysiological study. *Acta Neurologica Scandinavica,* **62**, Supplementum 78, 125 (1980)

14 FOX, J. C. and KLEMPERER, W. W. Vibratory sensibility. A quantitative study of its thresholds in nervous disorders. *Archives of Neurology and Psychiatry*, **48**, 622–645 (1942)

15 FRANZÉN, O. and LINDBLOM, U. Tactile intensity functions in patients with sutured peripheral nerve. In *Sensory Functions of the Skin in Primates*, **27**, edited by Y. Zotterman, 113–118. Oxford, Pergamon Press (1976)

16 FRUHSTORFER, H. Conduction in the afferent thermal pathways of man. In *Sensory Functions of the Skin in Primates*, **27**, edited by Y. Zotterman 355–366. Oxford, Pergamon Press (1976)

17 FRUHSTORFER, H. and DETERING, I. A simple thermode for rapid temperature changes. *Pflügers Archiv*, **349**, 83–85 (1974)

18 FRUHSTORFER, H. and LINDBLOM, U. (Unpublished observations)

19 FRUHSTORFER, H., GOLDBERG, J. M., LINDBLOM, U. and SCHMIDT, W. G. Temperature sensitivity and pain threshold in patients with peripheral neuropathy. In *Sensory Functions of the Skin in Primates*, **27**, edited by Y. Zotterman, 507–517. Oxford, Pergamon Press (1976)

20 FRUHSTORFER, H., GUTH, H. and PFAFF, U. Cortical responses evoked by thermal stimuli in man. In *Proceedings of the Third International Congress on Event-Related Slow Potentials of the Brain*, edited by W. C. McCallum and J. R. Knott, 30–33. Bristol, Wright and Sons (1976)

21 FRUHSTORFER, H., LINDBLOM, U. and SCHMIDT, W. G. Method for quantitative estimation of thermal thresholds in patients. *Journal of Neurology, Neurosurgery and Psychiatry*, **39**, 1071–1075 (1976)

22 GEORGOPOULOS, A. P. Functional properties of primary afferent units probably related to pain mechanisms in primate glabrous skin. *Journal of Neurophysiology*, **39**, 71–83 (1976)

23 GESCHEIDER, G. A. *Psychophysics. Method and Theory*, Chichester, John Wiley and Sons (1976)

24 GILLIATT, R. W. Sensory conduction studies in the early recognition of nerve disorders. *Muscle and Nerve*, Sept./Oct., 352–359 (1978)

25 GOFF, G. D., ROSNER, B. S., DETRE, T. and KENNARD, D. Vibration perception in normal man and medical patients. *Journal of Neurology, Neurosurgery and Psychiatry*, **28,** 503–509 (1965)

26 GOLDBERG, J. M. and LINDBLOM, U. Standardized method of determining vibratory perception thresholds for diagnosis and screening in neurological investigation. *Journal of Neurology, Neurosurgery and Psychiatry*, **42,** 793–803 (1979)

27 GRACELY, R. H. Psychophysical assessment of human pain. *Advances in Pain Research and Therapy*, **3,** 805–823 (1979)

28 GREGERSEN, G. Vibratory perception threshold and motor conduction velocity in diabetics and non-diabetics. *Acta Medica Scandinavica*, **183,** 61–65 (1968)

29 GYBELS, J. and VAN HEES, J. Unit activity from mechanoreceptors in human peripheral nerve during intensity discrimination of touch. In *Neurophysiology Studied in Man*, edited by G. G. Somjen, International Congress Series Number **253,** 198–206. Amsterdam, Excerpta Medica (1972)

30 HAEGERSTAM, G. and LINDBLOM, U. (Unpublished observations)

31 HALAR, E. M., MILUTINOVIV, J., BROZOVICH, F. V., DeLISA, J. A., INOUYE, V. L. and FOLLETTE, W. Uremic neuropathy: correlation of nerve conduction velocity and clinical findings. *Archives of Physical Medicine and Rehabilitation*, **59,** 564 (1978)

32 HALLIN, R. G., LINDBLOM, U. and WIESENFELD, Z. Psychophysical and neurophysiological methods to study patients with sensory disturbances. In *Sensory Functions of the Skin of Humans*, edited by D. R. Kenshalo, 23–37. New York, Plenum (1980)

33 HAMANN, H. D., HANDWERKER, H. O. and ASSMUS, H. Quantitative assessment of altered thermal sensation in patients suffering from cutaneous nerve disorders. *Neuroscience Letters*, **9,** 273–277 (1978)

34 HARDY, D. J., WOLFF, H. G. and GODELL, H. *Pain Sensations and Reactions*, Baltimore, Williams and Wilkins (1952)

35 HARRINGTON, T. and MERZENICH, M. M. Neural coding in the sense of pressure: human sensations of skin indentation compared with the responses of slowly adapting mechanoreceptive afferents innervating the hairy skin of monkeys. *Experimental Brain Research*, **10,** 251–264 (1970)

36 HEES, J. VAN and GYBELS, J. M. Pain related to single afferent C fibers from human skin. *Brain Research*, **48,** 397–400 (1972)

37 HULLIGER, M., NORDH, E., THELIN, A.-E. and VALLBO, Å. B. The responses of afferent fibres from the glabrous skin of the hand during

voluntary finger movements in man. *Journal of Physiology*, **291**, 233–249 (1979)

38 HUSKISSON, E. C. and HART, F. D. Pain threshold and arthritis. *British Medical Journal*, **4**, 193–195 (1972)

39 JOHANSSON, R. S. and VALLBO, Å. B. Detection of tactile stimuli, thresholds of afferent units related to psychophysical thresholds in the human hand. *Journal of Physiology*, **297**, 405–422 (1979)

40 JOHANSSON, R. S., VALLBO, Å. B. and WESTLIND, G. Thresholds of mechanosensitive afferents in the human hand as measured with von Frey hairs. *Brain Research*, **184**, 343–351 (1980)

41 JÄRVILEHTO, T. and HÄMÄLÄINEN, H. Touch and thermal sensations: psychophysical observations and unit activity in human skin nerves. In *Sensory Functions of the Skin of Humans*, edited by D. R. Kenshalo, 279–295. New York, Plenum (1979)

42 KEELE, K. D. Pain sensitivity tests. The pressure algometer. *Lancet*, **1**, 636–639 (1954)

43 KENSHALO, D. R. Improved method for the psychophysical study of the temperature sense. *Review of Scientific Instruments*, **34**, 883–886 (1963)

44 KENSHALO, D. R. Biophysics and psychophysics of feeling. *Handbook of Perception*, **VIB**, 30–74. New York, Academic Press (1978)

45 KENSHALO, D. R. and SCOTT, H. A. Temporal course of thermal adaptation. *Science*, **151**, 1095–1096 (1966)

46 KNIBESTÖL M. and VALLBO, Å. B. Intensity of sensation related to activity of slowly adapting mechanoreceptive units in the human hand. *Journal of Physiology*, **300**, 251–267 (1980)

47 KONIETZNY, F. and HENSEL, H. Response of rapidly and slowly adapting mechanoreceptors and vibratory sensitivity in human hairy skin. *Pflügers Archiv*, **368**, 39–44 (1977)

48 LAMOTTE, R. H. and CAMPBELL, J. N. Comparison of responses of warm and nociceptive C-fiber afferents in monkey with human judgements of thermal pain. *Journal of Neurophysiology*, **41**, 509–528 (1978)

49 LINDBLOM, U. Touch perception threshold in human glabrous skin in terms of displacement amplitude on stimulation with single mechanical pulses. *Brain Research*, **82**, 205–210 (1974)

50 LINDBLOM, U. Touch perception threshold in terms of amplitude and rate of skin deformation. In *Somatosensory and Visceral Receptor Mechanisms*, edited by A. Iggo and O. B. Ilyinski. *Progress in Brain Research*, **43**, 233–236. Amsterdam, Elsevier (1976)

51 LINDBLOM, U. Sensory abnormalities in neuralgia. In *Advances in Pain Research and Therapy*, edited by J. Bonica, J. Liebeskind and D. Albe-Fessard, **3**, 111–120. New York, Raven Press, (1979)

52 LINDBLOM, U. and GOLDBERG, J. M. Screening for neurological symptoms and signs after exposure of jet fuel. In *Symposia – Sixth International Congress of Electromyography* (Stockholm, Sweden, 1979) edited by A. Persson, Department of Clinical Neurophysiology, Huddinge Hospital, Sweden. 227 (1979)

53 LINDBLOM, U. and LINDSTRÖM, B. Tactile thresholds of normal and blind subjects on stimulation of finger pads with short mechanical pulses of variable amplitude. In *Sensory Functions of the Skin in Primates*, **27**, edited by Y. Zotterman, 105–112. Oxford, Pergamon Press (1976)

54 LINDBLOM, Y. and LUND, L. The discharge from vibration-sensitive receptors in the monkey foot. *Experimental Neurology*, **15**, 401–417 (1966)

55 LINDBLOM, U. and MEYERSON, B. A. Influence on touch, vibration and cutaneous pain of dorsal column stimulation in man, *Pain*, **1**, 257–270 (1975)

56 LINDBLOM, U. and MEYERSON, B. A. Mechanoreceptive and nociceptive thresholds during dorsal column stimulation in man. *Advances in Pain Research and Therapy*, **1**, edited by J. J. Bonica and D. Albe-Fessard. 469–474. New York, Raven Press (1976)

57 LINDBLOM, U. and VERRILLO, R. T. Sensory functions in chronic neuralgia. *Journal of Neurology, Neurosurgery and Psychiatry*, **42**, 422–435 (1979)

58 LYNN, B. and PERL, E. R. A comparison of four tests for assessing the pain sensitivity of different subjects and test areas. *Pain*, **3**, 353–365 (1977)

59 MERSKEY, H. Pain terms: A list with definitions and notes on usage, IASP Subcommittee on Taxonomy. *Pain*, **6**, 249–252 (1979)

60 MERSKEY, H. and SPEAR, F. G. The reliability of the pressure algometer. *British Journal of Social and Clinical Psychology*, **3**, 130–136 (1964)

61 MERZENICH, M. M. and HARRINGTON, T. The sense of flutter-vibration evoked by stimulation of the hairy skin of primates: Comparison of human sensory capacity with the responses of mechanoreceptive afferents innervating the hairy skin of monkeys. *Experimental Brain Research*, **9**, 236–260 (1969)

62 MEYER, R. A., WALKER, R. E. and MOUNTCASTLE, V. B. A laser stimulator for the study of cutaneous thermal and pain sensations. *IEEE Transactions on Biomedical Engineering*, **BME–23**, 54–60 (1976)

63 MOBERG, E. Methods for examining sensibility in the hand. In *Hand Surgery*, edited by J. E. Flynn, 435–449. Baltimore, Williams & Wilkins, (1966)

64 MOR, J. and CARMON, A. Laser emitted radiant heat for pain research. *Pain*, **1**, 233–237 (1975)

65 MOUNTCASTLE, V. B. Pain and temperature sensibilities. *Medical Physiology*, 13th ed., **1**, 348–381, C. V. Mosby, St Louis (1974)

66 NAKAHAMA, H. and YAMAMOTO, M. An improved radiant heat algo-meter and its application to pain threshold measurements in man. *Pain*, **6**, 141–148 (1979)

67 NIELSEN, V. K. Recovery from peripheral neuropathy after renal transplantation. *Acta Neurologica Scandinavica*, **46**, suppl. 43,207 (1970)

68 NIELSEN, V.K. The peripheral nerve function in chronic renal failure. *Acta Medica Scandinavica*, **191**, 287–296 (1972)

69 PROCACCI, P., ZOPPI, M. and MARESCA, M. Experimental pain in man. Review article, *Pain*, **6**, 123–140 (1979)

70 SCHAUMBURG, H. H., WISNIEWSKI, H. M. and SPENCER, P. S. Ultrastructu-ral studies of the dying-back process. 1. Peripheral nerve terminal and axon degeneration in systemic acrylamide intoxication. *Journal of Neuropathology and Experimental Neurology*, **23**, 260–284 (1974)

71 SEKULER, R., NASH, D. N. and ARMSTRONG, R. Sensitive, objective proce-dure for evaluating response to light touch. *Neurology*, **23**, 1282 –1291 (1973)

72 TALBOT, W. H. DARIAN-SMITH, I., KORNHUBER, H. H. and MOUNTCASTLE, V. B. The sense of flutter-vibration: Comparison of the human capacity with response patterns in mechanoreceptive afferents from the monkey hand. *Journal of Neurophysiology*, **31**, 301–334 (1968)

73 TOREBJÖRK, H. E. Afferent C units responding to mechanical, ther-mal, and chemical stimuli in human non-glabrous skin. *Acta Physiologica Scandinavica*, **92**, 374–390 (1974)

74 TSIRULNIKOV, E. M. and SHCHEKANOV, E. E. Temperature sensations among other sensations to the stimuli of focused ultrasound. The comparison with the temperature sensations by mechanical stimuli. In *Sensory Functions of the Skin in Primates*, **27**, edited by Y. Zotterman, 399–411, Oxford, Pergamon Press (1976)

75 VALLBO, Å. B., HAGBARTH, K.-E., TOREBJÖRK, H. E. and WALLIN, B. G. Somatosensory, proprioceptive, and sympathetic activity in human peripheral nerves. *Physiological Reviews*, **59**, 919–957 (1979)

76 VERRILLO, R. T. Age related changes in the sensitivity to vibration. *Journal of Gerontology*, **35**, 185–193 (1980)

77 VERRILLO, R. T. and ECKER, A. D. Effects of root or nerve destruction on vibrotactile sensitivity in trigeminal neuralgia. *Pain*, **3**, 239–255 (1977)

78 WESTLING, G., JOHANSSON, R. S. and VALLBO, Å. A method for mechanical stimulation of skin receptors. In *Sensory Functions of the Skin in Primates*, **27**, edited by Y. Zotterman, 151–158. Oxford, Pergamon Press, (1976)

79 ZOTTERMAN, Y. Studies in the peripheral nervous mechanism of pain. *Acta Medica Scandinavica*, **80**, 7–64 (1933)

9
Motor performance in normal human beings and patients with disorders of motor control

V. Dietz and R. R. Young

Introduction

Clinical neurophysiology plays an increasingly important role in studies of normal and pathological function of the motor system. It provides unique and often quantifiable methods for documentation of motor performance which, as techniques and understanding improve, will facilitate diagnosis and monitor any changes produced by physical, medical or surgical therapies. It is possible to record:

(1) electromyographic (EMG) activity (single unit or multi-unit activity in one or many muscles);
(2) mechanical events (joint angles, forces exerted, bodily position and changes in position – velocity and acceleration); and
(3) single or multi-unit Ia afferent activity coming from muscle spindles[83, 89].

Following a discussion of single motor unit activity during simpler voluntarily-controlled movements, the behavior of large numbers of motor units in different muscles, that is, 'innervation patterns', during more complex motor performances will be considered. Intensive investigation has been underway in these areas and in this brief review only certain important features of normal and abnormal behavior will be highlighted; the reader's interest, if aroused, will then be directed to more detailed analyses.

Motor unit behavior during simple voluntary movements

The size principle of Henneman

With slowly increasing tonic or ramp contractions, α-motoneurons are sequentially recruited beginning with the 'smallest' ones (*see* Chapter 2), that is to say, in any given functional area of a complex muscle, larger motor units are activated after smaller ones have been recruited. On the other hand, when contractions are progressively relaxed, larger motor units are derecruited before smaller ones (*Figure 9.1*). The 'smaller' the motor unit, the more easily it can be discharged; the larger, the greater the excitatory input required to activate it. This is the size principle defined by Henneman[46].

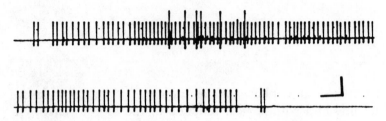

Figure 9.1 Recruitment of two motor units in a forearm muscle. The first unit increases in frequency and then, with progressive relaxation, decreases. The second, larger unit is recruited and derecruited first. Calibration is 1 s and 500 μV (From Henneman, Shahani and Young[45], courtesy of the publishers, *The Motor System – Neurophysiology and Muscle Mechanisms*)

During quick phasic or ballistic contractions, motor units of all sizes seem to be more or less synchronously recruited[10, 28]. For technical reasons, including the movement of wire or needle recording electrodes with regard to muscle fibers, it is difficult to be certain that the size principle describes the fastest ballistic movements but Desmedt's studies of masseter or intrinsic hand muscles[13, 14] support the size principle (*see also* Chapter 2).

In complex muscles, where different parts of the same gross anatomical structure function in different ways during different movements, units can be activated in one part by one particular movement and in another part of the muscle with a different movement without particular regard to the fine points of their size. Critical studies of the size principle should therefore be limited to muscles in which fibers insert on one long tendon so that they have one action, i.e. produce movement in one plane at one joint, for example, the tibialis anterior muscle.

Furthermore, the criteria for identification of different motor units must be strict. When attempting to 'rotate' activity between two units, there must be no change in the configuration of either unit, otherwise changes in the appearance of units is presumed to reflect movement of the intramuscular electrode.

When such critical studies have been undertaken[45], the recruitment order in humans for ramp contractions at low levels of tension has been found to be relatively fixed. Infrequent switching in the order of recruitment was possible only between motor units whose tension thresholds ('critical firing levels') and presumably, motor unit size, differed very slightly. Even this very restricted rotation of units is difficult – only a minority of subjects can do it and it is not clearly under conscious control. None could, on demand, immediately activate either of the units without the other.

Apparently the human nervous system cannot selectively activate ('isolate') from an available motoneuron pool, any motor unit desired according to the needs or wishes of the moment. That is to say, higher motor centers do not specify the activity of each motoneuron individually; they do control activities of motoneuron pools selectively, within which there is a natural rank-order determined by the size principle. Apart from suggestions that larger motor units may be preferentially involved in certain myoclonic activity[90], there is as yet no documentation of disease processes or lesions producing significant exceptions to the size principle.

Physiological and pathological motoneuron discharges and their mechanical effect

Statistical aspects
When a normal subject attempts to maintain a constant isometric force, intervals between discharges of any single motor unit are related in an interesting way. For a unit discharging at a mean rate of 10 Hz for example, compensatory mechanisms exist so that any interval which is longer than the mean (100 ms) tends to be followed by an interval shorter than the mean. This is called a 'negative serial correlation'. However, in patients with lesions of the 'upper motoneuron system'

producing 'spasticity', these compensatory mechanisms are much less prominent, so fluctuations or trends develop in tension and in length of successive intervals. That is to say, intervals longer than the mean tend to be followed by longer intervals and only after several seconds is the instantaneous firing frequency adjusted downwards[4, 30, 91].

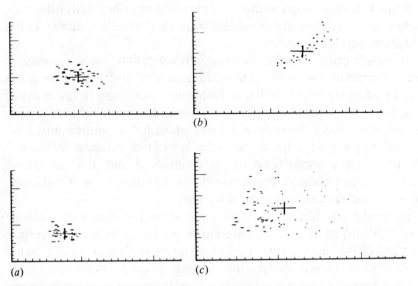

Figure 9.2 Joint-interval histogram of single motor unit discharges from finger extensor muscles – see text for details. Both *x* and *y* axes depict intervals from 0 to 250 ms, each small division representing 10 ms.
(*a*) Normal subjects with mean frequencies for single motor unit discharges 10 Hz (*above*) and 14 Hz (*below*). (*b*) Spastic-hemi-paretic limb. Note abnormal distribution with trends. (*c*) Patient with cerebellar ataxia. Tension could not be maintained constant and intervals are more randomly related. (From Young and Shahani[91], courtesy of the publishers, *Spasticity: Disordered Motor Control*)

Freund *et al.*[29, 30] demonstrated this relationship with a joint-interval histogram (JIH) which in normal circumstances tends to take the form of a circular clustering of dots, each representing the temporal relationship of the duration of two successive intervals (*Figure 9.2a*). In those paretic patients, where trends develop, dots tend to cluster along the 45° line from lower left to upper right[91] (*Figure 9.2b*). However, patients with cerebellar ataxia often produce JIHs in which dots are scattered in an apparently random fashion signifying that intervals between discharges of their single motor units have no apparent relationship (*Figure 9.2c*).

Though the CNS may not selectively activate individual motoneurons, mechanisms within the CNS do appear to regulate intervals between discharges of single motor units. This aspect of the control of timing of motoneuron discharge presumably minimizes moment-to-moment fluctuations in tension during contractions when the subject is meant to keep tension as stable as possible. The function of this mechanism, which can regulate firing frequency quickly enough to operate on a 'beat-to-beat' time scale, is more remarkable when two other aspects of single motor unit discharge which are affected by upper motor neuron lesions are considered. Naturally the number of motor units which can be voluntarily recruited in a paretic muscle is decreased. Furthermore those units which can be recruited voluntarily have, as a population, lower maximal firing rates than normal. Normally, as voluntarily-produced tension, and therefore motor unit firing rates, increase the variability in their interdischarge intervals decreases. This also occurs with paretic motor units, but even at low rates of discharge they have less variability in interdischarge intervals than normal motor units[4]. Also, the variability of interspike intervals depicted in JIHs is not simply a function of the mean interval, i.e. the firing rate, because in hemiparetic patients most interspike intervals fall outside the normal ratio of interspike to mean interval. This paradoxical finding of more variability of interdischarge intervals in normal subjects, plus the normal 'negative serial correlation' has led Andreassen[3] to postulate 'over-regulation' under normal circumstances, that is, to keep tension constant the instantaneous motor unit discharge frequency fluctuates continuously above and below the mean rather than maintaining a more constant rate.

All motoneurons in any one pool in a paretic patient are not equally abnormal. Many can be voluntarily recruited, can increase their firing rate as the patient tries harder, though usually not to normal, and then have decreased variability in interdischarge intervals. Some units, even in clearly paretic muscles, actually perform within normal limits for these paradigms. Whether this is due to incomplete lesions or something more basic is an important question; the answer will determine which strategies should be employed in neurological rehabilitation.

Asterixis appears to reflect, even at the single motor unit level, dysfunction in yet another mechanism which, it is hypothesized, is concerned with maintenance of sustained muscular contraction[80, 90].

Concomitants of voluntary contraction – physiological and pathological tremor

Normally, with slowly developing ramp contractions, human motor units begin firing irregularly at rates of approximately 4 Hz; as strength of contraction and firing rates increase, the pattern becomes fairly regular at 8–10 Hz, as noted above. Frequencies above about 15 Hz are rarely seen because with very strong contractions it is technically difficult to record single motor units. Normally with quick, ballistic or 'phasic' contractions or when the tension produced by a tonic contraction is suddenly increased, motor units may fire two or three times with a much higher instantaneous frequency (50–100 Hz)[59].

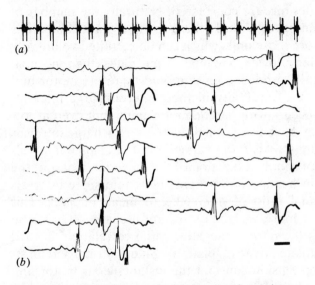

Figure 9.3 EMG from wrist extensors of a patient with tremor-at-rest of Parkinson's disease. (*a*) 5–6 Hz tremor bursts are seen (calibration is 200 ms). (*b*) Continuous recording of this activity with a faster sweep speed (calibration 10 ms). Note in (*b*) the same single unit often fires twice, with instantaneous frequencies up to 50 Hz

On the other hand, patients with Parkinson's disease have, as a common feature of their 'tremor-at-rest', double discharges of single motor units (*Figure 9.3*) with high instantaneous firing rates (50 Hz) even when they are in an attitude of repose and are not attempting to move[17]. Though the visible tremor itself is reflected by quick changes in tension under isotonic conditions, double discharges can be recorded in patients without visible tremor. During any single tremor burst in patients with essential–familial action tremors, instantaneous firing frequencies between 20 and 50 Hz may also be recorded though such double discharges are less prominent than in Parkinson's disease[81].

Essential–familial tremor and Parkinson's disease are entirely unrelated illnesses and their typical tremors (the former increased with voluntary muscle activity and the latter worse 'at rest') are not difficult to distinguish clinically or physiologically. Nevertheless more patients with Parkinson's disease than would be expected also have pre-existing essential–familial tremor[35]; the first sign of developing Parkinson's disease turns out to have been a significant worsening of that action tremor, at a time when there is no other evidence of Parkinson's disease. Physiologically, both tremors show high instantaneous frequency single motor unit discharges, 'double discharges', and both are also associated with increased synchronization of independent motor units (*see below*). This all suggests[79] that there may be tremor mechanisms common to the two disorders, i.e. the neurochemical abnormalities underlying Parkinson's disease also affect those functions involved in non-resting tremor. When any physiological overlap between these two diseases is clarified, it may serve as the focus for medical or other therapies less invasive than the ventrolateral thalamic lesions used now by surgeons to abolish both types of tremor.

In addition to this abnormal tendency for high instantaneous firing rates of a single motor unit under theoretically tonic circumstances, another important feature of tremors has to do with the exact timing of discharges in two independent single motor units. Normally, over the long run, discharges in one motor unit arise at a time which is statistically independent of those in another in the same pool (*Figure 9.4a*). However, when both units are firing at 8–12 Hz, 'short-term synchronization' of these independent motor units ('beating') will occur by chance. These temporarily synchronized discharges appear to have little significance; for example, there is no evidence that they produce the low-level physiological tremor found in all normal subjects. Dietz and coworkers[2, 16] have demonstrated it to be due, not to synchronization of motor units, but to mechanical factors inherent in the limb including poorly-fused contractions of units which have just been recruited and are firing at low frequencies. However, enhanced physiological tremor (*see below and*[39, 88]) which may increase a few minutes after the start of a tonic contraction, even though the subject

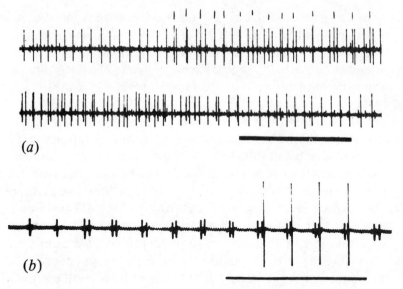

Figure 9.4 Single unit EMGs from wrist extensors. Three units from two separate subjects recorded simultaneously on one continuous tracing which uses both lines (*a*) and two units from a patient with Parkinson's disease (*b*). Note both 'double discharges' of the first-recruited unit and synchronization of the larger second-recruited unit and the first are in a 4–5 Hz tremor burst. Calibrations are 1 s

certainly does not yet feel fatigued, *is* due to synchronization of motor unit discharges. Differentiation of these tremors into physiological and enhanced physiological categories resolves debates in the literature about whether or not 'physiological tremor' is critically dependent upon the spinal stretch-reflex arc for its operation; enhanced physiological tremor is dependent, however ordinary physiological tremor is not.

In patients with several other types of tremor including Parkinson's tremor-at-rest, essential–familial action tremor or peripheral, β-adrenergic-induced 'nervous' tremor, synchronization of independent motor units also becomes more prominent and more important so that at the extreme, groups of independent motor units fire more or less at the same time producing bursts of multi-unit activity which are the EMG counterpart of the tremor itself (*Figure 9.4b*). Such 'long-term synchronization', particularly the β-adrenergic-induced variety, under-lies the various types of enhanced physiological tremor which can be produced in perfectly normal subjects, or in patients with various diseases, by maneuvers which produce grouping of muscle spindle Ia input to the spinal cord – these include 'fatigue', or even slight contraction of muscles for as little as a few minutes, vibration of muscle, 'nervousness', or β-adrenergic stimulation. The latter involves β-2 adrenergic receptors within the muscle; preliminary observations with fluorescence microscopy by Chan-Palay (unpublished observations) suggest these β-2 synapses may be on extrafusal muscle fibers themselves.

Slight alterations in mechanical properties of these fibers, time to reach peak tension following an EMG burst, for example, are common with 'fatigue' or adrenergic stimulation, both of which can shorten contraction time. Those alterations are very accurately sensed by primary muscle spindle endings in parallel with extrafusal fibers[39]. Stretch discharges arise from spindles when extrafusal fibers relax and unloading pauses in Ia input when extrafusal fibers contract – both are remarkably influential in timing discharges from an already discharging motoneuron pool (*Figure 9.5*). That is, Ia input from muscle can certainly synchronize discharges in independent motoneurons in the pool supplying that muscle[88].

Segmental stretch reflex mechanisms are therefore obviously involved in these tremors. Changes in timing of already discharging neurons are of concern here, not recruitment of previously silent ones,

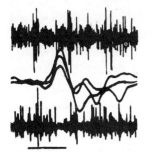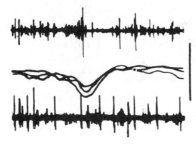

Figure 9.5 Superimposed recordings of multi-unit muscle spindle activity (*top*) from long flexor of index finger, goniometer on distal IP joint (*center*) and EMG from the same muscle (*bottom*). On the left are irregularities in the direction of flexion, on the right in extension. Notice Ia activity at the beginning of stretch phases with excessive recruitment (*left*) or decruitment (*right*) just before the movements. Calibrations are 200 ms and 0.5 degrees. (From Young and Hagbarth[88], courtesy of the Editor and publisher, *Journal of Neurology, Neurosurgery and Psychiatry*)

as with tendon jerks for example. When the timing of these EMG discharges, plus the relatively slow excitation–contraction coupling which eventually produces the tremor movement, is such that they reinforce inherent oscillatory tendencies in the limb, tremor amplitude is enhanced and clinicians speak of adrenergic tremor, fatigue tremor, thyrotoxic tremor, and so on.

These alterations in contractile properties, which happen to be associated with increased tremor amplitude, are evolutionarily adaptive insofar as they produce larger increments of tension more quickly. As noted above, sudden voluntary increases in output from a motoneuron pool are also reflected as both brief bursts of high instantaneous frequency discharges and synchronization of individual motor units. Training to increase 'muscle power' accentuates this tendency toward synchronization[67]. Both discharge patterns which are, in some sense, 'abnormal' during pathological tremors are normal mechanisms for increasing mechanical output from a muscle – as a 'side-effect' of their operation, tremors are produced.

Stereotyped ballistic and ramp movements of the arm

Centrally pre-programmed movements are of obvious importance in the human upper extremity as well as the lower (*see* p. 203). As first demonstrated by Wachholder[84] in 1923 and confirmed by the authors[41,51], quick flexion or extension movements of the human elbow or wrist are associated with a 'triphasic EMG pattern' (*Figure 9.6*) providing they are moved quickly from one precise position to another under visual control. This triphasic pattern consists of two EMG bursts in the prime mover or agonist muscle (AG 1 and AG 2) separated by a period of EMG silence. During that interval a burst of EMG activity is recorded from the antagonist muscle (AN 1). These triphasic EMG patterns are presumably useful for bringing the hand or forearm to a target with both speed and precision. AG 1 reflects muscular force accelerating the limb, AN 1 decelerates it and AG 2 is concerned with continuation of movement until the target is reached. This triphasic pattern was recorded from a de-afferented patient. For this and other reasons[41] this pattern appears to be a suprasegmental centrally pre-programmed one rather than a reflection of reciprocal inhibition and other spinal stretch reflex activity. For one thing, ballistic movements can reach their targets before peripheral feedback can have had time to be effective. However, it was subsequently

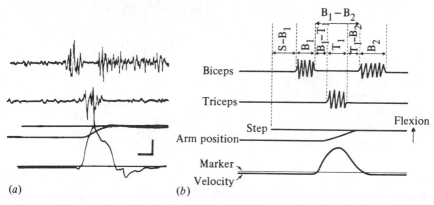

(a)   *(b)*

Figure 9.6 Triphasic EMG pattern in biceps and triceps brachii with fast, accurate elbow flexion. (*a*) Original recording; calibrations 50 ms and 500 μV. (*b*) Schematic diagram of this original with descriptions. See text for details. (From Hallett, Shahani and Young[41], courtesy of the Editor and publisher, *Journal of Neurology, Neurosurgery and Psychiatry*)

shown that changes in resistance which the limb encounters during its movement alter the amplitude and duration of AG 2 and also, to a lesser extent, of AN 1 and AG 1. Even these two early components, largely but not entirely pre-programmed, are not beyond the control of peripheral perturbations.

Recently it was demonstrated[82] that this EMG pattern is velocity-dependent. In slow 'smooth' movements, there is continuous EMG activity only in the agonist muscle and evidence suggests that the spinal servo-loop is continuously active and strongly influential even from the start of these movements. With slightly faster movements (75–125°/s), a two-burst pattern appears only in the agonist muscle. With greater angular velocity the antagonist burst appears and the duration of AG 1 and the interval between AG 1 and AG 2 becomes shorter. This timing becomes constant with velocities greater than 275°/s and a detailed study at these speeds[41] produced normal values for timing of the various parameters of these patterns.

Patients with cerebellar signs[42] tend to have an abnormally prolonged AG 1 or AN 1. The former could produce 'overshoot' and the latter 'undershoot' (hypometria) of the movement, providing other compensatory mechanisms also fail. These distortions of the initial part of this preprogrammed pattern, due to suprasegmental deficits, may be one objectification of clinical dysmetria.

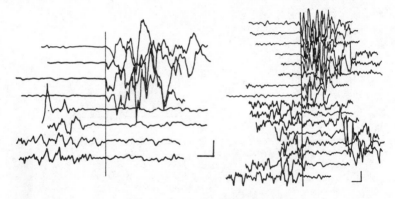

Figure 9.7 'Inhibition' of tonic triceps brachii activity before the onset of biceps activity with fast elbow flexion. These are composites of four (*left*) or eight (*right*) trials from a normal subject (*left*) and a patient with cerebellar ataxia (*right*). The top half of each record is biceps EMG and the bottom half triceps EMG. The first biceps and first triceps tracings were recorded simultaneously (and so on for the rest) – they are lined up so the vertical line is at the onset of biceps activity. Note triceps EMG stops 25 ms or so before biceps begins normally but not in the cerebellar patient. Time calibrations are 20 ms. (From Hallett, Shahani and Young[41, 42], courtesy of the Editor and publisher, *Journal of Neurology, Neurosurgery and Psychiatry*)

Studies in normals also showed that the first sign of a quick voluntary movement superimposed upon an ongoing contraction is cessation of tonic activity in the antagonist muscle, and also in the agonist itself, if it was previously active. This 'inhibition' occurs as much as 50 ms before the EMG producing the movement itself. In patients with cerebellar signs, this period is abnormally short – sometimes the antagonist EMG does not fall silent before the agonist begins (*Figure 9.7*). Naturally this failure to switch activity efficiently between antagonistic muscle groups would slow alternating movements (dysdiadochokinesia) and might also prevent rapid contraction of an antagonist when an isometric agonist contraction is unloaded ('rebound').

Interestingly, patients with Parkinson's disease do not have abnormalities of the length of AG 1, AG 2, AN 1 or the inhibitory period[43]. Their increased reaction time and decreased acceleration and velocity of movement once it starts ('bradykinesia') cannot be explained by failure of antagonistic muscles to relax or rigidity in those muscles.

Innervation patterns during complex motor performances

Preprogrammed versus stretch reflex-induced innervation of leg and arm muscles in normal subjects

Locomotion: significance of stretch-reflex activity in leg muscles

How are different phases of complex movements controlled and adapted to specific situations; which nervous system structures are involved in these control mechanisms? A movement-specific pattern of internal reflex controls is felt to be present prior to initiation of movements[6, 31, 57]. This concept of a hierarchical organization of movement control with purposeful innervation patterns, generated by the sensorimotor system and adapted to external conditions through specialized sub-systems, has been supported by a number of animal experiments[26, 31, 54] especially using spinal cats on treadmills[34, 87], which demonstrate specialized mechanisms within the cord that can produce stereotyped locomotor movements. Few investigations of the neural organization of complex movements have been done in man.

Innervation patterns in man were described by Melvill-Jones and Watt[65, 66] who first observed 'preprogrammed innervation' of foot extensor muscles 130–140 ms before contact with the ground during stepping and hopping movements. They emphasized the importance during stereotyped movements of such 'pre-innervation' in connection with the 'functional stretch-reflex', which appears about 120 ms after foot contact. However, the contribution of segmental myotatic stretch-reflex activity in leg extensor muscles to load compensation after landing from a fall[33] was controversial for a long time but was then investigated in man during running[22], hopping[20] and falling onto extended arms[19, 21]. As can be seen from gastrocnemius muscle EMG (*Figure 9.8*), pre-innervation is followed by a steep increase of activity at the beginning of the stance phase of a running cycle. This increase persists during the stretching phase of this muscle (dorsiflexion of the foot) and stops suddenly with its shortening, i.e. with extension of the foot for 'pushing-off' the body from the ground. Then, at the end of the stance phase, tibialis anterior EMG begins to counteract the forceful foot extension.

The increase in gastrocnemius activity after ground contact during running derives at least partly from spinal stretch-reflex activity. The steep increase in EMG following the plateau-like pre-innervation

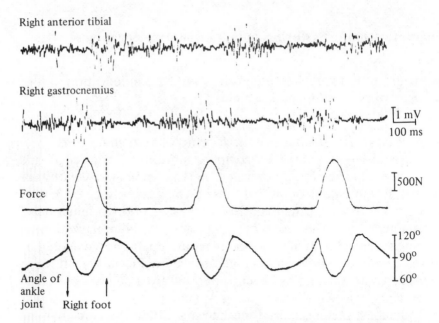

Right anterior tibial

Right gastrocnemius

1 mV
100 ms

Force

500N

Angle of
ankle
joint   Right foot

120°
90°
60°

Figure 9.8 EMG from leg muscles during three cycles of running in place, together with force exerted by the foot and the goniometer record of ankle angle. Arrows indicate beginning and cessation of platform contact. (From Dietz, Schmidtbleicher and Noth[22], courtesy of the Editor and publisher, *Journal of Neurophysiology*)

(*Figure 9.9*) begins about 40 ms after ground contact, i.e. when stretch of gastrocnemius begins, which is the latency of a segmental stretch-reflex. When leg muscle-spindle input is reduced by ischemic block of group I afferents, the gastrocnemius EMG peak is reduced, while the amplitude of gastrocnemius pre-innervation as well as tibialis anterior activity is unaffected. Peak activity of leg extensors, which in a sprint lasts about 50–60 ms, exceeds the EMG level reached during brisk maximum voluntary isometric muscle contraction (MVIC). This suggests full voluntary activation of gastrocnemius can only be reached with support of excitatory drive from muscle spindles via the segmental stretch-reflex pathway.

Its importance seems plausible because stereotyped complex movements such as running are largely executed automatically and adaptation to the environment is performed subconsciously. Such quick modifications of preprogrammed muscle innervation for a specific

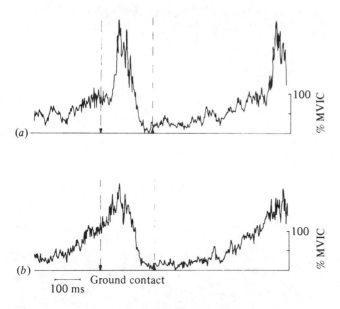

Figure 9.9 Rectified and averaged (50 trials) EMG activity
from right gastrocnemius during fast running in place. (*a*) The
control before ischemia shows the typical rapid increase in
EMG 35–40 ms after ground contact. In (*b*) after 20 min of
ischemia produced by a tourniquet around the thigh, this
stretch-induced EMG activity is reduced without a decrease in
activity prior to contact. (From Dietz, Schmidtbleicher and
Noth[22], courtesy of the Editor and publisher, *Journal of
Neurophysiology*)

running condition could only be provided individually for each stride
by the spinal stretch-reflex, which also reinforces the extensor activity
for pushing off during the stance phases of running. The functional
importance of a quick adjustment of innervation pattern can be
demonstrated, when the moment of ground contact is unknown to the
subject, by randomly altering the ground level (*Figure 9.10*). When the
ground is lower than expected, body balance is maintained by quick
enhancement of gastrocnemius activity produced by combined effects
of stronger pre-innervation, built up as a result of later ground contact,
and faster stretching of this muscle[76]. Dependency of spinal stretch-
reflex activity on the strength of pre-existing activity and velocity of
muscle stretch has also been demonstrated with a torque motor[32].

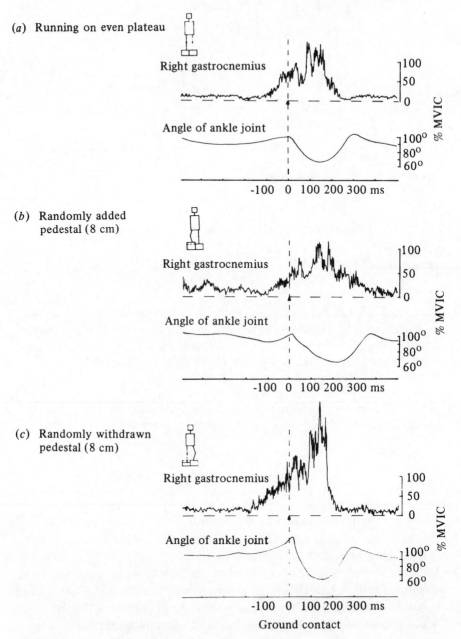

Figure 9.10 Rectified and averaged (30 trials) EMG activity from gastrocnemius together with the goniometer signal from ankle joint during running in place. During running on even plateau (*a*), the surface under the right leg was randomly lifted up (*b*) or lowered (*c*) by adding or withdrawing a pedestal of 8 cm height. Visual and acoustic clues for the running subject were excluded

Stretch reflex activity in arm muscles

Hammond, Merton and Sutton's hypothesis[44] that the spinal stretch-reflex is significantly less functional than long-loop stretch-reflexes, such as the functional stretch-reflex, has been widely accepted. However, the velocity of biceps brachii stretch in their experiments was one-fifth to one-tenth of that which can occur during natural complex movements. Also, evidence from recordings of human primary spindle afferent activity following such 100–200°/s stretches casts doubt upon the ability to define the function of long loops by recordings of EMG responses to muscle stretch[38, 40]. Each such stretch, because of non-linear mechanical properties of muscle, gives rise to three or four sequential bursts of Ia activity. When each Ia burst is then followed, at spinal stretch-reflex latency, by an EMG burst, the simplest explanation for this segmented EMG response is certainly not the operation of longer and longer reflex loops.

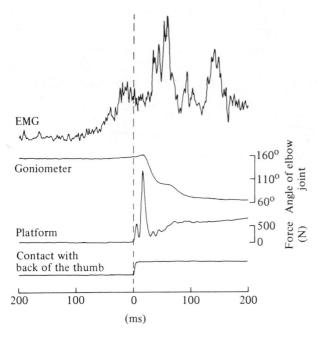

Figure 9.11 Comparison between averaged EMG from left triceps brachii (30 trials), goniometer signal from elbow joint and platform force during series of falls forward onto the hands. First contact with platform, made by ball of the thumb, indicated by interrupted line

The velocity of stretch in triceps surae with running[22] or hopping[20] and in triceps brachii during falls forward onto the hands with extended arms[21], is 400–1000°/s. EMG from arm extensors during this latter task showed that the segmental stretch-reflex is also able to contribute to activity, associated with stretching of triceps, which decelerates the body (over more than 200 ms). There is thus enough time for the segmental stretch-reflex to become mechanically effective for load compensation after impact (*Figure 9.11*). As with gastrocnemius EMG during running, this stretch-reflex induced activity is larger than triceps brachii EMG during MVIC.

Marsden, Merton and Morton[60,61] found no early EMG stretch responses during tracking movements of the human thumb. Their later stretch responses, which were thought to reflect long-loop activity, may merely represent spinal stretch-reflexes to repeated bursts of Ia afferent inputs[38, 40]. Failure to demonstrate a spinal stretch-reflex response to a single input could be explained by the very different motor tasks and abilities of arm and hand muscles versus leg muscles. The fingers especially may be much more under voluntary control of motor cortex and a low threshold spinal stretch-reflex contribution to EMG activity might be less advantageous for fine, goal-directed finger movements. In these muscle groups, unreinforced spinal stretch-reflex activity is probably suppressed with the growing importance of voluntary control. However, these 'primitive' reflexes are not eliminated as judged by postural, grasping and H reflexes normally present in human upper limbs in early infancy and reappearance of H reflexes in adults during voluntary contraction and with repetitive inputs; in leg muscles they are merely integrated more simply with central programs.

Control of posture

Normal stance. Normal upright stance is controlled with information from visual, vestibular and proprioceptive afferents[15, 55, 70–73] and the body sways slowly and irregularly without a predominant frequency[15]. During quiet standing, the stretch reflex system is not necessarily a fundamental mechanism for postural regulation after controlled perturbations in spite of the fact that during tilting of a supporting platform, changes in length of triceps surae were well above the very low threshold for activation of spinal stretch reflex mechanisms[36, 37].

Coordination of activity in muscles involved with control of posture may be achieved by interaction of central programs with information in various afferent signals[71, 73]. However, some subjects did use long-latency stretch-reflexes to reduce postural sway[73] and when rapid adjustment was needed after perturbations of posture all subjects showed EMG responses with the timing of long-latency stretch-reflexes. The absence of spinal stretch-reflex activity, mentioned above, has been ascribed to failure to reach necessary stretch velocity in leg muscles[32]. However, in the arm at least, stretch reflexes which as noted above are less easily obtained there, do appear in enhanced physiological tremor where a very small stretch is an adequate stimulus[39, 88].

Stance on an unstable base. Upright posture on an unstable base or with a minimal area on which to stand requires very quick control mechanisms to optimize stance regulation. This can be studied during balancing on a seesaw consisting of a platform with a curved base which swings in an anterior–posterior direction. Seesaw and body oscillations are then recorded with predominant frequency ranges between 4–5 Hz which cannot be suppressed or voluntarily modified; they are accompanied by short reciprocally-organized EMG bursts in leg muscles (*Figure 9.12*). These uncontrollable and unwanted oscillations result from spinal stretch-reflex mechanisms[18] and predominant sway frequency ranges of 4–5 Hz seem to be essential for relative stability of posture during balancing. When attempting to balance with impoverished proprioceptive function, during ischemic blockade of group I afferents from both legs or with the ankles fixed in plaster, body sway is larger, slower and the subject becomes increasingly more unstable[63]. These observations indicate the importance of stretch-reflex activity for balance but do not prove whether the reflex is mediated by a long-loop or segmental pathway. Calculations of reflex latencies and mechanical delays suggest fast balancing movements are due to spinal reflex activity. This hypothesis is also supported by the balancing reaction following a displacement produced by stimulation of the tibial nerves; its delay, about 40 ms before counterbalancing EMG actvity starts, is that of a fast-conducting segmental reflex[18].

Are these oscillations a basic mechanism for regulation of equilibrium during balancing or, to some extent, an unwanted side-effect of balancing movements? Following balancing practice for several days,

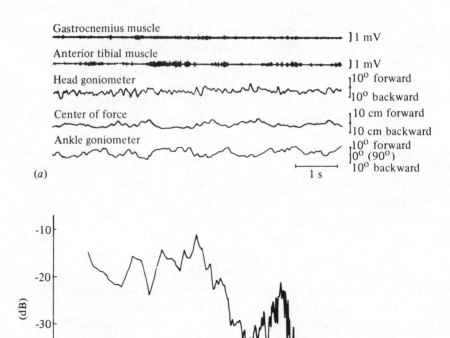

Figure 9.12 (*a*) EMG from leg muscles during balancing with eyes closed on a seesaw (12 cm height) together with goniometer records of head and ankle angle as well as the anterior–posterior displacement of the center of force exerted by seesaw on the platform. (*b*) Power spectrum of the force displacement. Fourier analysis was performed for a 60 s period of balancing

the oscillations decrease continuously, the subject becomes increasingly more stable and slower, larger body sway occurs less frequently (*Figure 9.13*). However, even after weeks of practice, fast balancing movements are still present as a smaller 4–5 Hz peak in the frequency power spectrum. At the beginning of this non-visual motor task, spinal stretch-reflex gain may be higher than during normal stance because of descending excitation from supraspinal centers to γ-motoneurons.

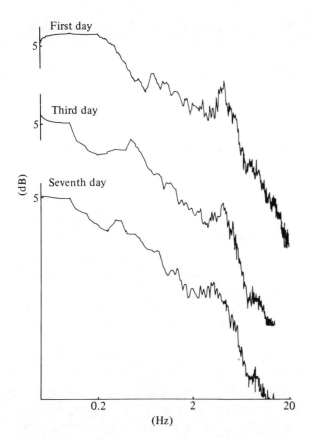

Figure 9.13 Power spectra of the anterior–
posterior displacement of force exerted by a
12 cm high seesaw with a subject balancing on the
first, third and seventh day of practice. The
Fourier analysis was performed for 60 s of balancing

This increase could maintain oscillations which are not necessary for
equilibrium. With practice, the gain may be increasingly adapted to
the task, so that spinal reflex activity is evoked only when advantageous for quick regulation of balance, when neural compensation
would not be fast enough with supraspinal reflex transmission or via
the vestibular system. However, slower components of body sway
during balancing in normals are needed to maintain equilibrium. Is

this larger slow-sway due to regulation via the vestibular system alone or in combination with long-loop reflexes?

Conclusions

Phylogenetically younger CNS motor centers prevail over older ones such as those responsible for spinal-stretch reflexes but these 'primitive' reflexes are not eliminated and tend to be usefully integrated with centrally preprogrammed innervation patterns. Short reaction time, an obvious advantage of the spinal stretch-reflex system, may be of greater signficance in leg muscles which appear to participate in more automatically executed movements. Supraspinal centers, also involved in regulation of these movements, adjust reflex gain to suit each specific motor task. The authors' balancing experiments support Welford's suggestion[86] that the motor system progressively and adaptively modifies the innervation pattern of a task with unexpectedly variable conditions by seeking to produce changes in the pattern of internal controls which will reduce executional errors in subsequent responses.

Analysis of innervation patterns in different complex movements also demonstrates that stretch-reflex activity is important primarily via close interaction with preprogrammed muscle innervation and mechanical properties of the activated muscle. Others[34, 65] stress the potential utility of pre-activated muscle, i.e. its specific visco-elastic properties, for quick compensations of external load changes. Hagbarth *et al.*[38-48, 87] have also stressed the functionally tight interplay between mechanical properties of muscle, Ia input and the outcome of spinal stretch-reflex activity.

Pre-innervation of extensor muscles during running, hopping or falling seems to be essential for two reasons. First, pre-activated muscle develops tension which minimizes overstretching just after ground contact before the onset of stretch-reflex activity. Second, many α-motoneurons are recruited during pre-innervation and can therefore respond more quickly with an increase in discharge frequency following a burst of excitatory spindle impulses produced by impact. When already active, they may also decrease their discharge rates with consequent bimodal, up-or-down alterations in timing depending on peripheral perturbations – a situation which would be impossible if they were quiescent. Muscle spindle primary endings, which happen also to respond to a physician's tendon tap, are thus seen to have more significant functions.

Innervation patterns in some disorders of motor control

Gait in patients with spasticity or Parkinsonism

For patients with lesions in the motor system, only slow walking is usually possible; it must be compared with normal gait at the same velocity. The basic difference between innervation patterns during walking and running is much less EMG activity in the leg muscles during the former; significant pre-innervation of calf muscles can rarely be distinguished during walking. Gastrocnemius activity during running or walking increases with forward bending of the leg (stretching of triceps surae) during the stance phase of a step cycle. The gastrocnemius EMG peak, during the second half of the stance phase, 'pushes off' the foot. At the end of the stance phase, when the foot is maximally extended, as during running (*Figure 9.14*), tibialis anterior EMG starts when gastrocnemius stops, so that at the beginning of the swing phase the foot is dorsiflexed to prevent the toes from dragging along the floor. In patients with supraspinal motor lesions, there are certain characteristic differences in this pattern of innervation during slow gait.

Gait in hemiparetic patients. Studies of movement patterns in hemiparetic patients[9, 23, 27, 56, 69, 78] have rarely been combined with EMG to analyse disturbed control of muscle activation. The few reported studies have found quite different and complex changes in leg muscle innervation patterns[7, 8, 12, 47–50, 58, 77]. Knutsson and Richards[53], in their investigation of patients with spastic hemiparesis of different severities due to various supraspinal lesions, described three different abnormal muscle activation patterns. In one, calf muscles were prematurely activated in the stance phase, supposedly due to enhanced stretch reflexes. In another, leg muscle EMG was either abolished or extremely small, and the third showed pathological co-activation of several or all muscles involved in locomotion. In other patients, activity was more complex and no specific pattern could be recognized. Different patterns could not be correlated with specific clinical symptoms, such as degree of paresis or spasticity, or with characteristics of the underlying lesion.

Because patients with predominantly paretic pattern (Knutsson and Richards' type II) do not show any spectacular EMG alterations, patients with muscular hypertonia were studied[21a]. EMGs recorded from patients with predominant spasticity during gait have features in common with Knutsson and Richards' first type. Because of circumduction of the extended leg, triceps surae is stretched very early after

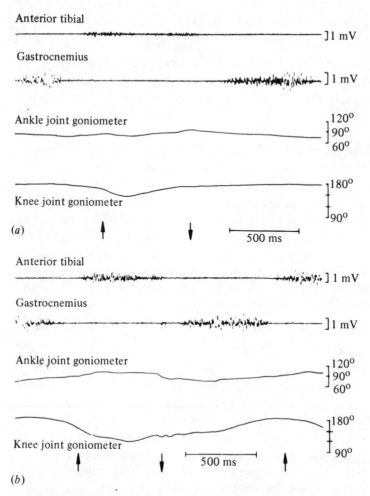

Anterior tibial

Gastrocnemius

Ankle joint goniometer

Knee joint goniometer

(*a*)   500 ms

Anterior tibial

Gastrocnemius

Ankle joint goniometer

Knee joint goniometer   500 ms

(*b*)

Figure 9.14 EMG from leg muscles of (*a*) normal subject and (*b*) patient with spastic paresis during walking on a treadmill, together with the goniometer record of ankle and knee angles. Arrows indicate beginning and cessation of contact

ground contact because of the pathologically plantar-flexed foot position; this results in an early increase of gastrocnemius EMG during the stance phase (*Figure 9.15*) which is usually not stronger than in normals. It was concluded that calf muscles in patients with spastic paresis are prematurely activated, not because of 'lowered threshold' for stretch reflexes, but because of earlier muscle stretch during the stance phase with an abnormally-placed foot lacking dorsiflexion[21a]. Because of the extreme and non-linear sensitivity of even normal

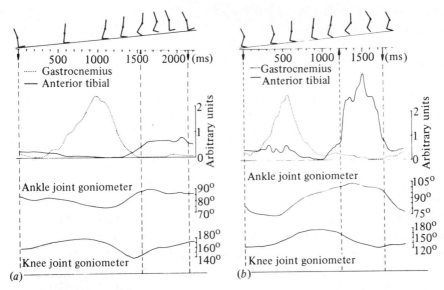

Figure 9.15 Comparison of rectified and averaged (30 trials) EMG from leg muscles together with goniometer records of ankle and knee joint in (*a*) normal subject and (*b*) patient with spastic paresis during walking on a treadmill with 10% incline. Arrows indicate beginning and cessation of ground contact

spindle primary endings in man to the onset of stretch[39], any lowering of threshold for stretch reflexes in spastic patients would presumably be due to increased CNS excitability to non-increased afferent inputs – Ia endings could hardly be more sensitive than normal. Furthermore, this same non-linear sensitivity would preclude the possibility of any reduction in reflex latency in spastic leg muscles.

In spastic patients, EMG activity in tibialis anterior during walking and in leg extensors during bicycling is strikingly stronger and of longer duration than in normals[5]. Although gastrocnemius EMG has ceased at the end of the stance phase and no mechanical obstruction of ankle joints was present, this increased tibialis activity is not sufficient to dorsiflex foot and toes[15, 21a]. Structural and histochemical changes in muscle fibers, which may occur during spasticity, could be partly responsible for increased muscle tone. Several biopsy studies[1, 24, 25] found distinct changes in muscle fiber filaments and enzymes; Edström[25] concluded selective disuse of high threshold motor units and increased usage of low threshold tonic units might be responsible for spasticity and rigidity.

Gait in patients with Parkinson's disease. Biomechanical analyses of Parkinsonian gait are very rare[52, 68] though clinical aspects are well known. Increased muscle tone (rigidity) can usually be observed and differentiated from spasticity – that Parkinsonian patients can more easily dorsiflex their feet and toes is demonstrable by goniometer recordings. The timing and coordination of leg muscle innervation during gait in these patients is, as in spastic patients, not significantly affected (*Figure 9.16*). They do show rather low gastrocnemius activity whereas tibialis EMG in untreated patients is clearly increased compared to normals or spastic patients[21a]. The physiological difference between spastic patients, who cannot dorsiflex their feet despite remarkable tibialis EMG, and untreated Parkinsonian patients, who counteract muscle rigidity by much stronger tibialis EMG, might be due to the paresis which is always connected with spasticity. Thus innervation patterns in leg muscles in both diseases are quite similar

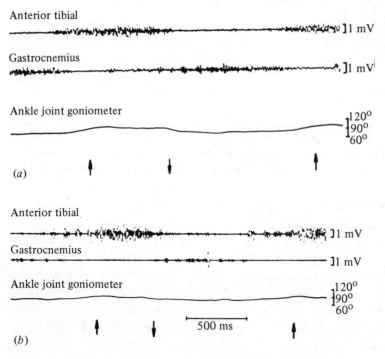

Figure 9.16 EMG from leg muscles together with goniometer record of ankle and knee joint in (*a*) a spastic and (*b*) a Parkinsonian patient walking on a treadmill. Note EMG-synchronization at a rate of about 5–6 per second. Arrows indicate beginning and cersation of contact

and muscle hypertonia cannot simply be explained by increased EMG activity in, or co-contraction of, antagonists[74, 75, 85]. There is also no direct evidence from recordings of Ia afferent discharges in man to support frequent suggestions that in spastic or rigid patients the spindle primary endings have increased sensitivity to stretch[11, 83].

Regulation of posture and balance in patients with motor system disorders

Posture. Upright stance is normally controlled by information from visual, vestibular and proprioceptive systems and when one of these afferent pathways is defective, its influence on postural stabilization can be compensated for. However, when two systems are impaired, stance is destabilized and regulating mechanisms due to the remaining control system can be investigated. In patients with tabes dorsalis, or normal subjects during ischemic blockade of group I afferents, stance

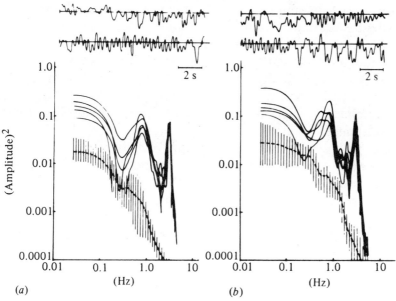

Figure 9.17 Fourier power spectra of anterior–posterior sway in a patient with late cortical cerebellar atrophy with (*a*) eyes open and (*b*) eyes closed. At the top are segments of the original recording. Recordings obtained on five consecutive days are shown and compared with the average (interrupted line) and the range of 15 normals (shaded area). (After Mauritz, Dichgans and Hufschmidt[62])

is relatively unstable[63]: while standing on a stable support with eyes closed, they have a large body-sway with predominant frequency of 1 Hz or less. Nashner[71] concluded that these slow oscillations are due to long latency (200–300 ms), vestibularly-induced leg muscle innervation.

Body sway of patients with postural ataxia due to cerebellar lesions[62] can be clearly distinguished from this pathognomonic 1 Hz sway of 'sensory ataxia'. Patients with late cortical atrophy of the anterior cerebellum have typical oscillations around 3 Hz in an anterior–posterior direction (*Figure 9.17*) which, if not present spontaneously, can be evoked by short sudden destabilization. Two other types of cerebellar lesion were seen. Patients with a lesion of cerebellar hemispheres showed only slight postural instability without directional preference. Patients with posterior vermal and flocculo-nodular lesions were very unstable without preferred axis or frequency of instability.

Balance. Analysis of postural sway during stance on solid ground is analogous to a Romberg test during a regular neurological examination. Patients with minor lesions in the motor system show no specific, pathognomonic disturbances of posture. A more provocative test involves the more demanding task of standing on a seesaw. As described (*see* p. 209), anterior–posterior body sway of normal subjects in this situation with a predominant frequency of 4–5 Hz is due to spinal stretch-reflex mechanisms for maintaining equilibrium when small disturbances occur[18].

Patients with slower nerve conduction velocities have prolonged stretch responses so their balancing oscillations should be slower compared with normals. Clinically 'healthy' relatives of patients with Charcot-Marie-Tooth disease, whose nerve conduction velocities were reduced to about half normal, have significantly slower balancing oscillations[64]. Their predominant body sway, around 3 Hz, naturally has larger amplitude and they are more unstable compared with normals (*Figure 9.18*). However, postural sway standing on solid ground was normal in these subjects who were still without clinical signs of their hereditary disease.

In patients with loss of sensation in both legs, the balancing test helped discriminate the type of underlying disturbance[64]. With impaired proprioceptive input from leg muscles, patients have very slow (around 0.5 Hz) large body sway; balancing oscillations around 4–5 Hz are lacking because of a defective reflex system. Patients with dorsal column lesions have nearly normal fast balancing movements. Patients with bilateral loss of vestibular function show no abnormality on the Romberg test and have normal fast balancing oscillations but are unable to stand on the seesaw without support when their eyes are closed. Beside spinal stretch-reflex mechanisms, other regulating systems must be needed to maintain equilibrium. In the dark or with eyes closed, the vestibular system, possibly in combination with long-loop reflexes, may be the regulating mechanism responsible for lower frequency ranges of body movement.

These convenient clinical neurophysiological tests of balance provide additional helpful information in patients who show no abnormality in the Romberg test. Quantitative analysis of body sway using both tests aids in differential diagnosis.

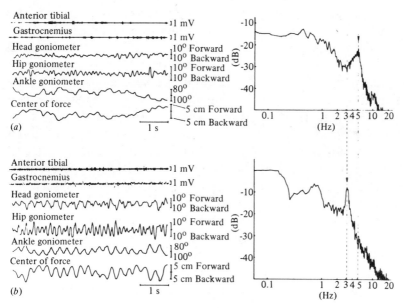

Figure 9.18 Original recording of EMG, anterior–posterior head and hip movements, ankle angle displacement and center of force (*left*) as well as the corresponding Fourier spectrum of the anterior–posterior displacements of center of force (*right*) in (*a*) typical normal subject and (*b*) patient with peroneal muscular atrophy. Characteristic frequency peak of the rapid balancing movements in the normal and the patients is indicated by interrupted lines. (From Mauritz, Dietz and Haller[64], courtesy of the Editor and publisher, *Journal of Neurology, Neurosurgery and Psychiatry*)

Conclusions

By careful application of discriminating clinical neurophysiological techniques to the study of movement and its disorders, we are beginning to get a glimpse of some of the mechanisms and strategies employed by the human CNS. Besides the obvious relevance of electrophysiological studies in normal human beings for understanding physiological mechanisms responsible for simple and complex movements, similar investigations are also important for demonstrating pathophysiological bases for disordered motor control.

In this review, the authors have tried to point out, on the basis of documented, reasonably specific dysfunctions, a number of 'mechanisms' – that is conceptualizations of hypothetical control systems which might constitute the building blocks of the motor system. Ideas are lacking about how the CNS uses all its known constituents to provide our manipulation of the outside world – which structures and pathways are of prime importance for which movements, what is its 'game plan'? Perhaps some of the mechanisms hypothesized will interest or guide neurophysiologists in designing their experiments. At the very least, studies such as those reviewed should limit speculation; both clinicians and physiologists can now speculate about clearly defined observations, for example, the statistical behavior of single motor units in a given condition, rather than on the basis of gross and subjective bedside impressions such as 'spasticity' or 'tremor'.

With increased knowledge of the pathophysiology of motor control, it is assumed that better treatments for patients will become possible. The electrophysiological studies described above, especially those which, after appropriate training, can be carried out by clinical neurophysiologists in a relatively simple and convenient fashion, also serve as improved diagnostic tools; earlier diagnoses are now possible and subtle alterations in performance, related to various therapeutic endeavors, or to the passage of time, can be documented.

References

1 AHLQUIST, G., LANDIN, S. and WROBLEWSKI, R. Ultrastructure of skeletal muscle in patients with Parkinson's disease and upper motor lesions. *Laboratory Investigation*, **32**, 673–679 (1975)

2 ALLUM, J. H. J., DIETZ, V. and FREUND, H.-J. Neuronal mechanisms underlying physiological tremor. *Journal of Neurophysiology*, **41**, 557–571 (1978)

3 ANDREASSEN, S. Single motor unit recording. In *Spasticity: Disordered Motor Control*, edited by R. G. Feldman, R. R. Young and W. P. Koella, 205–218. Chicago, Year Book Medical Publishers (1980)

4 ANDREASSEN, S. and ROSENFALCK, A. Impaired regulation of the firing pattern of single motor units. *Muscle and Nerve*, **1**, 416–418 (1978)

5 BENECKE, R. and CONRAD, B. Muscle activity patterns in spasticity during voluntary limb movements. *Acta Neurologica Scandinavica*, **60** (supplementum 73), 97 (1979)

6 BERNSTEIN, N. *Coordination and Regulation of Movements*. New York, Pergamon Press (1967)

7 BOGARDH, E. and RICHARDS, G. Gait analysis and re-learning of gait control in hemiplegic patients. In *Seventh International Congress, World Confederation for Physical Therapy*, (Montreal 1974), London, World Confederation for Physical Therapy, 443–453 (1974)

8 BRUNNSTROM, S. Recording gait patterns of adult hemiplegic patients. *Journal of the American Physical Therapy Association*, **44**, 11–18 (1964)

9 BRUNNSTROM, S. Motor testing procedures in hemiplegia. *American Journal of Physical Therapy*, **46**, 357–375 (1966)

10 BUDINGEN, H.-J. and FREUND, H.-J. The relationship between the rate of rise of isometric tension and motor unit recruitment in a human forearm muscle. *Pflügers Archiv*, **362**, 61–67 (1976)

11 BURKE, D. A reassessment of the muscle spindle contribution to muscle tone in normal and spastic man. In *Spasticity: Disordered Motor Control*, edited by R. G. Feldman, R. R. Young and W. P. Koella, 261–278. Chicago, Year Book Medical Publishers (1980)

12 CARLSÖÖ, S., DAHLLÖF, A.-G. and HOLM, J. Kinetic analysis of the gait in patients with hemiparesis and patients with intermittent claudication. *Scandinavian Journal of Rehabilitation Medicine*, **6**, 166–179 (1974)

13 DESMEDT, J. E. and GODAUX, E. Ballistic contractions in fast or slow human muscles: discharge patterns of single motor units. *Journal of Physiology*, **285**, 185–196 (1978)

14 DESMEDT, J. E. and GODAUX, E. Voluntary motor commands in human ballistic movements. *Annals of Neurology*, **5**, 415–421 (1979)

15 DICHGANS, J., MAURTIZ, K.-H., ALLUM, J. H. J. and BRANDT, TH. Postural sway in normals and ataxic patients: analysis of the stabilizing and destabilizing effects of vision. *Agressologie*, **17C,** 15–24 (1976)

16 DIETZ, V., BISCHOFBERGER, E., WITA, C. and FREUND, H.-J. Correlation between discharges of two simultaneously recorded motor units and physiological tremor. *Electroencephalography and Clinical Neurophysiology*, **40,** 97–105 (1976)

17 DIETZ, V., HILLESHEIMER, W. and FREUND, H.-J. Correlation between tremor, voluntary contraction and firing pattern of motor units in Parkinson's disease. *Journal of Neurology, Neurosurgery and Psychiatry*, **37,** 927–937 (1974)

18 DIETZ, V., MAURITZ, K.-H. and DICHGANS, J. Body oscillations in balancing due to segmental stretch reflex activity. *Experimental Brain Research*, **40,** 89–95 (1980)

19 DIETZ, V. and NOTH, J. Pre-innervation and stretch responses of triceps brachii in man falling with and without visual control. *Brain Research*, **142,** 576–579 (1978)

20 DIETZ, V. and NOTH, J. Spinal stretch reflexes of triceps surae in active and passive movements. *Journal of Physiology*, **284,** 180–181 (1978)

21 DIETZ, V., NOTH, J. and SCHMIDTBLEICHER, D. Interaction between pre-activity and stretch reflex in human triceps brachii during landing from forward falls. *Journal of Physiology*, **311,** 113–125 (1981)

21a DIETZ, V., QUINTERN, J. and BERGER, W. Electrophysiological studies of gait in spasticity and rigidity. Evidence that alterated mechanical properties of muscle contribute to hypertonia. *Brain* (in press)

22 DIETZ, V., SCHMIDTBLEICHER, D. and NOTH, J. Neuronal mechanisms of human locomotion. *Journal of Neurophysiology*, **42,** 1212–1222 (1979)

23 DRILLIS, R. Objective recording and biomechanics of pathological gait. *Annals of the New York Academy of Sciences*, **74,** 86–109 (1958)

24 EDSTRÖM, L. Histochemical changes in upper motor lesions, Parkinsonism and disuse; differential effect on white and red muscle fibres. *Experientia*, **24,** 916–918 (1968)

25 EDSTRÖM, L. Selective changes in the sizes of red and white muscle fibres in upper motor lesions and Parkinsonism. *Journal of Neurological Sciences*, **11,** 537–550 (1970)

26 ENGBERG, I. and LUNDBERG, A. An electromyographic analysis of muscular activity in the hindlimb of the cat during unrestrained locomotion. *Acta Physiologica Scandinavica*, **75,** 614–630 (1969)

27 FINLEY, F. R. and KARPOVICH, P. V. Electrogoniometric analysis of

normal and pathological gait. *Research Quarterly*, **35**, 379–384 (1964)

28 FREUND, H.-J. and BUDINGEN, H. J. The relationship between speed and amplitude of the fastest voluntary contractions of human arm muscles. *Experimental Brain Research*, **31**, 1–12 (1978)

29 FREUND, H.-J., BUDINGEN, H.-J. and DIETZ, V. Activity of single motor units from human forearm muscles during voluntary isometric contractions. *Journal of Neurophysiology*, **38**, 933–946 (1975)

30 FREUND, H.-J., DIETZ, V., WITA, C. W. and KAPP, H. Discharge characteristics of single motor units in normal subjects and patients with supraspinal motor disturbances. In *New Developments in Electromyography and Clinical Neurophysiology*, **3**, edited by J. E. Desmedt, 242–250. Basel, S. Karger (1973)

31 GELFAND, I. M., GURFINKEL, V. S., FOMIN, S. V. and TSTETLIN, M. L. (Editors) *Models of the Structural-Functional Organization of Certain Biological Systems*. Cambridge, MIT Press (1971)

32 GOTTLIEB, G. L. and AGARWAL, G. C. Response to sudden torques about ankle in man: the myotatic reflex. *Journal of Neurophysiology*, **42**, 91–106 (1979)

33 GREENWOOD, R. and HOPKINS, A. Landing from an unexpected fall and a voluntary step. *Brain*, **99**, 375–386 (1976)

34 GRILLNER, S. Locomotion in vertebrates: central and mechanisms and reflex interaction. *Physiological Reviews*, **55**, 247–304 (1975)

35 GROWDON, J. H., YOUNG, R. R. and SHAHANI, B. T. The differential diagnosis of tremor in Parkinson's disease. *Transactions of the American Neurological Association*, **101**, 197–199 (1976)

36 GURFINKEL, V. S., LIPSHITS, M. I., MORI, S. and POPOV, K. E. Postural reactions to the controlled sinusoidal displacement of the supporting platform. *Agressologie*, **17B**, 71–76 (1976)

37 GURFINKEL, V. S., LIPSHITS, M. I., MORI, S. and POPOV, K. E. The state of stretch reflex during quiet standing in man. In *Understanding the Stretch Reflex*, edited by S. Homma, *Progress in Brain Research*, **44**, 473–486 (1976)

38 HAGBARTH, K.-E., HÄGGLUND, J. V., WALLIN, E. U. and YOUNG, R. R. Grouped spindle and EMG responses to abrupt wrist extension movements in man. *Journal of Physiology*, (in press)

39 HAGBARTH, K.-E., YOUNG, R. R. Participation of the stretch reflex in human physiological tremor. *Brain*, **102**, 509–526 (1979)

40 HAGBARTH, K.-E., YOUNG, R. R., HÄGGLUND, J. and WALLIN, U. Spindle and EMG responses to sudden displacements of the human wrist. *Neurology*, **30**, 373 (1980)

41 HALLETT, M., SHAHANI, B. T. and YOUNG, R. R. EMG analysis of stereotyped voluntary movements in man. *Journal of Neurology, Neurosurgery and Psychiatry*, **38,** 1154–1162 (1975)

42 HALLETT, M., SHAHANI, B. T. and YOUNG, R. R. EMG analysis of patients with cerebellar deficits. *Journal of Neurology, Neurosurgery and Psychiatry*, **38,** 1163–1169 (1975)

43 HALLETT, M., SHAHANI, B. T. and YOUNG, R. R.Analysis of stereotyped voluntary movements at the elbow in patients with Parkinson's disease. *Journal of Neurology, Neurosurgery and Psychiatry*, **40,** 1129–1135 (1977)

44 HAMMOND, P. H., MERTON, P. A. and SUTTON, G. G. Nervous gradation of muscular contraction. *British Medical Bulletin*, **12,** 214–218 (1956)

45 HENNEMAN, E., SHAHANI, B. T. and YOUNG, R. R. Voluntary control of human motor units. In *The Motor System – Neurophysiology and Muscle Mechanisms*, edited by M. Shahani, 73–78. Amsterdam, Elsevier (1976)

46 HENNEMAN, E., SOMJEN, G. and CARPENTER, D. O. Functional significance of cell size in spinal motoneurones. *Journal of Neurophysiology*, **28,** 560–580 (1965)

47 HIRSCHBERG, G. G. and NATHANSON, M. Electromyographic recording of muscular activity of normal and spastic gait. *Archives of Physical Medicine*, **33,** 217–224 (1952)

48 HOEFER, P. F. A. Electromyographic study of the motor system in man. *Monatsschrift für Psychiatrie und Neurologie*, **117,** 241–256 (1949)

49 HOEFER, P. F. A. Physiological mechanisms in spasticity. *British Journal of Physical Medicine*, **15,** 88–90 (1952)

50 HOEFER, P. F. A. and PUTMAN, T. J. Action potentials of muscles in 'spastic' conditions. *Archives of Neurology and Psychiatry (Chicago)*, **43,** 704–725 (1940)

51 JUNG, R. and DIETZ, V. Übung und Seitendominanz der menschlichen Willkürmotorik. *Archiv für Psychiatrie und Nervenkrankheiten*, **222,** 87–116 (1976)

52 KNUTSSON, E. An analysis of Parkinsonian gait. *Brain*, **95,** 475–486 (1972)

53 KNUTSSON, E. and RICHARDS, C. Different types of disturbed motor control in gait of hemiparetic patients. *Brain*, **102,** 405–430 (1979)

54 KOTS, J. M. and ZHUKOV, V. I. Supraspinal control over segmental centers of antagonist muscles in man. III. Tuning of spinal reciprocal inhibition system during organization preceding voluntary movement. *Biophysics*, **16,** 1085–1091 (1971)

55 LESTIENNE, F., BERTHOZ, A., MASCOT, V. and KOITCHEVA, V. Effects postureaux induits par une scene visuelle en mouvement lineaire. *Agressologie*, **17C**, 37–46 (1976)

56 LIBERSON, W. T., HOLMQUEST, H. J. and HALLS, A. Accelerographic study of gait. *Archives of Physical Medicine and Rehabilitation*, **43**, 547–551 (1962)

57 MAREY, E. J. La machine animale. *Locomotion Terrestre et Aerienne*. Paris, Germer Bailliere (1873)

58 MARKS, M. and HIRSCHBERG, G. G. Analysis of hemiplegic gait. *Annals of New York Academy of Sciences*, **74**, 59–77 (1958)

59 MARSDEN, C. D., MEADOWS, J. C. and MERTON, P. A. Isolated single motor units in human muscles and their rate of discharge during maximal voluntary effort. *Journal of Physiology*, **217**, 12 (1971)

60 MARSDEN, C. D., MERTON, P. A. and MORTON, H. B. Servo action in human voluntary movement. *Nature*, **238**, 140–143 (1972)

61 MARSDEN, C. D., MERTON, P. A. and MORTON, H. B. Servo action in the human thumb. *Journal of Physiology*, **257**, 1–44 (1976)

62 MAURITZ, K.-H., DICHGANS, J. and HUFSCHMIDT, A. Quantitative analysis of stance in late cortical cerebellar atrophy of the anterior lobe and other forms of cerebellar ataxia. *Brain*, **102**, 461–482 (1979)

63 MAURITZ, K.-H. and DIETZ, V. Characteristics of postural instability induced by ischemic blocking of leg afferents. *Experimental Brain Research*, **38**, 117–119 (1980)

64 MAURITZ, K.-H., DIETZ, V. and HALLER, M. Balancing as a clinical test in the differential diagnosis of sensory-motor disorders. *Journal of Neurology, Neurosurgery and Psychiatry*, **43**, 407–412 (1980)

65 MELVILL-JONES, G. and WATT, D. G. D. Observations on the control of stepping and hopping movements in man. *Journal of Physiology*, **219**, 709–727 (1971)

66 MELVILL-JONES, G. and WATT, D. G. D. Muscular control of landing from unexpected falls in man. *Journal of Physiology*, **219**, 729–737 (1971)

67 MILNER-BROWN, H. S., STEIN, R. B. and LEE, R. G. Synchronization of human motor units: possible roles of exercise and supraspinal reflexes. *Electroencephalography and Clinical Neurophysiology*, **38**, 245–254 (1975)

68 MURRAY, M. P. Gait as a total pattern of movement. *American Journal of Physical Medicine*, **46**, 290–332 (1967)

69 MURRAY, M. P. and CLARKSON, B. H. The vertical pathways of the foot during level walking. II. Clinical examples of distorted pathways. *Journal of the American Physical Therapy Association*, **46**, 590–599 (1966)

70 NASHNER, L. M. Sensory feed-back in human posture control. *Sc.D. Thesis*, Center for Space Research, Massachusetts Institute of Technology, Boston, USA (1970)

71 NASHNER, L. M. Adaptive reflexes controlling human posture. *Experimental Brain Research*, **26,** 59–72 (1976)

72 NASHNER, L. M. and BERTHOZ, A. Visual contribution to rapid motor responses during posture control. *Brain Research*, **150,** 403–407 (1978)

73 NASHNER, L. M., WOOLLACOTT, M. and TUMA, G. Organization of rapid responses to postural and locomotor-like perturbations of standing man. *Experimental Brain Research*, **36,** 463–476 (1979)

74 NATHAN, P. Some comments on spasticity and rigidity. In *New Developments in Electromyography and Clinical Neurophysiology*, **3,** edited by J. E. Desmedt, 13–14. Basel, S. Karger (1973)

75 NOEL, G. Clinical changes in muscle tone. In *New Developments in Electromyography and Clinical Neurophysiology*, **3,** edited by J. E. Desmedt, 15–19. Basel, S. Karger (1973)

76 NOTH, J. and DIETZ, V. Spinal stretch reflexes in self initiated falls and in running movements. *Agressologie*, **20B,** 159–160 (1979)

77 PEAT, M., DUBO, H. I. C., WINTER, D. A., QUANBURY, A. O., STEINKE, T. and GRAHAME, R. Electromyographic temporal analysis of gait: hemiplegic locomotion. *Archives of Physical Medicine and Rehabilitation*, **57,** 421–425 (1976)

78 PERRY, J. The mechanics of walking in hemiplegia. *Clinical Orthopaedics and Related Research*, **63,** 23–31 (1969)

79 SHAHANI, B. T. and YOUNG, R. R. Physiological and pharmacological aids in the differential diagnosis of tremor. *Journal of Neurology, Neurosurgery and Psychiatry*, **39,** 772–783 (1972)

80 SHAHANI, B. T. and YOUNG, R. R. Asterixis – a disorder of the neural mechanisms underlying sustained muscle contraction. In *The Motor System – Neurophysiology and Muscle Mechanisms*, edited by M. Shahani, 301–306. Amsterdam, Elsevier (1976)

81 SHAHANI, B. T. and YOUNG, R. R. Action tremors: a clinical neurophysiological review. In *Physiological Tremor, Pathological Tremors and Clonus*, edited by J. E. Desmedt, *Progress in Clinical Neurophysiology*, **5,** 603–617. Basel, S. Karger (1978)

82 SHAHANI, B. T., YOUNG, R. R. and HARRISON, J. L. Velocity dependent centrally programmed human voluntary activity. *Society for Neuroscience Abstracts*, **6,** 464 (1980)

83 VALLBO, A. B., HAGBARTH, K.-E., TOREBJÖRK, H. E. and WALLIN, B. G. Proprioceptive, somatosensory and sympathetic activity in human peripheral nerves. *Physiological Reviews*, **59**, 919–957 (1979)

84 WACHHOLDER, K. Untersuchungen über Innervation und Koordination der Bewegung mit Hilfe der Aktionsströme. *Pflügers Archiv*, **199**, 595–625 (1923)

85 WEDDELL, G., FEINSTEIN, B. and PATTLE, R. E. The electrical activity of voluntary muscle in man under normal and pathological conditions. *Brain*, **67**, 178–257 (1944)

86 WELFORD, A. T. On sequencing of action. *Brain Research*, **71**, 381–392 (1974)

87 WETZEL, M. D. and STUART, D. G. Ensemble characteristics of cat locomotion and its neural control. In *Progress in Neurobiology*, **7**, 1–98, Oxford, Pergamon Press (1976)

88 YOUNG, R. R. and HAGBARTH, K.-E. Physiological tremor enchanced by manoeuvres affecting the segmental stretch reflex. *Journal of Neurology, Neurosurgery and Psychiatry*, **43**, 248–256 (1980)

89 YOUNG, R. R. and SHAHANI, B. T. Single unit behavior in human muscle afferent and efferent systems. In *The Extrapyramidal System and its Disorders*, edited by L. J. Poirier, T. L. Sourkes and P. J. Bedard, *Advances in Neurology*, **24**, 175–183. New York, Raven Press (1979)

90 YOUNG, R. R. and SHAHANI, B. T. Clinical neurophysiological aspects of post-hypoxic intention myoclonus. In *Cerebral Hypoxia and Its Consequences*, edited by S. Fahn, J. N. Davis and L. P. Rowland, *Advances in Neurology*, **26**, 85–105. New York, Raven Press (1979)

91 YOUNG, R. R. and SHAHANI, B. T. A clinical neurophysiological analysis of single motor unit discharge patterns in spasticity. In *Spasticity: Disordered Motor Control*, edited by R. G. Feldman, R. R. Young and W. P. Koella, 219–231. Chicago, Year Book Medical Publishers (1980)

10

Visual evoked potentials

A. M. Halliday and W. I. McDonald

Introduction

Before taking up any new electrophysiological technique for clinical testing it is sensible to ask what the method has to offer and what kind of investment in new equipment and training is required in order to make it available. This chapter will examine visual evoked potential (VEP) recording from both these points of view. At the outset, however, it can be said that VEP testing has already proved useful to the clinician in a number of areas, the most important of which are (1) the diagnosis of demyelinating disease, and in particular the detection of clinically 'silent' plaques in the optic nerve; (2) the detection of early compressive lesions affecting the visual pathways; (3) the differentiation of functional and organic visual loss; and (4) the elucidation of the underlying nature and site of the lesion in cases of undiagnosed visual impairment. Once the necessary equipment is installed and the technique established, it can be used to investigate a variety of other types of cases but the foregoing applications will in general provide the main current justifications for embarking on the use of the VEP for the first time.

The technique demands a good deal of additional equipment, not normally found in the traditional EEG department, including pattern stimulators, recording amplifiers with an adequate high frequency response, and averaging computers. Learning to read the VEP records produced with this equipment is a relatively easy task, although skill in dealing with the more difficult or equivocal records will only come with considerable experience. As with all other clinical methods, the amount of useful information obtained will depend on the degree of sophistication of the technique. A simple set-up with one or two recording channels will provide useful information in the 70 per cent or so straightforward records encountered in the responses from patients with demyelinating disease. To deal effectively with the minority of more difficult records requires a more elaborate technique, with multi-channel recording and a resort to recording the responses to more than one type of stimulus.

In either case, it is essential for the laboratory doing the tests to establish its own normal values at the outset. This is done by recording a group of healthy subjects (at least 20) using the identical set-up to that which it is intended to use on patients. In this way the variability of the normal mean latency and amplitude of the major components of the VEP can be determined, allowing one to set up a criterion, e.g. ± 2.5 standard deviations from the mean, to determine the upper or lower limit of normal. Since there are small, but significant, differences between the mean amplitude and latency of the pattern VEP in men and women[28, 52], it is worthwhile, if feasible, to do this separately for the two sexes if the maximum test sensitivity is to be achieved. Where elderly patients are to be tested, these normal controls should be extended to include a group of age-matched controls, since the normal latency increases somewhat in the elderly. Age-matched controls are not necessary, however, for recordings on patients between the ages of 16 and 50 years. The pattern of normal variability to be expected has already been well established by published data[29], but this does not preclude the need for each laboratory to establish its own norms, as the mean amplitude and latency of the response is sensitive to many stimulus parameters, such as field size, brightness, check size and contrast.

The technique of recording visual evoked potentials depends upon using an accurately timed and reasonably sharp-fronted visual stimulus to produce a synchronous afferent volley in the visual pathways from retina to visual cortex, where its arrival produces a detectable cortical potential of a few microvolts with a characteristic waveform. For a suitable stimulus under standardized conditions the cortical VEP is stereotyped and repeatable and a large number of these responses can be summed or averaged to give a clear record of the response, which would be otherwise obscured in single trial recording by the random background activity of the EEG. Typically one or two hundred summated trials are required to obtain an averaged VEP. Electromyographic activity, particularly from the paraspinal muscles attached to the inion, is best eliminated as far as possible by ensuring that the patient's neck is relaxed, e.g. by providing an adequate head rest if the subject is sitting, or recording the subject supine with either an overhead stimulating display or a display to one side viewed via a 45° mirror.

Visual stimulators

Suitable stimuli which have been employed in clinical testing include repetitive flashes from a gas discharge tube and abrupt changes of a viewed pattern, such as reversal of a black-and-white checkerboard or grating (*pattern reversal*) or the sudden appearance or disappearance of a pattern on a blank screen of equal mean luminance (*pattern onset* or *pattern offset*). Until 1970, flash stimulation was almost exclusively used for clinical VEP recording[24], but since the introduction of pattern stimulation[15, 23, 38] the flash stimulus has been largely superseded in clinical testing by the checkerboard reversal stimulus. Although a great variety of methods have been used to generate the pattern reversal stimulus[1], the three most commonly employed in the clinic have been:

(1) a slide projector and mirror;
(2) a television screen display; and
(3) an array of light-emitting diodes.

Translucent screen projector method

The slide of a black-and-white checkerboard is projected by way of a rotatable mirror onto the back of a translucent screen, viewed from in front by the patient at a distance of about 1 m[4, 33, 34, 35]. By rotating the mirror through a small angle, the checkerboard is abruptly displaced sideways by one square, so that the black squares become white and the white, black (pattern shift). Alternatively two projectors, fitted with fast, electrically-controlled shutters can be used, with a slide of a checkerboard and its photographic negative. Switching from one projector to the other provides true pattern reversal[38, 49]. There are problems, however, in getting adequate photographic registration of the two images over a large field, which make this two-projector technique more difficult to set up than the moving-mirror technique. Although pattern shift and pattern reversal stimuli differ in important respects, the two responses appear indistinguishable, provided the transition time is sufficiently short and well-matched, e.g. 10 ms.

Television display

A black-and-white checkerboard pattern is generated on the face of a television monitor by means of a pattern generator[2, 20, 41, 45, 52]. By inverting the pattern abruptly, the checkerboard reversal is completed in the time taken for the oscilloscope spot to completely traverse the screen (frame time). The reversal may be initiated at the start of the frame scan, but this has the disadvantage, where the frame rate is linked to the mains, of roughly synchronizing the stimulus with the main frequency, so that any mains hum picked up by the amplifiers is averaged with the response. Alternatively, the reversal of the display may be started at any point on the screen, unsynchronized with the frame rate or mains. This introduces some latency 'jitter' which slightly degrades the response, increasing the intra-trial variance[45, 52]. However, the mean peak latency between averages of 200 or more responses is still extremely consistent in any given individual[45, 52], with a test–retest reliability within 1–2 ms, even over a period of some months[52]. The TV method has the advantage of giving electronic control (at the touch of a switch) of many stimulus parameters, such as contrast, check size and field size. Independent half-field and quadrant stimulation is also easily available.

LED display

A display of a light-emitting diode (LED) matrix is wired in two sets, to come on alternately[21, 50, 52]. Although the contour of the individual diodes is usually round, square-faced diodes are obtainable, suitable for the construction of LED checkerboards. This method has the advantage that very rapid switching rates can be achieved. The colour is, however, limited to red or green and the maximum luminance levels are also somewhat restricted.

From the point of view of clinical testing, the optimal stimulus should provide low normal variability and high sensitivity to pathological changes. On both these counts the checkerboard pattern reversal stimulus is superior to the flash stimulus [20, 33, 34, 39, 45, 48]. The flash response has a much more variable waveform in different individuals than the pattern reversal response and also shows a less marked delay in patients with demyelinating disease affecting the optic nerve. However, the flash response possesses the merit of robustness, and is often obtainable in patients whose visual acuity is so much reduced that the pattern response is unobtainable. It can also be recorded through the closed lids and in uncooperative or comatose patients. Furthermore, in suspected retinopathy the flash electroretinogram (ERG) can give valuable additional evidence concerning retinal abnormalities[3, 5, 29, 42]. The merits of the pattern and flash VEPs are therefore in many respects complementary and the clinical neurophysiologist will be well advised to retain both stimuli in his armamentarium[39].

Recording technique

Electrode montages

The VEP can be recorded by scalp electrodes placed over the occiput. The response to either flash or pattern stimulation is usually of maximal amplitude in the midline about 5–6 cm above the inion and this is the optimal position for the active electrode where only one channel of recording is available. The response has a similar waveform, amplitude and spatial distribution whichever eye is stimulated[9], and this allows much subtler changes to be detected where the abnormality is limited to the response from one eye, since this can be directly compared with the response from the unaffected eye. This is a great advantage, particularly with regard to amplitude changes, since the variability of absolute amplitude in the healthy population is very large, whereas with well-controlled fixation the difference in amplitude between the responses from the two eyes in any one individual is very small. Comparison of the responses from each eye is therefore a powerful technique for detecting abnormalities secondary to lesions of the eye and the optic nerve on one side. In such cases, much of the relevant information will be obtainable by single-channel recording with an active electrode 5 cm above the inion.

With more posterior lesions, involving the fibres of the retino-cortical pathways in or behind the optic chiasma, the abnormality involves the responses from both eyes and affects differentially the cortical response generated by the left and right occipital lobes. Under these circumstances, the most significant changes are in the topography of the response over the back of the head[6, 7, 9, 10] and multichannel recording (preferably combined with a resort to half-field stimulation) is essential in order to make use of this information. In the authors' own practice, an electrode montage based on a transverse row of five occipital electrodes is used. The midline electrode is still placed 5 cm above the inion but additional pairs of electrodes are employed 5 cm and 10 cm out on each side. Three further channels are usually employed, with midline electrodes 2.5 cm above the inion, at the inion itself and 5 cm below, respectively. Other electrodes may also be used to record the response more anteriorly (e.g. 10 cm above the inion). All are recorded in monopolar mode with reference to a common mid-frontal electrode (Fz).

The choice of an indifferent reference electrode is important in recording the VEP. The earlobe or mastoid electrode often favoured by electroencephalographers is not to be recommended, as it is well within the area from which the response can be elicited and is, moreover, differentially affected by upper and lower field responses[38, 49]. Other references on the posterior half of the head have been recommended, such as the vertex or ipsilateral parietal electrodes, but these also are within the area from which the widespread VEP can be recorded[26, 30]. They are therefore liable to lead to a distortion of the response, particularly where the question of abnormal asymmetry is at issue. It is for these reasons that, in the authors' laboratory, all active electrodes are referred to a common mid-frontal electrode. This site is chosen to be well outside the area from which the occipital VEP can be recorded and to be situated in the midline, so that pathological asymmetries are minimally affected by the electrode montage. It is true that the mid-frontal reference is more vulnerable to eye movement artefact, but this is not a major problem in practice and such eye movements can easily be monitored by a pair of peri-orbital electrodes, which also provide a means of recording the ERG to both flash and pattern stimulation.

A ground electrode is also required and this can be conveniently located anywhere on the head (e.g. the vertex), the choice of location not being in any way critical.

Some laboratories have favoured bipolar recording, which displays the slope of the potential gradient between adjacent electrodes of the bipolar chain, but this approach obscures the common features of the underlying response at neighbouring electrodes[6, 26, 30]. Since the information provided by the bipolar montage can be easily derived from the monopolar records, but not vice versa, the latter recording technique is to be preferred.

Single or multichannel recording?

Where only one channel is available, the single active electrode should be placed 5 cm above the inion in the midline. Where only four channels are available, the midline channel can be combined with records from lateral electrodes 6 cm out on each side and a lower electrode situated at the inion. Where eight channels are available, the montage employing a transverse row of five electrodes, and three extra midline electrodes centred on the inion, is to be recommended.

Amplifiers

To adequately record the pattern or flash VEP, a band-width of *at least* 5–100 Hz is needed. In the authors' own laboratory, where a rather more conservative approach is adopted, the VEP is recorded with an amplifier time constant of one second and a high frequency cut of −3 dB at 2 kHz. It should be emphasized that with this arrangement the high frequency response of the amplifier does not represent the band-width of the final average, as the sampling rate used in the averager is either 400 or 800 Hz, giving a high frequency cut-off at approximately 160 Hz and 320 HZ respectively, There is a theoretical advantage, however, in having a higher frequency response from the recording amplifier than is used in the final average, since the high frequency noise helps in ensuring an effective cancellation of the random noise input in arriving at the final average.

Signal averagers

A variety of commercial averagers are now available, ranging from single-channel averagers designed for use in recording nerve action potentials to small on-line laboratory computers with a multi-channel facility. In almost all the current averagers, including the newer generation of microprocessor-based equipment, the input signal undergoes analogue-digital conversion before processing. Automatic rejection of inputs exceeding a certain predetermined size is often also provided as an artefact rejection facility. Most also provide the facility of measuring the amplitude and latency between points on the waveform, selected by manually adjustable cursors. Many averagers also have the facility of providing hard copy records by means of an XY plotter or an ink-writing, ultraviolet or photographic recorder.

Measurement of response parameters

Each record has to be calibrated for the amplifier gain setting used and this is best done by averaging a square wave signal of a size comparable to the VEP (e.g. 5 or 10 μV) using exactly the same filter and gain settings as are used in the VEP recording. This should preferably be done before each record, or at least at the beginning and end of each recording session. Where an automatic cursoring facility is available, the response parameters are then easily measured. Such a calibration provides a permanent record of the gain and frequency response actually achieved, as well as a rapid warning indication of any malfunction in the equipment or accidental alteration of the desired settings. The successive component peaks of the VEP are by convention labelled by their polarity (P or N) followed by their normal mean latency (e.g. $\overline{\text{P100}}$ or $\overline{\text{N145}}$). To distinguish this 'notational' latency from the actual latency recorded the component identifier is printed with a bar over it[19]. There is then nothing paradoxical about the statement that the $\overline{\text{P100}}$ component had a latency of 95, 110 or even 150 ms. Latencies are measured from the onset of the relevant stimulus transient (e.g. pattern reversal or onset, or flash). Amplitude is usually measured peak-to-peak between any two consecutive peaks of opposite polarity, but measurement from a prestimulus baseline is also possible. Waveform changes may also be relevant, but are difficult to quantify. The same applies to the changes in topography of the response recorded from multichannel arrays.

The effect of stimulus parameters on the normal response

Many of the features of the normal response, including amplitude, latency and waveform, are affected by changes in the character of the visual stimulus. Apart from the striking differences in waveform between the flash (luminance) EP and the pattern EP, there are also major differences in the components of the VEP to pattern reversal and pattern onset (the appearance of a checkerboard in a blank field of equal mean luminance)[44]. Even for the most commonly used black-and-white checkerboard reversal stimulus, where the waveform of the response is relatively stereotyped, the amplitude and latency of the individual components are sensitive to such stimulus parameters as brightness[35], contrast[20], check size and field size[11, 20, 28]. The pattern response to a full-field stimulus has a characteristic triphasic waveform

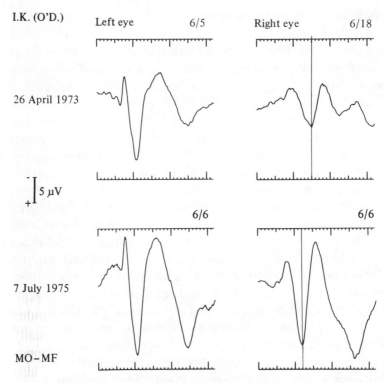

Figure 10.1 Pattern reversal responses recorded on two separate occasions from a patient with multiple sclerosis. The responses shown above were recorded at the age of 24, one month after the onset of an attack of right optic neuritis. The response from the affected eye, which still has a lowered visual acuity, is of reduced amplitude and delayed latency. The response from the unaffected left eye is within normal limits. The responses shown in the lower records were recorded two years later, by which time the VEP from the right eye has not only recovered in amplitude, paralleling the improvement in visual acuity, but has regained a peak latency almost within the normal range. Time scale in this and subsequent figures is in 10, 50 and 100 ms divisions. Sweep length 320 ms

with the major positivity preceded and followed by smaller negative peaks (*Figure 10.1*). The latency of the major positivity shows an increase of approximately 15 ms per log unit with reduction in the intensity of the checkerboard stimulus[35]. A parallel reduction in amplitude of approximately 15 per cent per log unit accompanies this latency change. At low contrast levels, the latency of the response is also sensitive to alterations in the relative brightness of the black-and-white checks, but this effect saturates at a level of about 20–40 per cent in the contrast, so that, provided the chosen contrast is greater than this, variation in this parameter will have little effect on the response. Field size and check size are important in determining which part of the retina is giving rise to the response. With very small checks, e.g. 10 or 15′, and a small field size, e.g. 2–4°, a centrally-fixated stimulus will produce a response predominantly from the macular area. This type of VEP is more sensitive to refractive errors than the larger stimuli more commonly used in clinical testing, e.g. a 32° field with 50′ checks[11, 16, 28]. For the latter, a refractive error will affect the amplitude of the major positivity, paralleling the reduction in visual acuity, but the latency is relatively unaffected. With the former, however, both amplitude and latency may be affected[11, 16, 28]. The choice of stimulus parameters appears to be an important factor determining the sensitivity and effectiveness of the VEP test[27].

Types of abnormality and the localization of lesions in the visual pathway

Abnormalities of the VEP may be reflected in changes of amplitude, latency or waveform of the mid-occipital response and also by changes in the topographical distribution of the response over the back of the head. Location of the site of the lesion is greatly aided by a knowledge of the anatomy of the visual pathways, combined with a resort to monocular and half-field stimulation[29]. Responses to stimulation of the left and right eye can be recorded separately and compared on the same occasion. In the healthy individual, the responses from the two eyes are normally nearly identical in amplitude, latency and waveform[9]. Even small amplitude differences therefore are significant. In a similar way, the responses from homonymous half-fields in the two eyes are also extremely similar, although there are more marked differences between the responses from heteronymous half-fields[9, 10]. This is probably due largely to anatomical differences in the spatial relationship between the visual cortical generator areas in each hemisphere and the scalp electrodes. Nonetheless, the limits of normal asymmetry can be determined for a given choice of stimulus and electrode array and will allow a criterion of abnormality to be set up[9, 10]. Lateralized lesions anterior to the chiasma are reflected in the difference of the responses from the two eyes, whereas more post-

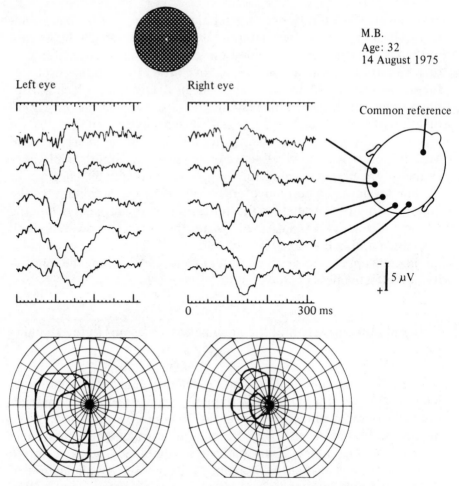

M.B.
Age: 32
14 August 1975

Figure 10.2 Example of an uncrossed asymmetry in a patient with demyelinating disease who developed a right hemiparesis and a right homonymous hemianopia. Full field stimulation of either eye produces a similar response showing the asymmetry characteristically associated with a left retrochiasmal lesion. The $\overline{P100}$ component is seen in the midline and left-sided channels, i.e. ipsilateral to the relatively preserved left half-field

eriorly-placed lesions affect the responses from both eyes and manifest themselves principally in the form of homonymous or heteronymous asymmetries in the amplitude, waveform and distribution of the response over the back of the head. In this way lateralized lesions of the retrochiasmal visual pathways and cortical generator areas can often be recognized and located by the typical *uncrossed asymmetry* with which they are characteristically associated [7, 9, 10, 25, 32]. This is by definition similar for the monocular responses from each eye (i.e. homonymous). Examples can be seen in *Figures 10.2* and *10.3*. In the case of chiasmal lesions, on the other hand, a *crossed asymmetry* is often encountered[7, 32]. Here, the asymmetric distribution of the response is reversed when the opposite eye is stimulated, reflecting the abnormality of the response from the opposite hemisphere, whose projection depends on the fibres subserving vision in the temporal half-fields of each eye, crossing in the chiasma (*Figure 10.5* on p. 247). For the detection of such asymmetries, associated with posterior lesions of the visual pathways, multichannel recording is essential (*see Figures 10.2 and 10.3* and *Figures 10.5 and 10.6* on pp. 247 and 248).

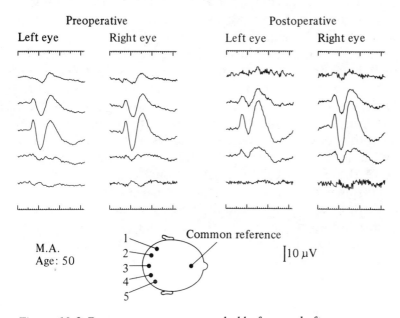

Figure 10.3 Pattern responses recorded before and after operation from a 50-year-old woman with a pituitary adenoma. The preoperative records show an uncrossed asymmetry of the type characteristic of a left retrochiasmal lesion. The patient had an incongruent right homonymous hemianopia. Postoperatively, when the field defect had disappeared, the VEPs regained their normal symmetry. However, the amplitude of the response from the left eye is significantly reduced, presumably from operative trauma, paralleling the reduction in the acuity of this eye from 6/5 to 6/9. (From Halliday *et al.*[32], courtesy of the Editor and publisher, *Brain*)

Amplitude changes

The normal variability of the pattern or flash EP is so large that absolute amplitude is seldom in itself enough to indicate an abnormality. Fortunately, however, this does not apply to the comparison of the amplitudes of the responses from the two eyes. The norms for the interocular difference in amplitude must be established for each laboratory by running a group of controls, but the ratio of amplitudes between the left and right eye is very near unity and the standard deviation extremely small. For the authors' stimulus, for instance, which consists of a 32° checkerboard of 50′ checks the interocular amplitude ratio is 1.03 ± 0.15 for a group of 50 healthy individuals. A difference of 7 µV is significant at the $P < 0.01$ level. The amplitude of the pattern reversal response tends to reflect fairly closely changes in the visual acuity level. Reduction in the size of the major positivity may therefore be encountered in such diverse conditions as refractive errors, amblyopia, opacities of the media, retinopathy and a variety of optic nerve lesions. Improvement of the visual acuity level by correcting for refractive errors[39], or during recovery following an acute attack of optic neuritis[35,37] are equally accompanied by an increase in the amplitude of the pattern response. However, as was originally demonstrated by Copenhaver and Perry[18] for the flash EP, the reduction of amplitude of the pattern EP for a given visual acuity level is more severe when this is produced by a neuro-retinal lesion rather than a refractive error or an opacity. The flash EP is much less sensitive to visual impairment than the pattern EP and may be well-preserved even in cases of gross visual impairment associated with cataract[39]. In severe lesions, however, the flash EP may also be reduced in amplitude or even abolished[39].

Although most pathological processes affecting the VEP are associated with a reduction in the response, an abnormal increase in amplitude is encountered in association with photosensitive epilepsy and in some patients with progressive myoclonic epilepsy[31].

Latency changes

An abnormal increase in the latency of the major positivity of the pattern response is very characteristic of demyelinating disease of the optic nerve. Even with quite prolonged latencies, the waveform of the response may be surprisingly well-preserved. Since the normal mean latency of the major positivity shows little variability, not exceeding a range of 20–30 ms or so in the healthy population[9,33,52], prolonged latency is the single most useful parameter of abnormality in clinical recording of the pattern EP. The normal variability of the flash EP is much greater and, as with amplitude, it is relatively insensitive to the effects of pathology. For both these reasons, the flash response shows a much smaller percentage of abnormal responses than the pattern response[20,27,34,35,45,48]. On the other hand, because of its robustness, it may still be obtainable after the pattern EP has been abolished. It is therefore of particular value in recording the VEP in association with severe or long-standing progressive lesions of the visual pathways.

Latency changes are not limited to demyelinating disease. They are also encountered in association with ischaemic optic neuropathy[4,39], axonal degeneration of the optic nerve fibres as in Friedreich's ataxia[12] and compressive lesions[32]. Long delays associated with a relatively well-preserved waveform are, however, characteristic of demyelinating disease.

Waveform changes

Waveform changes are easier to exemplify than to describe or define. Changes in the normal outline of the pattern EP may range from a slight blunting or loss of definition of the major positive peak to a total disorganization of the normal triphasic negative-positive-negative waveform. Among the changes commonly encountered in early compression, where waveform distortion is particularly frequently seen, are disappearance of the early negative wave ($\overline{N75}$) and broadening of the major positivity, probably associated with temporal dispersion of the afferent volley. In extreme cases this may lead to the replacement of the normal major positive peak by a broad, shallow, dish-shaped positive deflection of low amplitude, with no recognizable peak. The onset latency may in some cases still be within normal limits, although in other cases this too may be significantly delayed with a shift of the whole waveform to the right.

More complex waveform changes may also be associated with the topographical asymmetries characteristic of chiasmal and retrochiasmal lesions[9,10,30]. The mid-occipital electrode is in the area of maximal interaction between the independent half-field responses from the two hemispheres and is therefore particularly vulnerable to any alteration or abnormality in their relative contributions. Since the normal half-field response is highly asymmetric, with components of opposite polarity occurring at approximately the same latency on the two sides of the head[6, 8, 9], it is particularly difficult to interpret waveform changes in this 'transitional zone' between the two sides of the head, not only in the pathological response but also in the normal healthy individual. A further complication is provided by the striking changes in the waveform and polarity of the sub-components of the pattern responses produced by a central scotomatous field defect[30, 43], which is related to the existence of clearly differentiated macular and paramacular responses in the healthy subject[8, 30]. A fuller discussion of these changes is beyond the scope of this chapter, but will be found in the papers cited.

Optic neuritis

The outstanding finding in optic neuritis is a delay in the $\overline{\text{P100}}$, which is present in some 90 per cent of patients[4, 33, 41, 47, 51]. In 90 per cent of these the delay appears to persist indefinitely, although the authors have occasionally seen cases, such as that illustrated in *Figure 10.1*, in which a definite delay is later abolished. Delays of up to nearly 100 ms are seen but the mean is approximately 30–35 ms[33, 35, 51].

In acute cases the amplitude of the response is usually reduced but tends to return to normal as the acuity improves[33, 35, 51]. Group data suggest that there may be a small persistent reduction in amplitude even when the visual acuity returns to normal[47], but the variability in amplitude in normal subjects is such that this finding is helpful only occasionally.

The serial study of individual patients and the pooling of data from groups of patients with a history of optic neuritis, has shown that visual evoked potential abnormalities may persist when all the usual tests of visual function have returned to normal[4, 34]. The commonest persistent clinical deficit is an abnormality of colour vision, which may occasionally be present when the VEP is normal (Wray, personal communication).

When normal or equivocal results are obtained using the standard 32° pattern reversal stimulus, definite abnormalities may be revealed by using other techniques. For instance, Hennerici, Wenzel and Freund[41] found that pattern appearance in the central 4° could reveal abnormalities when the larger field stimulus gave normal results and Nilsson[50] found the same for a LED display presented in the central field. Occasionally half-field stimulation may provide convincing evidence of a delay when the full-field stimulus produces equivocal results[25].

In addition to a comparison of the amplitude between the two eyes, a comparison of latency may be helpful when the absolute values are within normal limits. In the authors' own laboratory a difference of 8 ms in latency is outside the normal range at the $P < 0.01$ level.

The explanation of the abnormal interocular evoked potential differences in these otherwise normal cases probably lies in the occurrence of unusually small lesions within the visual pathways. With regard to the foveal abnormalities, it would not be surprising if damage to a small proportion of the fibres activated by a large stimulus resulted in an abnormal contribution to the evoked potential too small to be discerned within the response evoked by the remaining normal fibres.

Indications

In the majority of patients with acute optic neuritis, the diagnosis is clear from the clinical picture and VEPs are not necessary to confirm it. The observation of a delay in the apparently unaffected eye, of course, provides evidence of a second lesion and increases the probability of a diagnosis of multiple sclerosis[17]. But since the management of the patient with isolated optic neuritis will not be altered thereby, this consideration does not in itself constitute an indication for an evoked potential examination. The main indication is in patients with atypical clinical features, in particular failure to improve. In such cases the possibility of tumour must always be considered and a VEP examination including half-field stimulation is important (*see below*). The finding of a strictly unilateral abnormality with a substantial delay considerably increases confidence in the diagnosis of optic neuritis.

Multiple sclerosis

A common problem in the diagnosis of MS is difficulty in demonstrating more than one necessarily separate lesion in the central nervous system in patients whose history suggests a diagnosis of demyelinating disease. The observation that VEPs may be abnormal when the usual tests of visual function are not, suggested that this technique might be helpful[33]. There is now a mass of evidence to show that it is.

The incidence of VEP abnormalities in multiple sclerosis has varied in different published reports, but all are agreed that it is high in clinically definite disease[27]. It seems likely that variations in stimulus parameters (*see above*), as well as variations in patient population and in the strictness with which diagnostic criteria are applied, contribute to the variations in incidence of VEP abnormality. Overall, abnormalities are likely to be found in approximately three quarters of patients who are referred with the presumptive diagnosis of MS. In patients with clinically definite MS a similar proportion will be found to have abnormal VEPs despite having normal optic discs, although again, different figures have been reported from different laboratories[4, 27, 34, 41, 47, 51].

The characteristic VEP abnormality is a delay in the $\overline{\text{P100}}$, but any of the abnormalities already described in isolated optic neuritis may be found in multiple sclerosis. So striking and so common are the VEP abnormalities in demyelinating disease that there is a tendency to regard them as specific and diagnostic. They are not. The high incidence of VEP abnormalities simply reflects the frequency of involvement of the optic nerves in multiple sclerosis[46]. Just as in rare cases of MS coming to post mortem the optic nerves are spared (Blackwood, personal communication), so in otherwise typical cases of established disease, the visual evoked potentials may be normal. Moreover, as *Figure 10.1* shows, a delayed evoked potential may occasionally revert to normal.

In some patients with otherwise typical multiple sclerosis the evoked potentials, though not delayed, may show abnormalities in waveform or distribution. An example of the latter is shown in *Figure 10.2* which illustrates the typical uncrossed asymmetry of a retrochiasmal lesion, indistinguishable from that produced by a tumour (*Figure 10.3*). This patient illustrates three important principles. First, that while an evoked potential abnormality may be characteristic of a particular disease it is neither specific to it, nor essential for its diagnosis. Secondly, the form of an evoked potential abnormality is influenced by the location of the lesion. In these two respects the evoked potential resembles an abnormal physical sign elicited by clinical examination of the central nervous system – its presence indicates that there is something wrong with the part of the nervous system being studied but not the cause, which must be determined by a consideration of the whole clinical picture. Thirdly, if recordings are made from only a single midline channel, significant abnormalities may be missed.

Indications

While the VEP examination may provide interesting information, it is not necessary in patients in whom the diagnosis is clear as a result of the clinical examination. Its chief use is in the assessment of patients with what appears to be an isolated lesion of the spinal cord or brainstem. In progressive spastic paraplegia in middle life a quarter to a half of the patients with normal optic discs have VEP abnormalities from one or both eyes[4, 36, 50]. The same is true for a rather smaller proportion of patients with acute brainstem lesions[4, 41], although some studies have failed to find them[34, 47]. A note of caution must be sounded in relation to patients in the former group. Spinal cord compression cannot of course be excluded by VEP examination. The authors have themselves seen one patient with an operatively proved Arnold-Chiari malformation who had abnormal evoked potentials. The delays characteristic of multiple sclerosis were, however, not present and the waveform was markedly distorted. The ventricular system, including the occipital horns, was dilated and it seems likely that the VEP abnormalities were at least in part attributable to secondary damage to the visual pathways. Their own policy with patients with progressive spastic paraplegia is not to carry out myelography when the VEPs show a typically delayed, well-formed $\overline{P100}$, and CSF protein electrophoresis reveals an oligoclonal pattern in the γ-globulins, provided there are no other signs suggesting a focal compressive lesion. Fortunately these criteria cover the majority of patients, but when there are atypical features in the VEPs or in the spinal fluid, or when clinical doubt remains, myelography is often necessary.

Tumours

In detecting early compression of the visual pathways, as in the case of demyelinating disease, abnormalities may be detected before there is any clinical evidence of visual impairment[32]. None of the VEP changes is specific to compression and the different pathological types of tumour cannot be distinguished electrophysiologically. Alterations in waveform and in the distribution of the VEP over the scalp without marked changes in latency are common but there are rare cases in which there is a fairly long delay in a well-preserved $\overline{P100}$. This result is interesting in the light of the recent observations of Clifford-Jones,

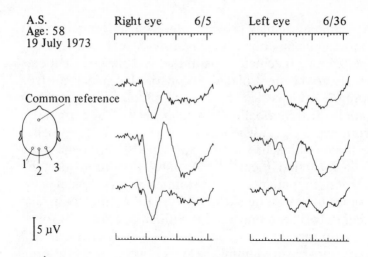

Figure 10.4 Pattern responses from a 58-year-old man with a neurilemmoma of the left optic nerve. The response from the left eye shows a $\overline{P100}$ of reduced amplitude and significantly delayed latency, in contrast to the normal response from the other eye

Landon and McDonald[14] who found that experimental chronic compression of the optic nerve in the orbit can produce a predominantly demyelinating lesion.

Tumours confined to the optic nerve, of course, produce uniocular VEP abnormalities. *Figure 10.4* shows a typical response from a patient with an orbital neurilemmoma. The amplitude of the response is reduced and the latency is significantly increased.

Chiasmal and retrochiasmal lesions can be distinguished by the patterns of asymmetry they produce (*see above*). The pure chiasmal lesion results in a crossed asymmetry (*Figure 10.5*) while the retrochiasmal produces an uncrossed asymmetry (*Figure 10.3*) corresponding with the bitemporal and homonymous hemianopic field defects respectively. In some cases, however, where the response from one eye is abolished by optic nerve compression on that side, the only clue to retrochiasmal involvement may be an asymmetry typical of a temporal hemianopia from the contralateral eye (*Figure 10.6*). Tumours in the chiasmal region commonly involve more than one part of the visual pathway. In patients with compression of the intracranial optic nerve, it is not uncommon to find evoked potential evidence of a

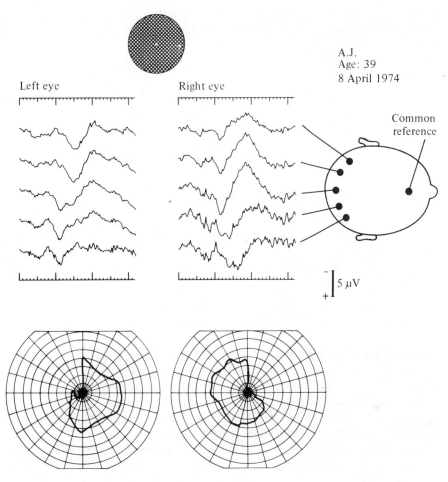

Figure 10.5 Pattern EPs from each eye of a 39-year-old man with a pituitary adenoma, associated with an incomplete bitemporal hemi-anopia. The responses show the crossed asymmetry characteristically associated with compression of the fibres crossing in the chiasma, the P100 component being seen in the midline and ipsilateral to the preserved nasal field, i.e. on the right for the left eye and on the left for the right eye

temporal defect in the apparently normal eye indicating that the crossing nasal fibres are already involved. Systematic half-field ·stimulation is particularly helpful in the investigation of such patients and may play an important part in deciding on management. In optic nerve glioma, for example, the finding of such a defect, (which may precede

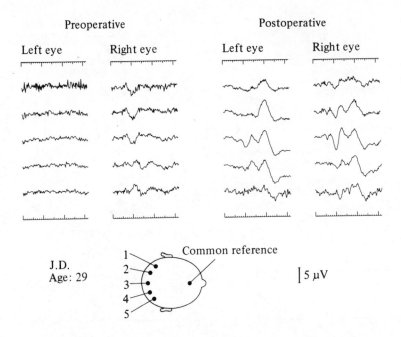

Figure 10.6 Pattern responses recorded before and after operation in a patient with a craniopharyngioma. Preoperatively there was no response from the left eye, in which the visual acuity was reduced to the perception of hand movements. The response from the right eye is of reduced amplitude and shows an asymmetry typical of a right temporal field defect, the $\overline{\text{P100}}$ being relatively preserved ipsilaterally to the nasal field of that eye. Visual acuity in the right eye was better than 6/12 and there was a temporal field defect sparing the midline. Postoperatively both responses are markedly improved, paralleling the return of normal acuity. (From Halliday *et al.*[32], courtesy of the Editor and publisher, *Brain*)

a field defect to standard methods of examination) indicates that radical surgical cure is not possible[29, 54].

Surgical removal of a tumour often results in a prompt return of the evoked potentials to a more normal appearance, particularly in those patients in whom there is good recovery of acuity and resolution of the field defect (*Figures 10.3 and 10.6*). Flash evoked potentials recorded during operation may recover promptly following relief of the compression[22]. The possible mechanisms underlying such rapid recovery have been discussed elsewhere[14].

Indications

The main role of the VEP is in determining the presence or absence of involvement of the visual pathways in cases of suspected tumour and in determining the localization of the lesion. It is obvious from the normal responses recorded from the midline channels in many cases (e.g. *Figures 10.3 and 10.5*) that for these purposes multichannel recording is essential.

Other optic neuropathies

Abnormalities of the VEP have been reported in a variety of less common optic neuropathies. Some cases of ischaemic optic neuropathy are associated with a delay of the same order as that seen in MS[4, 39, 41]. The authors, however, have seen a patient who presented at the age of 40 with a unilateral ischaemic optic neuropathy in whom there was a reduction in amplitude of the VEP without a delay. The second eye was subsequently involved and the amplitude of the response from this eye fell to that of the first affected eye, again without the development of a delay.

Tropical amblyopia

Tropical amblyopia has been reported as being associated with delayed responses[4] or with a triphasic PNP waveform replacing the normal NPN complex, giving an apparent delay[40]. Ikeda, Tremain and Sanders[42] found no delay, but a subnormal ERG and a reduced amplitude of the VEP.

Pernicious anaemia

In pernicious anaemia without visual symptoms, delayed VEPs have been reported in three cases[53]. The defects were, however, marginal and if the upper limit of normal is defined as 2.5 SD above the mean, i.e. 112.4 ms in this study, instead of 2.0 SD above it, only one of the six eyes had an abnormal VEP (latency 121.4 ms).

Toxic amblyopia

Toxic amblyopia, due to tobacco and/or alcohol excess, has been investigated by Ikeda, Tremain and Sanders[42] and Kriss *et al.*[43]. As in tropical amblyopia there was little change in the latency of the $\overline{\text{P100}}$.

The amplitude of the response was, however, reduced, and in contrast to the findings in demyelinating disease and compressive optic neuropathy, the flash evoked ERG was subnormal, particularly with respect to the cone-mediated retinal function. In three out of four patients studied by Ikeda[42], treatment by abstinence and vitamin B12 injections resulted in improvement in visual acuity, and in both the VEP and the ERG. There was evidence that the fourth patient continued to drink to excess. Kriss *et al.*[43] in a study of 18 patients found the pattern reversal response exhibiting the characteristic changes typical of a dense central scotoma, the macular NPN complex being largely replaced by the phase-reversed PNP complex originating from stimulation of the paramacular retina[8, 30]. Although much attenuated the $\overline{P100}$ was usually of normal latency and showed an increase in amplitude following treatment[43].

Hereditary optic neuropathies

Leber's optic atrophy
In Leber's optic atrophy gross abnormalities from the affected eyes are usual. Carroll and Mastaglia[13] investigated a six generation family with the disease. Fourteen members were clinically affected. The pattern evoked potential was frequently absent, in keeping with the marked impairment of acuity. In those with less severe involvement, the VEPs had positivities of increased latency, abnormal waveform and much reduced amplitude. Mild or atypical VEP features were fairly frequent, being found in 16/40 of asymptomatic family members and 50 per cent of the descendants from the female lineage who were at risk of developing the disease. A surprising result was the presence of similar abnormalities in 30 per cent of the descendants from the male line who were not at risk.

Friedreich's ataxia
In Friedreich's ataxia there is a high incidence, approximately 70 per cent, of asymptomatic visual pathway involvement as judged clinically and by VEP[12]. The VEP abnormalities, present in 15/22 patients, were always binocular and comprised increased $\overline{P100}$ latencies and decreased amplitudes, usually with a normal waveform. The response was occasionally absent. Comparison with a matched group of patients with demyelinating optic neuritis showed that the delays tended to be

somewhat smaller and the decrease in amplitude somewhat greater, possibly reflecting greater nerve fibre loss in Friedreich's ataxia.

There is little information available about the other forms of hereditary ataxia. However, Carroll *et al.*[12] refer briefly to a study of 16 members of a family with autosomal dominant cortical cerebellar degeneration with four clinically affected members. None had VEP abnormalities. Harding, Crews and Good[40] report an abnormal triphasic PNP response in dominant optic atrophy similar to that seen by them in Leber's optic atrophy and West Indian amblyopia.

Hysteria

The VEP may be useful in two quite different ways in the management of patients in whom there is a possibility that some of the deficit may be hysterical. A visual acuity of 6/36 (20/120) or less is incompatible with a well-formed pattern evoked potential. *Figure 10.7* illustrates a patient with a personality disorder who produced entirely normal pattern responses after presenting with a complaint of blindness in both eyes for four weeks.

On the other hand, a VEP abnormality may constitute the crucial evidence for an underlying organic defect in patients with undoubted

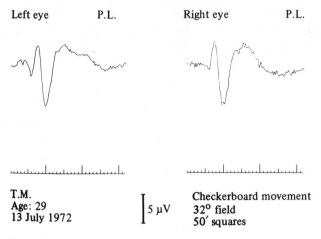

Left eye   P.L.   Right eye   P.L.

T.M.
Age: 29   5 µV   Checkerboard movement
13 July 1972   32° field
                                               50′ squares

Figure 10.7 Pattern responses of normal waveform and latency recorded in a 29-year-old man presenting with a four weeks' history of blindness in both eyes and severe personality problems

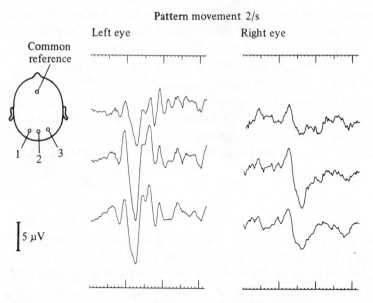

Figure 10.8 Pattern EPs in a 33-year-old woman with numerous hospital admissions for investigation over the previous five years for a variety of fluctuating symptoms, including vertigo, deafness, right-sided numbness and weakness, blurring of vision and depression. There was gross hysterical elaboration of many of the symptoms and a paucity of objective neurological signs. The pattern response from the right eye is grossly delayed

hysterical features. *Figure 10.8* shows the responses recorded from a patient who had been seen intermittently over several years with a vague history of impairment of balance and paraesthesiae. No confirmed abnormality on examination had been found in the past. She was referred again with a complaint of acute unilateral visual loss which was thought at first to be hysterical. The optic discs were normal but there was a delay in the VEP from the affected side, typical of that seen in acute optic neuritis. Her subsequent course has included a number of undoubtedly organic episodes, leading to a diagnosis of multiple sclerosis.

Conclusion

The VEP technique provides a sensitive means of detecting damage to the visual pathways. In the clinic its chief uses are in the early diagnosis of multiple sclerosis, by virtue of its ability to reveal subclinical abnormalities, and in the assessment of unexplained visual failure because of the influence that the location of the lesions has on the type of abnormality occurring in the evoked potentials. The VEPs may also give a guide to the pathology, but none of the changes is specific.

As the authors have always emphasized[32, 34, 37] the evoked potential has the status in neurology of an abnormal physical sign. Its presence indicates that something is wrong with the corresponding part of the nervous system but its significance must be interpreted in the light of the rest of the clinical picture.

References

1 ARDEN, G. B., BODIS-WOLLNER, I., HALLIDAY, A. M., JEFFREYS, A, KULI-KOWSKI, J. J., SPEKREIJSE, H. and REGAN, D. Methodology of patterned visual stimulation. In *Visual Evoked Potentials in Man: New Developments*, edited by J. E. Desmedt, 3–15. Oxford, Clarendon Press (1977)

2 ARDEN, G. B., FAULKNER, D. J. and MAIR, C. A versatile television pattern generator for visual evoked potentials. In *Visual Evoked Potentials in Man: New Developments*, edited by J. E. Desmedt, 90–109. Oxford, Clarendon Press (1977)

3 ARMINGTON, J. C. Electroretinography. In *Electrodiagnosis in Clinical Neurology*, edited by M. J. Aminoff, 305–347. New York, Churchill Livingstone (1980)

4 ASSELMAN, P., CHADWICK, D. W. and MARSDEN, C. D. Visual evoked responses in the diagnosis and management of patients suspected of multiple sclerosis. *Brain*, **98**, 261–282 (1975)

5 BABEL, J., STANGOS, N., KOROL, S. and SPIRITUS, M. *Ocular Electrophysiology: A Clinical and Experimental Study of Electroretinogram, Electro-oculogram, Visual Evoked Response*, 1–172. Stuttgart, Thieme (1977)

6 BARRETT, G., BLUMHARDT, L., HALLIDAY, A. M., HALLIDAY, E. and KRISS, A. A paradox in the lateralisation of the visual evoked response. *Nature*, **261**, 253–255 (1976)

7 BLUMHARDT, L. D., BARRETT, G. and HALLIDAY, A. M. The asymmetrical visual evoked potential to pattern-reversal in one half-field and its significance for the analysis of visual field defects. *British Journal of Ophthalmology*, **61**, 454–461 (1977)

8 BLUMHARDT, L. D., BARRETT, G., HALLIDAY, A. M. and KRISS, A. The effect of experimental 'scotomata' on the ipsilateral and contralateral responses to pattern-reversal in one half-field. *Electroencephalography and Clinical Neurophysiology*, **45**, 376–392 (1978)

9 BLUMHARDT, L. D. and HALLIDAY, A. M. Hemisphere contributions to the composition of the pattern-evoked potential waveform. *Experimental Brain Research*, **36**, 53–69 (1979)

10 BLUMHARDT, L. D. and HALLIDAY, A. M. Cortical abnormalities and the visual evoked response. *Proceedings of the Eighteenth ISCEV Symposium*, edited by H. Spekreijse and P. Apkarian. *Documenta Ophthalmologica*, **27**, 347–365. The Hague, Junk (1981)

11 CARROLL, W. M. and KRISS, A. (Unpublished observations)

12 CARROLL, W. M., KRISS, A., BARAITSER, M., BARRETT, G. and HALLIDAY, A. M. The incidence and nature of visual pathway involvement in Friedreich's ataxia. A clinical and visual evoked potential study of 22 patients. *Brain*, **103**, 413–434 (1980)

13 CARROLL, W. M. and MASTAGLIA, F. L. Leber's optic neuropathy: A clinical and visual evoked potential study of affected and asymptomatic members of a six generation family. *Brain*, **102**, 559–580 (1979)

14 CLIFFORD-JONES, R. E., LANDON, D. N. and McDONALD, W. I. Remyelination during optic nerve compression. *Journal of Neurological Science*, **46**, 239–243 (1980)

15 COBB, W. A., MORTON, H. B. and ETTLINGER, G. Cerebral potentials evoked by pattern reversal and their suppression in visual rivalry. *Nature*, **216**, 1123–1125 (1967)

16 COLLINS, D. W. K., CARROLL, W. M., BLACK, J. L. and WALSH, M. Effect of refractive error on the visual evoked response. *British Medicial Journal*, **1**, 231–232 (1979)

17 COMPSTON, D. A. S., BATCHELOR, J. R., EARL, C. J. and McDONALD, W. I. Factors influencing the risk of multiple sclerosis developing in patients with optic neuritis. *Brain*, **101**, 495–511 (1978)

18 COPENHAVER, R. M. and PERRY, M. W. Factors affecting visually evoked cortical potentials such as impaired vision of varying etiology. *Investigative Ophthalmology*, **3**, 665–675 (1964)

19 DONCHIN, E., CALLAWAY, E., COOPER, R., DESMEDT, J. E., GOFF, W. R., HILLYARD, S. A. and SUTTON, S. Publication Criteria for Studies of Evoked Potentials (EP) in Man. Report of a Committee. In *Attention, Voluntary Contraction and Event-Related Cerebral Potentials*, edited by J. E. Desmedt, 1–11. Basel, S. Karger. (1977)

20 DUWAER, A. L. and SPEKREIJSE, H. Latency of luminance and contrast

evoked potentials in multiple sclerosis patients. *Electroencephalography and Clinical Neurophysiology*, **45**, 244–258 (1978)

21 EVANS, B. T., BINNIE, C. D. and LLOYD, D. S. L. A simple visual pattern stimulator. *Electroencephalography and Clinical Neurophysiology*, **37**, 403–406 (1974)

22 GUTIN, P. H., KEMME, W. M., LAGGAR, R. L., MacKAY, A. R., PITTS, L. H. and HOROBUCHI, Y. Management of the unresectable cystic craniopharyngioma by aspiration through an Ommaya reservoir drainage system. *Journal of Neurosurgery*, **52**, 36–40 (1980)

23 HALLIDAY, A. M. Changes in the form of cerebral evoked responses in man associated with various lesions of the nervous system. In *Recent Advances in Clinical Neurophysiology*, edited by L. Widén, 178–192. Amsterdam, Elsevier (1967)

24 HALLIDAY, A. M. The effect of lesions of the visual pathway and cerebrum on the visual evoked response. In *Evoked Responses. Handbook of Electroencephalography and Clinical Neurophysiology*, **8a**, 119–129. Amsterdam, Elsevier (1975)

25 HALLIDAY, A. M. Commentary: evoked potentials in neurological diagnosis. In *Event-Related Brain Potentials in Man*, edited by E. Callaway, S. H. Koslow, and P. Tueting, 197–213. New York, Academic Press (1978)

26 HALLIDAY, A. M. Discussion of a paper by G. E. Holder: Abnormalities of the pattern visual evoked potential in patients with homonymous visual field defects. In *Evoked Potentials*, edited by C. Barber, 292–298. Lancaster, MTP Press (1980)

27 HALLIDAY, A. M. Event-related potentials and their diagnostic usefulness. In *Motivation, Motor and Sensory Processes of the Brain: Electrical Potentials, Behaviour and Clinical Use*, edited by H. H. Kornhuber and L. Deecke, *Progress in Brain Research*, **54**, 469–485. Amsterdam, Elsevier/North Holland (1980)

28 HALLIDAY, A. M. Problems in defining the normal limits of the VEP. *Proceedings of the Symposium on Clinical Applications of Evoked Potentials in Neurology*, (Lyon, 16–17th October 1980) New York, Raven Press (in press)

29 HALLIDAY, A. M. (Editor) *Evoked Potentials in Clinical Testing*. Edinburgh, Churchill Livingstone (in press)

30 HALLIDAY, A. M., BARRETT, G., BLUMHARDT, L. D. and KRISS, A. The macular and paramacular sub-components of the pattern evoked response. In *Human Evoked Potentials: Applications and Problems*, edited by E. Callaway and D. Lehmann, 135–151. London, Plenum Press (1979)

31 HALLIDAY, A. M. and HALLIDAY, E. Cerebral somatosensory and visual evoked potentials in different clinical forms of myoclonus. In *Clinical Uses of Cerebral, Brainstem and Spinal Somatosensory Evoked Potentials*, edited by J. E. Desmedt, *Progress in Clinical Neurophysiology*, **7**, 292–311. Basel, S. Karger (1980)

32 HALLIDAY, A. M., HALLIDAY, E., KRISS, A., McDONALD, W. I. and MUSHIN, J. The pattern evoked potential in compression of the anterior visual pathways. *Brain*, **99**, 357–374 (1976)

33 HALLIDAY, A. M., McDONALD, W. I. and MUSHIN, J. Delayed visual evoked response in optic neuritis. *Lancet*, **1**, 982–985 (1972)

34 HALLIDAY, A. M., McDONALD, W. I. and MUSHIN, J. The visual evoked response in the diagnosis of multiple sclerosis. *British Medical Journal*, **4**, 661–664 (1973)

35 HALLIDAY, A. M., McDONALD, W. I. and MUSHIN, J. Delayed pattern-evoked responses in optic neuritis in relation to visual acuity. *Transactions of the Ophthalmological Society of the UK*, **93**, 315–324 (1973)

36 HALLIDAY, A. M., McDONALD, W. I. and MUSHIN, J. Delayed pattern-evoked responses in progressive spastic paraplegia. *Neurology (Minneapolis)*, **24**, 360–361 (1975)

37 HALLIDAY, A. M., McDONALD, W. I. and MUSHIN, J. Visual evoked potentials in patients with demyelinating disease. In *Visual Evoked Potentials in Man: New Developments*, edited by J. E. Desmedt, 438–449. Oxford, Clarendon Press (1977)

38 HALLIDAY, A. M. and MICHAEL, W. F. Changes in pattern-evoked responses in man associated with the vertical and horizontal meridians of the visual field. *Journal of Physiology*, **208**, 499–513 (1970)

39 HALLIDAY, A. M. and MUSHIN, J. The visual evoked potential in neuro-ophthalmology. In *Electrophysiology and Psychophysics: Their Use in Ophthalmic Diagnosis*, edited by S. Sokol, *International Ophthalmology Clinics*, **20**(1), 155–183. Boston, Little Brown (1980)

40 HARDING, G. F. A., CREWS, S. J. and GOOD, P. A. The VEP in neuro-ophthalmic disease. In *Evoked Potentials*, edited by C. Barber, 235–241. Lancaster, MTP Press (1980)

41 HENNERICI, M., WENZEL, D. and FREUND, H.-J. The comparison of small-size rectangle and checkerboard stimulation for the evaluation of delayed visual evoked responses in patients suspected of multiple sclerosis. *Brain*, **100**, 119–136 (1977)

42 IKEDA, H., TREMAIN, K. E. and SANDERS, M. D. Neurophysiological investigation in optic nerve disease: combined assessment of the

visual evoked response and electroretinogram. *British Journal of Ophthalmology*, **62**, 227–239 (1978)

43 KRISS, A., CARROLL, W. M., BLUMHARDT, L. D. and HALLIDAY, A. M. Changes in the pattern evoked potential in toxic optic neuropathy. *Proceedings of the Symposium on Clinical Applications of Evoked Potentials in Neurology*, (Lyon, 16–17th October 1980) New York, Raven Press (in press)

44 KRISS, A. and HALLIDAY, A. M. A comparison of occipital potentials evoked by pattern onset, offset and reversal by movement. In *Evoked Potentials*, edited by C. Barber, 205–212. Lancaster, MTP Press (1980)

45 LOWITZSCH, K., RUDOLPH, H. D., TRINCKER, D. and MÜLLER, E. Flash and pattern-reversal visual evoked responses in retrobulbar neuritis and controls: A comparison of conventional and TV stimulation techniques. In *EEG and Clinical Neurophysiology*, edited by H. Lechner, and A. Aranibar, 451–463. Amsterdam, Excerpta Medica (1980)

46 LUMSDEN, C. E. The neuropathology of multiple sclerosis. In *Handbook of Clinical Neurology*, edited by G. W. Bruyn and P. J. Vinker, **9**, 217–309. Amsterdam, Elsevier/North Holland (1970)

47 MATTHEWS, W. B., SMALL, D. G., SMALL, M. and POUNTNEY, E. The pattern reversal evoked visual potential in the diagnosis of multiple sclerosis. *Journal of Neurology, Neurosurgery and Psychiatry*, **40**, 1009 –1014 (1977)

48 MAUGUIERE, F., MITROU, H., CHALET, E., POURCHER, E. and COURJON, J. Intérêt des potentiels évoqués visuels dans la sclérose multiloculaire (S. M.): étude comparative des résultats obtenus en stimulation par éclair lumineux et inversion de damier. *Revue EEG Neurophysiologie*, **9**, 209–220 (1979)

49 MICHAEL, W. F. and HALLIDAY, A. M. Differences between the occipital distribution of upper and lower field pattern evoked responses in man. *Brain Research*, **32**, 311–324 (1971)

50 NILSSON, B. Y. Visual evoked responses in multiple sclerosis: Comparison of two methods for pattern reversal. *Journal of Neurology, Neurosurgery and Psychiatry*, **41**, 499–504 (1978)

51 SHAHROKHI, F., CHIAPPA, K. H. and YOUNG, R. R. Pattern shift visual evoked responses. *Archives of Neurology (Chicago)*, **35**, 65–71 (1978)

52 STOCKARD, J. J., HUGHES, J. F. and SHARBROUGH, F. W. Visually evoked potentials to electronic pattern reversal: latency variations with gender, age, and technical factors. *American Journal of EEG Technology*, **19**, 171–204 (1979)

53 TRONCOSO, J., MANCALL, E. L. and SHATZ, N. J. Visual evoked responses in pernicious anaemia. *Archives of Neurology* (Chicago) **36,** 168–169 (1979)

54 WRIGHT, J. E., McDONALD, W. I. and CALL, N. B. Management of optic nerve gliomas. *British Journal of Ophthalmology*, **64,** 545–552 (1980)

11
Brainstem auditory evoked potentials

Keith H. Chiappa

Introduction

In 1970 it was demonstrated[15, 16] that the auditory evoked response produced by a brief click contained brainstem components which could be recorded from the scalp. These brainstem auditory evoked potentials (BAEPs) are sometimes termed 'far-field' because the electrical activity of the small anatomical structures involved is recorded at a relatively greater distance away on the scalp, whereas previously, activity in these same structures had been recorded only from depth electrodes. BAEPs, as recorded at the scalp, have an amplitude of about $0.25\,\mu V$, as compared with $30-60\,\mu V$ for normal α-activity and $5-20\,\mu V$ for a pattern shift visual EP (PSVEP). Thus, reliable recording of BAEPs presents technical problems the solution to which requires experience, careful attention to the details of the recording procedure and the use of averaging computers.

Methods

BAEPs are obtained using monaural (one ear at a time) stimulation and recording, since abnormalities are often seen only unilaterally and the normal response produced in the good ear during binaural stimulation masks the abnormality (*see Figure 4 in reference 7*). For example, 45 percent of the BAEP abnormalities seen in a group of 200 patients with multiple sclerosis (MS) were unilateral[7] (e.g. *Figure 11.3* on p. 296). Furthermore, human clinicopathological correlations in patients with brainstem tumors and infarctions suggest that, in spite of the abundance of crossing fiber tracts in the auditory system, the BAEP waves are generated primarily by structures ipsilateral to the ear being stimulated[3, 8], as is discussed in more detail below.

Click stimuli

Monaural clicks are produced by applying 100 µs electrical square waves to earphones. This produces a sound of almost equal intensity over a wide frequency range (at least 400–4000 Hz) so that much of the cochlea is stimulated. Filtering of the click can produce more discrete stimulation[11]. Click polarity influences the shape of the IV–V complex and, to a minor degree, interwave separation, so it must be kept constant[9, 10, 37, 38]. Rarely, excessive stimulus artifact partially obscures wave I and alternating polarity clicks can reduce the size of the artifact[37] (see *Figure 11.1c and d*). The click repetition rate used is 10/s. In normal subjects faster stimulus rates increase absolute and interwave latencies and cause loss of resolution of waves[7, 12, 37] making accurate measurements difficult. In patients, faster rates occasionally worsen abnormalities evident at 10/s but only very rarely have revealed abnormalities if the BAEP was normal at 10/s, so that the faster rates have little clinical utility[8].

When BAEPs are used to study the central nervous system (CNS) rather than the peripheral hearing apparatus, click intensity is adjusted to 65 to 70 dB above the click hearing threshold for that ear, i.e. 70 dB above sensation level (SL). Decreased effective stimulus intensity, secondary to peripheral hearing loss or lowered earphone output, causes the absolute latency (time from stimulus to waveform) of all waves to increase equally. The interwave separation, i.e. the time interval between waveforms, does not change. It also decreases amplitude of all waves so that waves II, IV and VI disappear first, then III, I, and lastly V, which often can still be seen at 10 or 20 dBSL. The decreased amplitude of the waves, which hinders recognition and accurate measurements, is avoided by adjusting the effective stimulus intensity relative to the individual ear. When waveform recognition is a problem, the manoeuvre of decreasing click intensity with subsequent BAEP simplification can be used. Conductive and cochlear hearing losses produce the same effect on the BAEP as decreasing stimulus intensity[9], unless intensity versus latency curves are studied[10], although cochlear lesions may induce minor changes in interwave latencies[10].

Masking noise

A masking white noise is usually presented to the ear not being stimulated with the clicks since there is a significant amount of cross-stimulation via bone and air conduction. This is roughly 30 or

40 dB less than the click intensity at the stimulated ear and thus is sufficient to produce recognizable waveforms. In this manner a non-functioning ear may appear to be producing BAEP waves (e.g. *Figure 4 in reference 7*). Under more normal circumstances, the impulses from the stimulated, ipsilateral ear arrive in the brainstem before those from the contralateral ear, stimulated by cross-conduction and probably set up inhibitory influences, so that these considerations are then less important.

Recording parameters

Differential amplifier inputs are taken from electrodes on the earlobe ipsilateral to stimulation and the vertex, filtered for a bandpass of 100–3000 Hz, and amplified 500 000 to 1 000 000 times. Hearing loss often renders wave I identification difficult and the use of an external ear canal electrode can produce a higher amplitude wave I (e.g. *Figure 11.1* on p. 265). This is a conventional EEG needle electrode inserted a few millimetres below the skin surface in the easily accessible anterior wall of the superficial segment of the external ear canal. Other techniques employ electrodes closer to the tympanic membrane; placement of these is technically much more difficult.

The signal for 10 ms poststimulus is averaged for 1000 to 2000 clicks. BAEP waveform amplitudes are much smaller than those of the PSVEP (0.25 versus 5 µV) and great care must be taken to minimize muscle and movement artifact. The test is often performed as a sleep study, using appropriate premedication with chloral hydrate (chloral betaine) and/or diphenhydramine, as necessary. Averaging must be halted manually or automatically when excessive artifact is present, such as during a swallow. Repeat trials must be superimposed to ensure waveform validity, and the grand average of the separate trials also recorded. Concentration on a single set of stimulus and recording parameters with repetition of trials until reliable and consistent results are obtained is much more important than varying stimulus parameters. The test takes about 45 min to perform.

Normal findings

Normal human adult BAEPs are shown in *Figure 11.3* (AS) on p. 269 and *Figure 11.4a* on p. 270; the waves are usually labelled I–VII, as shown. Since the activity recorded is being generated in the primary sensory pathways, it is very resistant to alteration. Patients under general anesthesia and high-dose barbiturate therapy for increased intracranial pressure show little change in the first five waves of the BAEP and a patient who almost met the clinical and EEG criteria of brain death secondary to a barbiturate overdose had normal BAEPs[39]. Thus, subject attentiveness and drowsiness are not factors in the clinical interpretation of BAEPs.

Measurements are made of interwave separations and the wave I to wave V amplitude ratio. Absolute latencies are not usually used in interpretation since they are affected by stimulus intensity changes and other factors sometimes difficult to control[7, 37], all of which induce excessive variability. Neurologically the major concerns are central conduction times which are accurately reflected in the interwave latency separations. These are affected by audiogram shape[9, 10], age [22, 23, 32, 37, 38], sex[37], temperature[37] and various other parameters[37] although most of these effects are demonstrable only by statistical comparisons between large groups of subjects. When BAEPs are interpreted clinically, the important parameters are age if less than 2 years, temperature if below 33°C, and click polarity.

Thus, great effort is put into producing a clear wave I (VIIIth nerve activation potential) so that all measurements can be made relative to this peak and thereby rendering unnecessary considerations of effective stimulus intensity. Absolute amplitudes are not used because of their extreme variabililty. An abnormality of interwave latency separation, and perhaps the I:V amplitude ratio, is an indication of a conduction defect in that segment of the pathway.

BAEP normative data have been reported[2, 7, 12, 21–23, 29, 34, 37, 38]. In the author's laboratory[7] the upper limits of normal – the normal mean plus 3 standard deviations – and mean/SD for 50 normal subjects, for interwave separations were: I–III = 2.6 ms (2.1/0.15), III–V = 2.4 ms (1.9/0.18), I–V = 4.7 ms (4.0/0.23). The upper limit of normal (mean/SD) for the I/V amplitude ratio (expressed as a percentage) was: I/V = 218 percent (73/48). It should be noted that these values, particularly the amplitude ratio, are subject to some alteration by technical factors[7, 37, 38] and each laboratory should confirm their agreement with these tables before undertaking the interpretation of data obtained from patients. The experience gained during the testing of the normal subjects will also result in a greater confidence in abnormal findings in patients.

Anatomic correlations

The probable origins of BAEP waveforms have been partially determined by animal microelectrode and lesion experiments and human clinicopathological correlations.

In humans, wave I is:

(1) the same wave as N1 of electrocochleography;
(2) a negative wave recorded in the immediate region of the ear being stimulated; and
(3) primarily the VIIIth nerve activation potential.

In animals, waves II and III may be generated in the cochlear nucleus and superior olivary complex, respectively[1,4]. In humans, isolation of a functioning cochlear nucleus by a lesion must be exceedingly rare and has not yet been encountered in patients who have had BAEP testing. However, occasional patients with pontine hemorrhages or infarctions have had BAEP testing and subsequent neuropathological examination. In some of these cases there was a transection of the auditory pathways in the medial pons but sparing of the lower one-third of the pons with the superior olivary complexes (*Figure 11.6* on p. 272). The latter patients had had intact waves I–III in the BAEPs, supporting the hypothesis that the generators of waves II and III are in the lower one-third of the pons and are probably the cochlear nucleus and superior olivary complex.

In animals, there is some dispute over the generator sources of waves IV and V. Buchwald and Huang[4] performed experiments with lesions in cats and found that the fifth wave was abolished by removal of the inferior colliculi. Achor and Starr[1] made discrete lesions in the inferior colliculi of cats and found no significant change in the fifth wave. Nor is there agreement on the effects of lesions in cats on the fourth wave[1,4]. The difficulty in making a human correlation is that the latency separation between waves I and V in their cats (approximately 5.3 ms) is greater by far than that between the waves labelled I and V in humans (4.0 ms). However, humans with clinical and neuroradiological evidence of midbrain lesions, usually pinealomas, sometimes have wave V absent or only partially present. The single reported case of a restricted collicular lesion in a human had perhaps some loss of wave V amplitude unilaterally[33]. The origin of wave IV in humans is similarly conjectural.

In humans, waves VI and VII are not seen in all subjects and are of little clinical utility, Wave VI was absent unilaterally in 16 percent and bilaterally in 8 percent of 52 normal subjects[7]. Wave VII was found in only 43 percent of the ears of 20 normal subjects[7]. It is speculated that wave VI arises in the medial geniculate body and VII in the auditory radiations and temporal lobe but there are few data that bear on this point. Recordings from intrathalamic depth electrodes in humans (*see Figure 6 in reference 5*) have thus far provided inconsistent data.

In summary, waves I–V can reasonably be considered for clinical purposes as being the scalp-recorded manifestation of the successive activation of the brainstem auditory pathways ipsilateral to the ear being stimulated – VIIIth nerve, cochlear nucleus, superior olivary complex, lateral lemniscus (tracts and/or nuclei) and inferior colliculus, respectively.

The relationship between abnormalities of BAEP waves II–VII and functional hearing as tested by conventional audiometric methods is not fully understood. Known lesions of the auditory tracts usually produce abnormalities of the expected BAEP waveforms. However, one commonly sees, e.g. in multiple sclerosis (MS) patients, absence of wave V without clinical evidence of auditory system dysfunction as reported by patients and on conventional behavioural audiometry[8]. Only when detailed tests of auditory localization capabilities are performed can other manifestations of the disturbance be seen[14].

Clinical applications

Screening for acoustic neuromas

The use of BAEPs in the evaluation of peripheral hearing loss is outside the scope of this discussion which deals with the use of the BAEP in clinical neurology. However, the BAEP is the most sensitive screening test for acoustic neuromas[20, 26, 28], which commonly present with progressive hearing loss. Occasionally the BAEP shows abnormalities when all routine audiologic tests are normal and the CT scan is unrevealing. In a group of 25 patients with acoustic neuromas and five with cerebellopontine angle (CPA) meningiomas all had abnormal BAEPs on the side of the tumor, five had normal computed tomography (CT) scans and five had normal standard audiometry[20]. Twelve had no recognizable BAEPs, five had prolonged I–III interwave

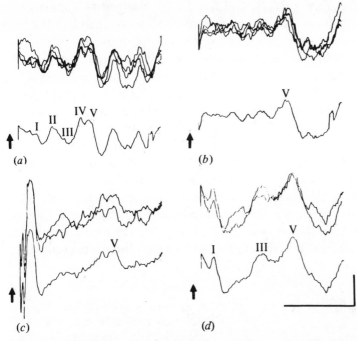

Figure 11.1 BAEPs from monaural stimulation of each ear of a patient with an acoustic neuroma. (*a*) Unaffected AS showing the normal waveforms, labelled I through V, although I is often seen as a more discrete peak than is the case here. (*b*), (*c*) and (*d*) are all from the affected ear (AD). (*b*) was obtained by conventional recording from the earlobe (and vertex) – note the absence of all waves except V. (*c*) was obtained by recording from a needle electrode in the external ear canal – note the large wave I which is, however, partially obscured by stimulus artifact. In (*a*), (*b*) and (*c*) click polarity was constant, whereas in (*d*) click polarity was alternated – note loss of stimulus artifact which leaves wave I as a discrete peak. Both the I–V and I–III separations are markedly abnormal suggesting a lesion between peripheral VIIIth nerve and lower pons; the CT scan was normal but a posterior fossa contrast study showed a tumor and a 15 mm acoustic neuroma was found at surgery. The superimposed trials have n = 1024 clicks each; the single trace below each set of superimposed trials is the grand average of the superimposed trials. For this and all subsequent figures the recording derivation was earlobe ipsilateral to monaural stimulation referred to vertex (CZ); relative positivity of the vertex is an upward trace deflection. The calibration marks are 5 ms and 0.25 µV. (From Chiappa[6], courtesy of the Editor and publisher, *Weekly Update: Neurology and Neurosurgery*)

separations (e.g. *Figure 11.1*), and five had prolonged I–V interwave separations with normal I–III separations or no recognizable wave III. All acoustic neuroma patients with interwave separation abnormalities had small to moderate sized tumors, two had normal hearing by standard audiometry and two had normal CT scans, e.g. patients whose BAEPs are shown in *Figures 11.1* and *11.2*. Four patients with large acoustic neuromas had wave I, but no subsequent waves. Three patients had no wave I, but a prolonged wave V absolute latency or an inter-ear wave V absolute latency difference abnormality. One meningioma patient had normal waves I, II and III with no waves IV or V. Five patients with large tumors had abnormalities of BAEPs on the side opposite the tumor as well as on the ipsilateral side. This contralateral abnormality is thought to be due to cross-compression of the brainstem. One patient was tested two years after tumor removal and the contralateral BAEP abnormality was no longer present[20].

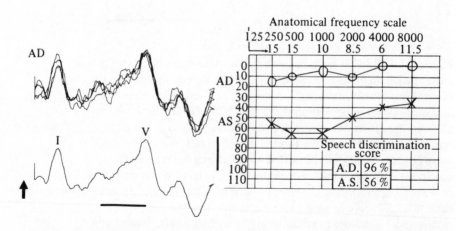

Figure 11.2 BAEPs and audiogram from patient tested because of progressive hearing loss in left ear (AS). AS audiogram shows a 40–50 dB pure tone hearing loss with 56 percent speech discrimination; BAEPs in AS (not shown) were normal. AD pure tone audiogram and speech discrimination were normal; BAEPs in AD (above) show a clear abnormality with only waves I and V present at a markedly abnormal latency separation of 5.0 ms (normal mean + 3 standard deviations = 4.7 ms). CT scan was normal but posterior fossa contrast study showed a tumor and surgery revealed an acoustic neuroma. BAEPs have four separate trials (n = 1024 each) superimposed, with the average of those below. Calibration marks are 0.25 μV and 2.5 ms

Abnormal interwave separations (I–III or I–V) are the most specific and sensitive abnormalities seen with CPA tumors. Increased absolute latency of waves II–V (when I is absent), inter-ear wave V absolute latency difference abnormalities, and absence of all waves are less specific and may be seen with peripheral hearing loss. Strict attention to wave I facilitates the localization of conduction abnormalities as being central to the inner ear, and the use of the external ear canal electrode can help to define this wave (*Figure 11.1*). Thus far, in over 200 patients tested with BAEPs in the author's own laboratory because of a clinical suspicion of acoustic neuroma, there have been no false negative BAEPs in patients who have been proven to have acoustic neuromas (25 patients). There have been rare instances (less than 5 percent) where there is an abnormal I–III separation but no abnormality on posterior fossa contrast study – the lesions in these cases are not yet known.

Demyelinating disease

The BAEP is also useful in the evaluation of patients suspected of having demyelinating disease. The finding of abnormal BAEPs can be helpful in three ways:

(1) in patients who present with a non-brainstem locus of CNS involvement, the abnormal BAEP provides evidence of another clinically unsuspected site of involvement;

(2) in those in whom the clinical findings are subjective, historical, or otherwise uncertain, the abnormal BAEP can provide objective evidence of disturbed function; and

(3) by monitoring abnormal BAEPs, various modes of treatment can be followed and objectively evaluated.

Patients with demyelinating diseases have been studied in detail[8, 19, 21, 29, 35, 36, 39]. *Tables 11.1* and *11.2* present the incidence of abnormal BAEPs and the relationship of these abnormalities to symptoms and signs in a large group of MS patients[8]. The abnormalities were unilateral in 45 percent of the patients with abnormal BAEPs and the

Table 11.1 Incidence of abnormal BAEPs in multiple sclerosis*. (From Chiappa *et al.*[8], courtesy of the Editor and publisher, *Annals of Neurology*)

	Number (percent) of patients†			
	Definite	*Probable*	*Possible*	*Total*
With symptoms and/or signs of brainstem lesion	34/60 (57)	8/38 (21)	7/33 (21)	49/131 (37)
Without symptoms and/or signs of brainstem lesion	4/21 (19)	6/29 (21)	5/21 (24)	15/71 (21)
All patients	38/81 (47)	14/67 (21)	12/54 (22)	64/202 (32)

*MS classifications by McAlpine's criteria[18].
†The second number is the number of patients who fit the clinical criteria irrespective of BAEP results, e.g. there were 60 patients with definite MS who had symptoms and/or signs of brainstem lesions and 34 of these (57 percent) had abnormal BAEPs.

Table 11.2 Incidence of abnormal BAEPs in multiple sclerosis with respect to various symptoms and/or signs of brainstem lesions. (From Chiappa *et al.*[8], courtesy of the Editor and publisher, *Annals of Neurology*)

	Number (percent) of patients*			
	Definite	*Probable*	*Possible*	*Total*
Internuclear ophthalmoplegia	14/20 (70)	1/6 (17)	1/4 (25)	16/30 (53)
Diplopia	16/28 (57)	2/12 (17)	2/14 (14)	20/54 (37)
Nystagmus	17/32 (53)	5/20 (25)	2/17 (12)	24/69 (35)
Other	15/31 (48)	5/15 (33)	2/8 (25)	22/54 (41)

*The second number is the number of patients who fit the clinical criteria irrespective of BAEP results, e.g. there were 20 patients with definite MS who had an internuclear ophthalmoplegia and 14 of these (70 percent) had abnormal BAEPs. Note that the symptoms and/or signs were not necessarily present when the BAEP was performed and some patients had more than one symptom.

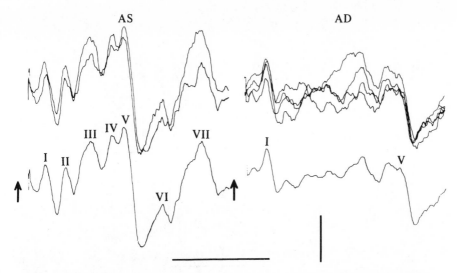

Figure 11.3 BAEPs from stimulation of each ear of one patient with MS showing the marked asymmetry which can be present with monaural stimulation. AS is normal. AD shows another type of BAEP abnormality seen in MS – a lack of wave III and markedly abnormal I–V separation of 6.7 ms demonstrating a conduction defect in the pontine auditory tracts. AS superimposed trials have n = 1024 clicks each; in AD, n = 2048 clicks each. The single trace below each is the sum of the superimposed trials. Calibration marks are 0.25 µV and 5 ms. (From Chiappa *et al.*[8], by courtesy of the Editor and publisher, *Annals of Neurology*)

asymmetry was often striking, as in *Figure 11.3*. Loss of amplitude of waves IV and V was seen in 88 percent of the patients with abnormal BAEPs and progressive examples of this are shown in *Figure 11.4*. Thirteen percent of the BAEP-abnormal patients had only interwave latency abnormalities, 55 percent had only wave V amplitude ratio abnormalities and 33 percent had both.

As well as documenting the presence of clinically unsuspected lesions and confirming the presence of clinically suspected lesions in MS patients, as shown in *Table 11.2*, the BAEP can help to localize the source of nystagmus, or other symptom, e.g. dysphonia[27], in any patient as central or peripheral. Since the vestibular system tracts and nuclei are contiguous with those of the auditory system, a lesion which produces abnormal function in one system might well affect the other. For example, 37 percent of the MS patients who presented with nystagmus at the time of testing had central BAEP abnormalities

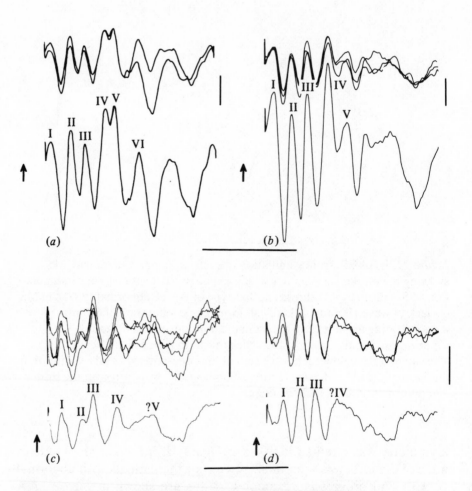

Figure 11.4 Spectrum of IV–V complex abnormalities seen in MS. (*a*) and (*b*) are following stimulation of the same ear of the same patient, (*b*) two months after (*a*). The IV–V separation increased from 0.5 ms to 1.1 ms and the I/V amplitude ratio percentage went from 90 percent to 20 percent; both measures in (*b*) are at the upper limit of normal. (*c*) and (*d*) are from different patients, showing further progression of the abnormality. In (*c*) wave IV is clearly visible but wave V is difficult to recognize – note poor reproducibility in repeated trials. In (*d*) wave V is absent and wave IV is not present as a distinct peak. In (*a*), (*b*) and (*c*) the superimposed trials have n = 1024 clicks each; in (*d*) n = 2048 clicks each. The single trace below each is the sum of the superimposed trials. Calibrations as for *Figure 11.3*. (From Chiappa *et al.*[8], by courtesy of the Editor and publisher, *Annals of Neurology*)

whereas no patient in a group of 21 with Meniere's disease, labyrinthitis or vestibular neuronitis had central BAEP abnormalities. It is interesting to note that, in spite of obvious BAEP abnormalities, few MS patients have symptomatic hearing difficulty or abnormal conventional behavioural audiometry. However, abnormal function can be demonstrated in those patients by detailed auditory localization tests[14].

It should be obvious from a consideration of the generator sources involved, that BAEPs cannot be equated with total brainstem function. There can be gross lesions in the brainstem with normal BAEPs. For example, some patients with 'locked-in' syndrome from basilar artery occlusion have normal BAEPs[3]. This situation is simply a reflection of the fact that the infarcted territory is most commonly in the ventral pons where the motor tracts lie, whereas the auditory tracts lie in the pontine tegmentum. Similarly, patients with internuclear ophthalmoplegias can have normal BAEPs (*see Table 11.2*) in spite of the relative proximity of the medial longitudinal fasciculus to the brainstem auditory tracts.

Intrinsic brainstem tumors

Most patients with mass lesions involving the brainstem, e.g. gliomas (*see Figure 11.5*) have abnormal BAEPs[3, 5, 10, 20, 26–29, 31, 33–35, 39]. In cases where the clinical history and/or findings are equivocal, the BAEP can demonstrate the presence of a central lesion, i.e. suggest that the symptoms and signs in question are being produced by a central lesion. Of 22 patients with intrinsic brainstem lesions studied[3], in three with brainstem gliomas the clinical examinations and neuroradiologic studies indicated a predominant laterality of the tumor. This was verified at autopsy in one case, and the BAEPs were most abnormal on stimulation of the ear ipsilateral to the tumor (*Figure 11.5*). Another 13 cases (four with autopsies) agreed with these findings, albeit with somewhat less marked correlations. This suggests that auditory impulses generating BAEP waves I–V may ascend the brainstem ipsilateral to the ear stimulated, whereas neuroanatomic and behavioral studies suggest that the pathways are primarily contralateral. Thus, the BAEP waves may not necessarily be related directly to functional hearing; involvement in auditory localization is a possibility. Two patients with rostral tegmental pontine hemorrhages

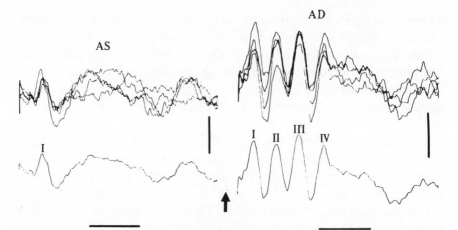

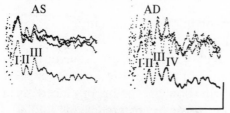

Figure 11.5 BAEPs from a patient with a brainstem glioma; at the time of BAEP testing the left corneal reflex was absent, there was numbness of the entire left face (maximum in V2) and the jaw deviated to the left on opening, in addition to other non-lateralized neurological findings. Note the marked asymmetry between the ears. Clinical, radiological and subsequent neuropathological findings consistently demonstrated a marked asymmetry of tumor involvement with the left brainstem most severely affected, corresponding to the asymmetry of the BAEPs. Calibrations as for *Figure 11.2*

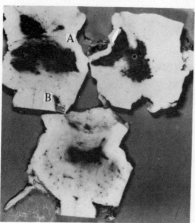

Figure 11.6 BAEPs and brainstem neuropathology of a patient with a pontine hemorrhage. Both ears show normal waves I–III, only AD shows a subsequent wave (probably IV). Frontal coronal sections of pons (A is at pontomesencephalic border, B is at pontomedullary border) show a hemorrhage transecting the pons, sparing the lower one-third and the superior olivary nuclei. Calibrations as for *Figure 11.3*

confirmed by CT scan (and autopsy in 1 case) (*Figure 11.6*) had normal BAEP waves I–III bilaterally, with bilaterally abnormal or absent waves IV and absent waves V. This is consistent with the localization of the generator of wave III in the superior olivary complex, and of the generator of waves IV and V above that level. Of four patients with 'locked-in' syndromes secondary to basilar artery occlusion, one had normal BAEPs, reflecting the predominantly ventral pontine involvement usually seen in that lesion. Three patients with lateral medullary syndromes had normal BAEPs.

In both brainstem mass lesions and MS, BAEPs offer a means by which the disease process and therapeutic effectiveness can be objectively documented. However, at present, there is little clinical data available with respect to these uses of the BAEP, although it has been used to follow the clinical course of central pontine myelinolysis[36].

Brain death

It has been suggested[13,30,39] that BAEPs can assist in the clinical definition of brain death since an absence of BAEP waveforms would provide additional evidence of a significant lack of brainstem function. For example, in deep coma secondary to drug overdose, the BAEP is relatively unchanged[39]. Six (22 percent) of a group of 27 patients who met clinical and EEG criteria for brain death had wave I but no waves thereafter present[13]. This confirmed a loss of function in the brainstem auditory pathways; however, 21 of these patients (78 percent) did not have wave I visible (in addition to having no subsequent waves), even when external ear canal needle electrodes were used. The absence of wave I in cases of brain death cannot yet be adequately explained although it is thought to be on the basis of interference with the blood supply to the VIIIth nerve and cochlea which is derived primarily from the posterior intracranial circulation via the internal auditory artery. Without an identifiable wave I no inferences can be made as to the localization of the interruption of the auditory signal since the integrity of the peripheral hearing apparatus in an individual patient is often not known. For example, a traumatic transverse fracture of the temporal bone might have damaged the cochlea, or in a case where the clinical history is poor, the patient might had a pre-existing deafness in the only ear available for BAEP testing.

In comparison, in 50 patients who were clinically poorly-responsive but had some preservation of brainstem and CNS function, i.e. in coma but not brain dead, BAEPs were found to be normal in 26 (52 percent)[13]. Of these patients, four died, 10 remained in coma or other neurovegetative state, and 12 regained some degree of function. All except eight patients (16 percent) had wave I present at least unilaterally. In general, there was no correlation between BAEP results and clinical outcome, although those patients with bilaterally absent BAEP waves, thought not to be secondary to peripheral hearing loss or a difficult recording situation, had a higher likelihood of not surviving, and those who had absent waves after III had a poor outcome. BAEPs have been reported in other groups of patients in coma with diverse etiologies[25, 29, 31, 34, 39, 40].

Surgical monitoring

The BAEP can also be used to monitor the function of the VIIIth nerve and brainstem auditory structures during neurosurgical procedures in the posterior fossa. Preservation of hearing is sometimes a goal in surgery for removal of acoustic neuromas and the BAEP provides a means of relating manipulations of the tumor and nerve to loss of function[17].

The BAEP can be reliably recorded from infants of all ages, including prematures, and correlations of BAEP parameters with age[5, 23, 32, 37, 38] and various diseases of the CNS[24, 35] are now becoming available so that the test provides another tool for investigation of this age-group and their distinctive set of pathologic processes.

References

1 ACHOR, L. J. and STARR, A. Auditory brain stem responses in the cat. I. Intracranial and extracranial recordings. II. Effects of lesions. *Electroencephalography and Clinical Neurophysiology*, **48**, 154–190 (1980)

2 ALLISON, T., GOFF, W.R. and WOOD, C. C. Auditory, somatosensory and visual evoked potentials in the diagnosis of neuropathology: recording considerations and normative data. In *Human Evoked Potentials*, edited by D. Lehmann and E. Callaway. New York, Plenum (1979)

3 BROWN, R. H., CHIAPPA, K. H. and BROOKS, E. B. Brainstem auditory evoked responses in 22 patients with intrinsic brainstem lesions: Implications for clinical interpretations. *Electroencephalography and Clinical Neurophysiology*, **51**, 38P (1981)

4 BUCHWALD, J. S. and HUAN, C. M. Fair-field acoustic response: origins in the cat. *Science*, **189**, 382–384 (1975)

5 CHIAPPA, K. H. Physiologic localization using evoked responses: pattern shift visual, brainstem auditory and short latency somatosensory. In *Barrow Neurological Institute Symposium on New Techniques in Cerebral Localization* (February 1980, Phoenix, Arizona). New York, Raven Press (1981)

6 CHIAPPA, K. H. Evoked responses II: brainstem auditory. In *Weekly Update: Neurology and Neurosurgery*, **2**, 129–135 (1980)

7 CHIAPPA, K. H., GLADSTONE, K. J. and YOUNG, R. R. Brainstem auditory evoked responses: studies of waveform variations in 50 normal human subjects. *Archives of Neurology*, **36**, 81–87 (1979)

8 CHIAPPA, K. H., HARRISON, J. L., BROOKS, E. B. and YOUNG, R. R. Brainstem auditory evoked resonses in 200 patients with multiple sclerosis. *Annals of Neurology*, **7**, 135–143 (1980)

9 COATS, A. C. and MARTIN, J. L. Human auditory nerve action potentials and brain stem evoked responses. Effects of audiogram shape and lesion location. *Archives of Otolaryngology*, **103**, 605–622 (1977)

10 COATS, A. C. Human auditory nerve action potentials and brain stem evoked responses. Latency-intensity functions in detection of cochlear and retrocochlear abnormality. *Archives of Otolaryngology*, **104**, 709–717 (1978)

11 DON, M. and EGGERMONT, J. J. Analysis of the click-evoked brainstem potentials in man using high-pass noise masking. *Journal of the Acoustic Society of America*, **63**, 1084–1092 (1978)

12 DON, M., ALLEN, A. R. and STARR, A. Effect of click rate on the latency of auditory brain stem responses in humans. *Annals of Otolaryngology*, **86**, 186–195 (1977)

13 GOLDIE, W. D., CHIAPPA K. H. and YOUNG, R. R. Brainstem auditory evoked responses and short-latency somatosensory evoked responses in the evaluation of deeply comatose patients. *Neurology*, **29**, 551 (1979)

14 HAUSLER, R. and LEVINE, R. A. Brainstem auditory evoked potentials are related to interaural time discrimination in patients with multiple sclerosis. *Brain Research*, **191**, 589–594 (1980)

15 JEWETT, D. L., ROMANO, M. N. and WILLISTON, J. S. Human auditory evoked potentials. Possible brainstem components detected on the scalp. *Science*, **167**, 1517–1518 (1970)

16 JEWETT, D. L. and WILLISTON, J. S. Auditory-evoked far fields averaged from the scalp in humans. *Brain*, **94**, 681–696 (1971)

17 LEVINE, R. A. Monitoring auditory evoked potentials during acoustic neuroma surgery. In *Neurological Surgery of the Ear*, edited by H. Silverstein and H. Norell. Birmingham, Alabama, Aesculapius Publishing Co. (1977)

18 McALPINE, D., LUMSDEN, C. E. and ACHESON, E. D. *Multiple Sclerosis: A Reappraisal*. Edinburgh, Churchill Livingstone (1972)

19 OCHS, R., MARKLAND, O. N. and DeMYER, W. E. Brainstem auditory evoked responses in leukodystrophies. *Neurology*, **29**, 1089–1093 (1979)

20 PARKER, S. W., CHIAPPA, K. H. and BROOKS, E. B. Brainstem auditory evoked responses in patients with acoustic neuromas and cerebello-pontine angle meningiomas. *Neurology*, **30**, 413 (1980)

21 ROBINSON, K. and RUDGE, P. Abnormalities of the auditory evoked potentials in patients with multiple sclerosis. *Brain*, **100**, 19–40 (1977)

22 ROWE, M. J. Normal variability of the brain-stem auditory evoked response in young and old adult subjects. *Electroencephalography and Clinical Neurophysiology*, **44**, 459–470 (1978)

23 SALAMY, A. and McKEAN, C. M. Postnatal development of human brainstem potentials during the first year of life. *Electroencephalography and Clinical Neurophysiology*, **40**, 418–426 (1976)

24 SATYA-MURTI, S., CACACE, A. T. and HANSON, P. A. Abnormal auditory evoked potentials in hereditary motor-sensory neuropathy. *Annals of Neurology*, **5**, 445–448 (1978)

25 SEALES, D. M., ROSSITER, V. S. and WEINSTEIN, M. E. Brainstem auditory evoked responses in patients comatose as a result of blunt head trauma. *Journal of Trauma*, **19**, 347–353 (1979)

26 SELTERS, W. A. and BRACKMANN, D. E. Acoustic tumor detection with brainstem electric response audiometry. *Archives of Otolaryngology*, **103**, 181–187 (1977)

27 SHARBROUGH, F. W., STOCKARD, J. J. and ARONSON, A. E. Brainstem auditory-evoked responses in spastic dysphonia. *Transactions of the American Neurological Association*, **103**, 198–201 (1978)

28 SOHMER, H., FEINMESSER, M. and SZABO, G. Sources of electrocochleographic responses as studied in patients with brain damage. *Electroencephalography and Clinical Neurophsyiology*, **37**, 663–669 (1974)

29 STARR, A. and ACHOR, J. Auditory brain stem responses in neurological disease. *Archives of Neurology*, **32**, 761–768 (1975)

30 STARR, A. Auditory brain-stem responses in brain death. *Brain*, **99**, 543–554 (1976)

31 STARR, A. and HAMILTON, A. E. Correlation between confirmed sites of neurological lesions and abnormalities of far-field auditory brain-stem responses. *Electroencephalography and Clinical Neurophysiology*, **41**, 595–608 (1976)

32 STARR, A., AMLIE, R. N., MARTIN, W. H. and SANDERS, S. Development of auditory function in newborn infants revealed by auditory brainstem potentials. *Pediatrics*, **60**, 831–839 (1977)

33 STARR, A. and ACHOR, L. J. Anatomical and physiologic origins of auditory brain stem responses (ABR). In *Human Evoked Potentials: Applications and Problems*, edited by D. Lehmann and E. Callaway. New York, Plenum Press (1978)

34 STOCKARD, J. J. and ROSSITER, V. S. Clinical and pathologic correlates of brain stem auditory response abnormalities. *Neurology*, **27**, 316–325 (1977)

35 STOCKARD, J. J. STOCKARD, J. E. and SHARBROUGH, F. W. Detection and localization of occult lesions with brainstem auditory responses. *Mayo Clinics Proceedings*, **52**, 761–769 (1977)

36 STOCKARD, J. J. ROSSITER, V. S. and WIEDERHOLT, W. C. Brain stem auditory evoked responses in suspected central pontine myelinolysis. *Archives of Neurology*, **33**, 726–728 (1976)

37 STOCKARD, J. J. STOCKARD, J. E. and SHARBROUGH, F. W. Nonpathologic factors influencing brainstem auditory evoked potentials. *American Journal of EEG Technology*, **18**, 177–209 (1978)

38 STOCKARD, J. E., STOCKARD, J. J. WESTMORELAND, B. F. and CORFITS, J. L. Brainstem auditory-evoked responses. Normal variations as a function of stimulus and subject characteristics. *Archives of Neurology*, **36**, 823–831 (1979)

39 STOCKARD, J. J. and SHARBROUGH, F. W. Unique contributions of short-latency sensory evoked potentials to neurologic diagnosis. In *Clinical Uses of Cerebral, Brainstem and Spinal Somatosensory Evoked Potentials. Progress in Clinical Neurophysiology*, **7**, 231–263 (1980)

40 UZIEL, A. and BENEZECH, J. Auditory brain-stem responses in comatose patients: relationship with brain-stem reflexes and levels of coma. *Electroencephalography and Clinical Neurophysiology*, **45**, 515–524 (1978)

12

Somatosensory evoked potentials

E. M. Sedgwick

Introduction

The study of human CNS evoked potentials began in 1947 with Dawson's use[11] of photographic superimposition of the poststimulus EEG to demonstrate a waveform following peripheral nerve stimulation. He observed that a patient with myoclonic epilepsy had a somatosensory evoked potential (SEP) of much higher amplitude than normal[12]. As amplifiers have improved and computers have become more easily obtainable to carry out signal averaging, more laboratories have studied evoked potentials, especially the small *short latency* ones which are of particular clinical interest.

A volley of impulses evoked by electrical stimulation of a nerve can be recorded along the course of the nerve especially where it lies close to the skin. These potentials are used clinically to measure peripheral nerve conduction velocities and initially were not considered in evoked potential (EP) studies. They should be recorded routinely however as they confirm an adequate stimulus has been given and, if recorded close to the spinal cord (at Erb's point or over the sciatic notch), can be used as a time mark from which interwave latencies are measured. Latency variability of later waves due to differing limb lengths and conduction velocities can thereby be minimized.

Normal values

Spinal cord potentials

Spinal cord potentials using intrathecal or epidural electrodes have been recorded in animals[2, 3, 33] and man[29, 30, 44, 59-62]. Shortly after arrival of a volley in low threshold cutaneous afferents, a negative

278

wave, the N1 or cord dorsum potential, develops over the spinal cord and spreads two or three segments rostral and caudal to those which the volley enters. This potential arises from synaptic activation of dorsal horn neurons in Rexed's lamina III and IV by collaterals of afferent fibres.

Use of intrathecal and epidural electrodes, involving risk and discomfort, is clinically unjustifiable. Liberson[40] succeeded in recording a potential from the skin of the neck following median nerve stimulation at the wrist and Cracco[9] began the systematic analysis of these surface recorded potentials. Four distinct peaks on the negative waves were soon identified[38, 49]. They are called by their latency and polarity $\overline{N9}$, $\overline{N11}$, $\overline{N13}$ and $\overline{N14}$ (*see Figure 12.1*).

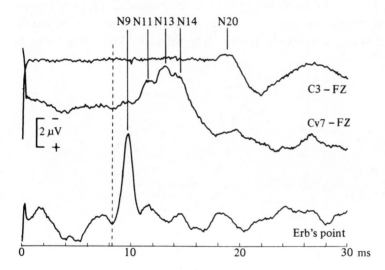

Figure 12.1 The afferent volley in brachial plexus following a median nerve stimulus is shown in a recording from Erb's point (lower trace). Cervical cord potentials (N11, N13 and N14) can be seen in the middle trace and the cerebral potential (N20) is shown on the upper trace. The interrupted line marks the beginning of the Erb's point potential and it is useful to time subsequent events from this point thus eliminating variations due to different arm lengths or slowing of peripheral conduction. Normal subject, right median nerve stimulation (0.2 ms duration at 3 × sensory threshold); 128 sweeps averaged. Cv7 = Seventh cervical vertebra. (After Dimitrijevic *et al.*[20], courtesy of the Editor and publisher, *Journal of Physiology*)

The origin of these peaks is not resolved but the major peak, $\overline{\text{N13}}$, may correspond to N1 or the cord dorsum potential; although some favour an origin at about the foramen magnum[5, 39] and others claim the afferent volley in dorsal columns is the source. Shimoji, Shimizu and Marugama[62] and Ertekin[31] recording simultaneously from the epidural space and from the skin surface, found good correspondence between the cord dorsum potential and $\overline{\text{N13}}$. $\overline{\text{N13}}$ has also been recorded in patients with high clinically-complete cervical cord lesions[20, 25, 57]. Jones[38] has shown $\overline{\text{N9}}$ to be a brachial plexus potential; $\overline{\text{N11}}$ is possibly a dorsal root or presynaptic potential and $\overline{\text{N14}}$ may arise in more rostral structures, perhaps in the medulla oblongata.

Recording over the lumbar cord is technically more difficult because of the greater mass of muscle between the electrode and the cord. Two negative peaks $\overline{\text{N10}}$ and $\overline{\text{N13}}$ have been identified after stimulation of the tibial nerve at the popliteal fossa[13, 19, 25] (*Figure 12.2*); their spatial distribution and other properties suggest they are generated by cauda equina and spinal cord respectively. An additional travelling wave at

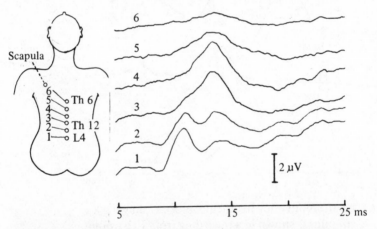

Figure 12.2 Lumbar somatosensory evoked potentials (following tibial nerve stimulation at the popliteal fossa) consisting of two waves, N10 and N14. N10 is recorded primarily by the caudal electrode at L4 and N14 is of highest amplitude at Th12 vertebral level where spinal lumbar cord segments are located. The reference electrode was placed on the scapula, stimulation to R tibial nerve, 0.2 ms, 2 × sensory threshold, 256 sweeps averaged. (From El-Negamy and Sedgwick[25], courtesy of the Editor and publisher, *Journal of Neurology, Neurosurgery and Psychiatry*)

successively higher levels of the cord, presumed to be an ascending volley in the long sensory tracts, can be recorded following stimulation of tibial or peroneal nerve[10, 43, 66].

Subcortical potentials

Figure 12.1 shows a positive wave between $\overline{N14}$ and $\overline{N20}$. This $\overline{P15}$ component, seen best with a noncephalic reference electrode, is widely distributed over the scalp and can even be recorded from the ear and mastoid, sites often used for the reference electrode. It is larger over the contralateral scalp[8] and Desmedt and Brunko[15] claim it has two components which can be differentially affected by changes in location of the reference electrode. Allison *et al.*[1] who reviewed properties of this potential and evoked potentials which have been recorded at surgery by depth electrodes, concluded that $\overline{P15}$ has properties indicating a subcortical origin but there is no satisfactory demonstration of the generators. However a positive potential of appropriate latency can be recorded from the ventroposterolateral nucleus (VPL) of thalamus, the lemniscal relay nucleus. Many other subcortical structures are undoubtedly also being activated at this time and $\overline{P15}$ may well be a composite potential with several different generators.

The same arguments apply to $\overline{N20}$ (*see below*); at least two groups have recorded a negative potential in VPL at about 20 ms latency[6, 36].

Cortical somatosensory potentials

Following median nerve stimulation, a sharp-peaked negative wave of 20 ms latency ($\overline{N20}$) is recorded maximally over contralateral scalp. *Figure 12.3* shows this potential to be followed by several others which will be discussed below. Initially there was confusion about $\overline{N20}$ because it was not adequately recorded by early equipment. Direct recordings from cortex at surgery suggest its generator is in the postcentral gyrus resulting from synaptic activity evoked by the volley as it travels in thalamocortical fibres to activate cortical neurons in the appropriate area[15] (*Figure 12.3*). Direct cortical recording shows $\overline{N20}$ is produced in a small area of sensory cortex and the cortical SEP is quite different when recorded nearby[53]. From the scalp, $\overline{N20}$ can be recorded over a wide region including the parietal region and an area anterior to the central sulcus.

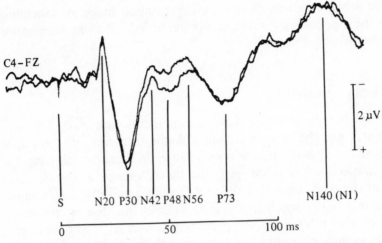

Figure 12.3 The cortical somatosensory evoked potential following left median nerve stimulation at 3 × sensory threshold. The reference electrode is at FZ and the two electrodes were isoelectric for the $\overline{P15}$ component which therefore cannot be seen. The final component (N1) is the first of the so-called 'vertex potentials' or 'late potentials' and is altered by changes in cognitive state. Normal subject, 256 sweeps, two separate runs are superimposed to indicate the reproducibility of the potentials

Subsequent potentials vary in latency from subject to subject but are consistent in any one subject. The descending limb of N20 continues to swing positive and forms a sharp, positive peak at about 30 ms (P30); there is then a negative peak (N42) which in some subjects does not reach the baseline and then becomes P48 which is small in this recording. The form of the SEP is sometimes referred to as a 'W' made up of P30 and P48 but this characteristic profile is not always seen as the intermediate negative wave ($\overline{N42}$) may be absent. These potentials are best recorded from parietal locations; from frontal regions a single consistent $\overline{N30}$ peak can be recognized. These constitute the early components of the SEP, are little affected by changes in attention or sleep and relate most directly to sensory inputs along the fast-conducting lemniscal pathway[35]. After $\overline{N20}$, parallel processing occurs in different cerebral areas as afferent volleys travelling in slower pathways begin to impinge on cortex. To look for single generators of these waves is probably not realistic but their physiological properties may offer insights into cortical neurophysiology. Studies of the interaction of two closely applied stimuli in the same or related nerves help define the recovery time after one volley and the extent to which different nerves share the same generator[65].

Late potentials, often called vertex potentials, may be evoked by somatosensory, visual or auditory stimuli and have common properties. Their latencies are more variable than short latency potentials. Somatosensory stimuli elicit a negative potential N1 at 120–160 ms, and two positive potentials, P2 at 170–220 ms and P3 at 300 ms, which are modified in amplitude according to the subjects' cognitive state[14]. N1 is enhanced by stressing the subject and asking him to attend to some stimuli and not others, i.e. count the stimuli to one finger and ignore stimuli to any other fingers. If the task is made difficult by using low-strength stimuli and forcing the pace, N1 is enhanced[18]. The P3 or P300 component is produced when the subject detects a targer stimulus – if he makes an error or misses one of the target stimuli, no P300 is seen. P300 can also arise in situations where one of a regular series of stimuli is omitted. These late potentials and their relationships to different cognitive states are receiving much attention from psychologists but they have not yet made great impact in medicine or psychiatry. They may assist investigation of psychiatric disease or neurological dysfunction after head injury or encephalitis and during neurological rehabilitation.

The discovery by Eccles and his colleagues[23] of presynaptic inhibition acting at primary sensory relay nuclei, apparently under cortical control, led to an hypothesis that this may account for selective attention. It was suggested that all primary sensory afferents, except those being attended to, would be suppressed by presynaptic inhibition. Indeed experiments seemed to show that early evoked potentials in animals were of lower amplitude if the animal was attending an interesting stimulus presented to another modality. Experiments in humans show clearly that abrupt stimuli evoke identical early potentials regardless of the state of attention. It appears that selective filtering of important from non-important stimuli can first be detected by evoked potentials some 70 ms after the stimulus which suggests the sensory volley is admitted to cortex and undergoes some form of processing before being assigned as relevant or not.

Central conduction time

Low threshold afferent fibres producing these potentials conduct at about 60 m/s in the arm. From spinal cord to cortex, conduction velocity is about 50 m/s after allowance is made for a delay of 0.3 ms at each synapse along the pathway[15]. As axons of four separate neurons are traversed, one cannot speak of conduction velocity in the same way as in a peripheral nerve – *conduction time* is a better parameter and was found to be 5.6 ± 0.5 ms[36] in normal subjects. Latency between the Erb's point potential and $\overline{\text{N13}}$ at the cervical cord gives an estimate of conduction time through certain dorsal roots. To date, this is the most direct method of estimating conduction primarily in the dorsal roots although less direct methods using reflexes and the F wave, which utilizes only ventral roots, have been available previously[21] and are being increasingly widely used (*see* Chapter 6).

Conduction velocity in dorsal column fibres, determined directly by Ertekin[30] who used widely separated intrathecal electrodes, stimulating through one and recording from the other, was 45.8 ± 4.7 m/s. Recording from two intrathecal sites following tibial nerve stimulation however, he found a dorsal column conduction velocity of 37.7 ± 5.2 m/s. Both techniques were employed in the same subjects so the discrepancy is puzzling unless they measure different populations of fibres. Studies on four multiple sclerosis patients[24] with closely spaced epidural electrodes placed for spinal cord stimulation but temporarily used to stimulate and record, gave conduction velocities of 10, 14, 25 and 50 m/s. Conduction velocity of the travelling wave over the spine recorded with surface electrodes[9, 10, 43] is about 65 m/s; conduction may be slower over the cauda equina and faster more rostrally[9]. Studies on young children[7] showed a wave travelling at 25 m/s in the newborn. Its velocity increased quickly in the first two years and then slowly to reach adult values by 4–5 years of age. Studies of central conduction from cervical cord to cortex in children[16] gave a velocity of 10 m/s in neonates rising slowly during the first 8 years of life to an adult value of 49 m/s. At the other end of life's scale, octogenarians were found to have normal adult central conduction velocities (49 m/s) even though conduction velocity in peripheral sensory fibres had fallen by 20 per cent[17]. $\overline{\text{N20}}$ had a longer duration and higher amplitude in the elderly.

Another approach is to measure the latency between lumbar cord and cortex potentials and subtract from it the cervical cord to cortex time determined by median nerve stimulation. The figure obtained is closely related to the time taken for a volley to travel from Th12 vertebral level to Cv7 vertebral level. Conduction velocity of dorsal columns determined by this method is 55 m/s, with a range of 47–68 m/s (Sedgwick and Fayaz, unpublished observations.)

An outdated indirect method of determining spinal cord conduction velocity depends upon determining the latency of the waveform equivalent to $\overline{N20}$ when a leg nerve is stimulated to get total conduction time. The time of arrival of the *sensory* volley at the cord is estimated from measurement of F and direct motor (M) responses from a muscle supplied by the nerve stimulated. Chapter 6 deals with details of the F response. After subtraction of M response latency and allowing an arbitrary 1 ms for re-exciting the motoneuron, the hypothetical time taken for the impulses to travel from the stimulus site to the cord and back again is arrived at. Half this time is taken to represent the arrival of the motor volley at the spinal cord. If this motor conduction time is determined for arm and leg, together with sensory latency to the cortex, a 'conduction time' from lumbar to cervical cord can be estimated. Using this method, Dorfman[21] found a conduction velocity in dorsal column fibres of 55.1 ± 9.9 m/s; in one subject with a Brown-Sequard syndrome, conduction velocities were 23.1 m/s on the affected side but 43.8 m/s on the other side. Clearly this method involves a number of assumptions not least of which is that sensory and motor peripheral fibres conduct at the same velocity, clearly erroneous. Errors in individual measurements can compound to give a total error estimation as high as 24 per cent[21]. This technique therefore is of little use and since one can now record potentials at Erb's point, the spinal segmental level and in the lumbar roots, it should be discarded.

Table 12.1 summarizes the results of different methods. Despite the wide range of velocities, central fibres appear to conduct more slowly

Table 12.1 Estimation of conduction velocity of dorsal column fibres

Author	Method	Conduction velocity (m/s)	Comment
Ertekin[30]	Intrathecal	45.8 ± SD 4.7	Intrathecal stimulation and recording
El-Negamy[24]	Epidural	Range 10–50	Epidural stimulation and recording (MS patients)
Ertekin[30]	Intrathecal	37.7 ± SD 5.2	Stimulation of posterior tibial nerve
Cracco[9]	Spinal travelling wave	About 65	
Jones and Small[43]	Spinal travelling wave	60–65	
Sedgwick and Fayaz (unpublished)	Spinal and cortical SEP	55.2 ± SD 8.9	10 subjects
Dorfman[21]	Indirect	55.1 ± SD 9.9	Error up to 25%

than peripheral fibres, which is to be expected, as they are of smaller diameter.

Somatosensory potentials in disease

Brachial plexus lesions

In traumatic brachial plexus lesions which are difficult to evaluate early when multiple injuries are present, prognosis depends on whether roots have been avulsed from the cord or whether damage has been sustained distal to dorsal root ganglia, in which case some regeneration may be expected. Such lesions are on the increase as motorcycle riders survive accidents which would have killed them had they not been wearing protective helmets.

Jones[41] studied 26 cases, 10 of which were subsequently explored surgically. Erb's point potentials (peripheral nerve at the clavicle corresponding to spinal cord evoked potential $\overline{N9}$), spinal cord potentials ($\overline{N13}$ at cervical 7) and cortical potentials ($\overline{N20}$) were recorded. A normal $\overline{N9}$ potential with absent or much reduced $\overline{N13}$ indicated a root avulsion proximal to the ganglion. $\overline{N13}$ was reduced approximately in proportion to the extent of the injury and was more sensitive to this than the cortical ($\overline{N20}$) potential. Preoperative assessment by evoked potentials was found to correspond reasonably well with the operative findings.

Cervical spondylosis

Delayed cervical somatosensory responses have been reported in some patients with cervical spondylosis[26] while others showed normal potentials or, in a significant number, no clear potential could be detected.

In a more recent study, low amplitude as well as delayed cord potentials were noted and delay between spinal and cortical potentials was also seen in some subjects[32]. No abnormalities were seen in patients with symptoms only, without neurological signs; even some patients with signs of radiculopathy and myelopathy had normal potentials. The most characteristic feature of evoked potentials in this condition is increased $\overline{N9}$–$\overline{N13}$ delay showing slowed conduction between the brachial plexus and cord. Further studies are needed to determine whether the findings in radiculopathy or myelopathy due to spondylosis are sufficiently characteristic to aid in its documentation and differentiation from multiple sclerosis for example.

Multiple sclerosis

Demyelination results in slowed or blocked conduction in affected fibres and delayed evoked potentials reflect the slowed conduction which does not always result in symptoms. Namerow first reported a delayed $\overline{N20}$ in MS in 1968[51]. Abnormal cervical potentials were recorded in a high proportion of MS patients by Small, Matthews and Small[63] who pointed out that stimulation of clinically normal limbs frequently gave abnormal potentials and the abnormalities could persist even during complete remission. Sometimes one of the three components $\overline{N11}$, $\overline{N13}$ or $\overline{N14}$ was absent or separated from its neighbour by a longer than normal interval, but delayed response was much less common than an absent or reduced amplitude wave. The cervical SEP which is more often abnormal than the cortical SEP[28] is useful clinically to determine the presence of subclinical lesions. It remains abnormal but stable during remission but can worsen during a relapse and recover somewhat afterwards[50]. The use of spinal cord stimulation in the management of MS was accompanied by an improvement of the cervical SEP in some patients[37, 58].

Concerning the relative clinical usefulness of cervical SEPs compared with visual EP in patients suspected of having MS, most reports are of more positives with the visual EP though both together increased the positives still further. Careful use of EPs can save patients the risk and discomfort of contrast myelography, not to mention the expense[45-47]. Matthews[48], using the SEP, could not predict which patients would develop MS after an attack of retrobulbar neuritis. Though SEPs recorded after stimulation of the leg test a greater length of the neuraxis, they were not felt to be diagnostically helpful in MS[27]. Dorfman, Bosley and Cummins[22], using indirect techniques to determine spinal conduction velocity[21], were able to show slowed conduction in the thoracic cord of two subjects.

Spinal trauma

Cervical and lumbar cord potentials can be present with normal latency and form after complete or partial cord transection[20, 57]. They are also present during spinal shock when reflex function is completely depessed. When the lesion was only a few segments above the generator site, potentials were frequently absent presumably because damage extended several segments along the cord to involve the generators.

Patients with clinically complete lesions show no cortical potentials from a stimulus delivered to a nerve entering the cord below the level of the lesion. In only half the patients with an incomplete lesion could a cortical response be recorded and these patients tended to make a good recovery[54, 55]. Rowed, McLean and Tator[56] showed that recovery of the cortical SEP could precede clinical recovery and was a good prognostic sign. Evoked potentials can therefore be usefully exploited in spinal injury to assess the completeness of a lesion in the early stages when the patient may be unconscious. Techniques routinely used are of little help in defining the level of a lesion but modifications to stimulate at successively higher levels can sometimes demonstrate the upper limit of a lesion.

Charcot-Marie-Tooth disease

Eight patients with this hereditary motor-sensory neuropathy were studied by Noël and Desmedt[52], in some of whom, because of demyelination, remyelination and axonal loss, sensory nerve action potentials were unrecordable. In others, low amplitude delayed potentials showed conduction velocities in peripheral nerves as low as 10 m/s. Despite that, they were able to record very delayed cervical spinal potentials ($\overline{N13}$ had a latency of 35 ms in one subject). Cortical potentials however were always present and followed spinal potentials by about 6 ms, a normal central conduction time, indicating that conduction is not slowed centrally in this condition.

Spinocerebellar degeneration

In Friedreich's ataxia, large myelinated fibres in peripheral nerves degenerate. Remaining fibres produce low amplitude potentials at Erb's point and over the cervical cord which are delayed slightly if at all. $\overline{N20}$ was, however, delayed with a prolonged rise time suggesting slowed conduction in central pathways[42]. In another study[52], $\overline{N20}$, small but not delayed, was followed by similar wavelets leading to a wave with the appearance of $\overline{N20}$ but developing almost 10 ms later than normal. In this study, central conduction time was assessed as normal and the delayed wave thought to reflect axonal loss.

Subarachnoid haemorrhage

Subarachnoid haemorrhage is frequently complicated by hemisphere ischaemia due to arterial spasm and it has been suggested that central conduction time ($\overline{N13}$ to $\overline{N20}$) may serve as a useful monitor of ischaemia[64]. In patients who developed hemiplegia, central conduction time to the affected hemisphere was prolonged while to the other hemisphere a normal time was maintained. Conduction time normalized on recovery. In serial studies, prolonged conduction time paralleled the reduction in cerebral blood flow but preceded the onset of clinical signs. This technique seems an interesting and possibly useful alternative to determinations of cerebral blood flow.

Localized structural lesions

Changes seen in SEPs with structural lesions have recently been reviewed[4, 5, 52]. Structural lesions which interrupt fast ascending sensory pathways will alter or obliterate those components of the EP which are generated by structures rostral to the lesion. Evoked potential studies should play an increasing part in assessing the functional extent of a lesion and its progression or regression.

Myoclonus

The Hallidays[34] have recently published their findings concerning SEPs and VEPs in a large series of patients with myoclonus. Of the cortical SEP components, $\overline{P30}$ wave is the one most enhanced. In the Hallidays' heterogeneous group of 22 progressive myoclonic epileptics, $\overline{P30}$ was 0.8–44 μV (mean 13.6 μV) in amplitude compared with 3.0 ± 1.9 μV in normals; it was enlarged in 13 out of 22 cases but its latency was normal. The SEP varied within each case and was largest when the patient suffered myoclonus, becoming smaller, perhaps within the normal range, when jerks abated or were suppressed by clonazepam. There may be a strong somatotopic relationship between the limb or part affected by myoclonus and the area of cortex showing an enhanced potential. Visual evoked potentials also tend to be large but there is more overlap with the normal range. In benign essential myoclonus, SEPs and usually EEGs are within normal limits – these two investigations can be of practical help should there be doubt about the diagnosis.

Outlook

The EP technique opens up new dimensions for human neurophysiology and neurology, giving insights into the pathophysiology of disease which were not previously thought possible. EPs have barely penetrated neurological rehabilitation but their use in assessing neurological damage and progress of disease can be confidently forecasted. From the point of view of neurological practice, thorough appraisals of EPs are required to determine just how reliable they are when used for diagnosis and in what situations they can replace or, at least, guide invasive investigations. They will not replace the basic clinical skills of history-taking and physical examination but EPs already represent significant and sensitive extensions of the neurologists' clinical examination; also, when taken alone, they are no more aetiologically ecific.

References

1 ALLISON, T., GOFF, W. R., WILLIAMSON, P. D. and VAN GELDER, J. C. On the neural origin of early components of the human somatosensory evoked potential. In *Clinical uses of Cerebral, Brainstem and Spinal Somatosensory Evoked Potentials*, edited by J. E. Desmedt, *Progress in Clinical Neurophysiology*, **7**, 51–68. Basel, S. Karger (1980)

2 BEALE, J. E., APPLEBAUM, A. E., FOREMAN, R. D. and WILLIS, W. D. Spinal cord potentials evoked by cutaneous afferents in the monkey. *Journal of Neurophysiology*, **40**, 199–211 (1977)

3 BERNHARD, C. G. The cord dorsum potentials in relation to peripheral source of afferent stimulation. *Cold Spring Harbour Symposium in Quantitative Biology*, **17**, 221–232 (1952)

4 CHIAPPA, K. H. *Evoked Potentials in Clinical Neurology*, New York, Raven (in press)

5 CHIAPPA, K. H., CHOI, S. and YOUNG, R. R. Short-latency somatosensory evoked potentials following median nerve stimulation in patients with neurological lesions. In *Clinical Uses of Cerebral, Brainstem and Spinal Somatosensory Evoked Potentials*, edited by J. E. Desmedt, *Clinical Neurophysiology*, **7**, 264–281. Basel, S. Karger (1980)

6 CHIAPPA, K. H., YOUNG, R. R. and GOLDIE, W. D. Origins of the components of human short-latency somatosensory evoked responses (SER). *Neurology*, **29**, 598 (1979)

7 CRACCO, J. B., CRACCO, R. Q. and GRAZIANI, L. J. The spinal evoked response in infants and children. *Neurology*, **25**, 31–36 (1975)

8 CRACCO, R. Q. The initial positive potential of the human scalp recorded somatosensory evoked response. *Electroencephalography and Clinical Neurophysiology*, **32**, 623–629 (1972)

9 CRACCO, R. Q. Spinal evoked response: peripheral nerve stimulation in man. *Electroencephalography and Clinical Neurophysiology*, **35**, 379–386 (1973)

10 CRACCO, R. Q., CRACCO, J. B., SARNOWSKI, R. and VOGEL, H. B. Spinal evoked potentials. In *Clinical Uses of Cerebral, Brainstem and Spinal Somatosensory Evoked Potentials*, edited by J. E. Desmedt, *Progress in Clinical Neurophysiology*, **7**, 87–104. S. Karger, Basel (1980)

11 DAWSON, G. D. Cerebral responses to electrical stimulation of peripheral nerve in man. *Journal of Neurology, Neurosurgery and Psychiatry*, **10**, 134–140 (1947)

12 DAWSON, G. D. Investigations on a patient subject to myoclonic seizures after sensory stimulation. *Journal of Neurology, Neurosurgery and Psychiatry*, **10**, 141–149 (1947)

13 DELBEKE, J., McCOMAS, A. J. and KOPES, S. J. Analysis of evoked lumbosacral potentials in man. *Journal of Neurology, Neurosurgery and Psychiatry*, **41**, 293–302 (1978)

14 DESMEDT, J. E. Editor. Cognitive Components in Cerebral Event-Related Potentials and Selective Attention. *Progress in Clinical Neurophysiology*, **10**, Basel, S. Karger (1979)

15 DESMEDT, J. E. and BRUNKO, E. Functional organization of far field and cortical components of somatosensory evoked potentials in normal adults. In *Clinical Uses of Cerebral, Brainstem and Somatosensory Evoked Potentials*, edited by J. E. Desmedt, *Progress in Clinical Neurophysiology*, **7**, 27–50. Basel, S. Karger (1980)

16 DESMEDT, J. E., BRUNKO, E. and DEBECKER, J. Maturation, aging and the somatosensory evoked potentials. In *Clinical uses of Cerebral Brainstem and Spinal Somatosensory Evoked Potentials*, edited by J. E. Desmedt, *Progress in Clinical Neurophysiology*, **7**, 146–161. Basel, S. Karger (1980)

17 DESMEDT, J. E. and CHERON, G. Somatosensory pathway and evoked potentials in human normal aging. In *Clinical Uses of Cerebral, Brainstem and Spinal Somatosensory Evoked Potentials*, edited by J. E. Desmedt, *Progress in Clinical Neurophysiology*, **7**, 162–169. Basel, S. Karger (1980)

18 DESMEDT, J. E. and ROBERTSON, D. Differential enhancement of early and late components of the cerebral somatosensory evoked potentials during force paced cognitive tasks in man. *Journal of Physiology*, **271**, 761–782 (1977)

19 DIMITRIJEVIC, M. R., LARSSON, L. E., LEHMKUHL, D. and SHERWOOD, A. Evoked spinal cord and nerve root potentials in humans using a non-invasive recording technique. *Electroencephalography and Clinical Neurophysiology*, **45**, 331–340 (1978)

20 DIMITRIJEVIC, M. R., SEDGWICK, E. M., SHERWOOD, A. and SOAR, J. S. A spinal cord potential in man. *Journal of Physiology*, **303**, 37 (1980)

21 DORFMAN, L. J. Indirect estimation of spinal cord conduction velocity in man. *Electroencephalography and Clinical Neurophysiology*, **42**, 742–753 (1977)

22 DORFMAN, L. J., BOSLEY, T. M. and CUMMINS, K. L. Electrophysiological localization of central somatosensory lesions in patients with multiple sclerosis. *Electroencephalography and Clinical Neurophysiology*, **44**, 742–753 (1978)

23 ECCLES, J. C. *The Physiology of Synapses*, 220–238. Berlin, Springer Verlag (1964)

24 EL-NEGAMY, E. Subcortical Somatosensory evoked potentials studied in man. *Doctoral Thesis*, University of Southampton (1978)

25 EL-NEGAMY, E. and SEDGWICK, E. M. Properties of a spinal somatosensory evoked potential recorded in man. *Journal of Neurology, Neurosurgery and Psychiatry*, **41**, 762–768 (1978)

26 EL-NEGAMY, E. and SEDGWICK, E. M. Delayed cervical somatosensory potentials in cervical spondylosis. *Journal of Neurology, Neurophysiology and Psychiatry*, **42**, 238–241 (1979)

27 EISEN, A. and ODUSOTE, K. Central and peripheral conduction times in multiple sclerosis. *Electroencephalography and Clinical Neurophysiology and Psychiatry*, **48**, 253–265 (1979)

28 EISEN, A., STEWARD, J., NUDLEMAN, K. and COSGROVE, J. B. R. Short latency somatosensory responses in multiple sclerosis. *Neurology*, **29**, 827–834 (1979)

29 ERTEKIN, C. Studies on the human evoked electrospinogram. I. The origin of the segmental evoked potentials. *Acta Neurologica Scandinavia*, **53**, 3–20 (1976)

30 ERTEKIN, C. Studies on the human electrospinogram. II. The conduction velocity along the dorsal funiculus. *Acta Neurologica Scandinavia*, **53**, 21–38 (1976)

31 ERTEKIN, C. Comparison of the human evoked electrospinogram recorded from the intrathecal, epidural and cutaneous levels. *Electroencephalography and Clinical Neurophysiology*, **44**, 683–690 (1978)

32 GANES, T. Somatosensory conduction times and peripheral, cervical and cortical evoked potentials in patients with cervical spondylosis.

Journal of Neurology, Neurosurgery and Psychiatry, **43**, 683–689 (1980)

33 GASSER, H. S. and GRAHAM, H. T. Potentials produced in the spinal cord by stimulation of dorsal roots. *American Journal of Physiology*, **103**, 303–320 (1933)

34 HALLIDAY, A. M. and HALLIDAY, E. Cerebral somatosensory and visual evoked potentials in different clinical forms of myoclonus. In *Clinical Uses of Cerebral, Brainstem and Spinal Somatosensory Evoked potentials*, edited by J. E. Desmedt, *Progress in Clinical Neurophysiology*, **7**, 292–310. Basel, S. Karger (1980)

35 HALLIDAY, A. M. and WAKEFIELD, G. S. Cerebral evoked potentials in patients with dissociated sensory loss. *Journal of Neurology, Neurosurgery and Psychiatry*, **26**, 211–219 (1963)

36 HUME, A. L. and CANT, B. R. Conduction time in central somatosensory pathways in man. *Electroencephalography and Clinical Neurophysiology*, **45**, 361–375 (1978)

37 ILLIS, L. S., SEDGWICK, E. M. and TALLIS, R. C. Spinal cord stimulation in multiple sclerosis; clinical results. *Journal of Neurology, Neurosurgery and Psychiatry*, **43**, 1–14 (1980)

38 JONES, S. J. Short latency potentials recorded from the neck and scalp following median nerve stimulation in man. *Electroencephalography and Clinical Neurophysiology*, **43**, 853–863 (1977)

39 LESSER, R. P., HAHN, J. F., KLEM, G. and LENDERS, H. The origin of the early somatosensory potentials evoked by median nerve stimulation. *Electroencephalography and Clinical Neurophysiology*, **51**, 40P (1981)

40 LIBERSON, W. T. and KIM, K. C. The mapping out of evoked potentials elicited by stimulation of the median and peroneal nerves. *Electroencephalography and Clinical Neurophysiology*, **15**, 721 (1963)

41 JONES, S. J. Investigation of brachial plexus traction lesions by peripheral and spinal somatosensory evoked potentials. *Journal of Neurology, Neurosurgery and Psychiatry*, **42**, 107–116 (1979)

42 JONES, S. J., BARAITSER, M. and HALLIDAY, A. M. Peripheral and central somatosensory nerve conduction defects in Friedreich's ataxia. *Journal of Neurology, Neurosurgery and Psychiatry*, **43**, 495–503 (1980)

43 JONES, S. J. and SMALL, D. G. Spinal and sub-cortical evoked potentials following stimulation of the posterior tibial nerve in man. *Electroencephalography and Clinical Neurophysiology*, **44**, 299–306 (1978)

44 MAGLADERY, M. W., PORTER, W. E., PARK, A. M. and TEASDALE, R. D. Electrophysiological studies of nerve and reflex activity in normal

man. IV. The two neurone reflex and identification of certain action potentials from spinal roots and cord. *Bulletin of the Johns Hopkins Hospital*, **99**, 499–519

45 MASTAGLIA, F. L., BLACK, J. L., CALA, L. A. and COLLINS, D. W. K. Evoked potentials, saccadic velocities and computerised tomography in diagnosis of multiple sclerosis. *British Medical Journal*, **1**, 1315–1317 (1977)

46 MASTAGLIA, F. L., BLACK, J. L., CALA, L. A. and COLLINS, D. W. K. Electrophysiology and avoidance of invasive neuroradiology in multiple sclerosis. *Lancet*, **1**, 144 (1980)

47 MASTAGLIA, F. L., BLACK, J. L. and COLLINS, D. W. K. Visual and spinal evoked potentials in diagnosis of multiple sclerosis. *British Medical Journal*, **1**, 732 (1976)

48 MATTHEWS, W. B. Somatosensory evoked potentials in retrobulbar neuritis. *Lancet*, **1**, 443 (1978)

49 MATTHEWS, W. B., BEAUCHAMP, M. and SMALL, D. G. Cervical somatosensory evoked response in man. *Nature*, **252**, 230–231 (1974)

50 MATTHEWS, W. B. and SMALL, D. G. Serial recording of visual and somatosensory evoked potentials in multiple sclerosis. *Journal of the Neurological Sciences*, **40**, 11–21 (1979)

51 NAMEROW, N. S. Somatosensory evoked responses in multiple sclerosis patients with varying sensory loss. *Neurology*, **18**, 1197–1204 (1968)

52 NOËL, P. and DESMEDT, J. E. Cerebral and far-field somatosensory evoked potentials in neurologic disorders involving the cervical spinal cord, brainstem, thalamus and cortex. In *Clinical Uses of Cerebral, Brainstem and Spinal Somatosensory Evoked Potentials*, edited by J. E. Desmedt, *Progress in Clinical Neurophysiology*, **7**, 205–230. Basel, S. Karger (1980)

53 PAPAKOSTOPOULOS, D. and CROW, J. J. Direct recording of the somatosensory evoked potentials from the cerebral cortex of man and the difference between precentral and post central potentials. In *Clinical Uses of Cerebral, Brainstem and Spinal Somatosensory Evoked Potentials*, edited by J. E. Desmedt, *Progress in Clinical Neurophysiology*, **7**, 15–26. Basel, S. Karger (1980)

54 PEROT, P. L. The clinical use of somatosensory evoked potentials in spinal cord injury. *Clinical Neurosurgery*, **20**, 367–381 (1973)

55 PEROT, P. L. Somatosensory evoked potentials in the evaluation of patients with spinal cord injury. In *Current Controversies in Neurosurgery*, edited by T. P. Morley, 160–167. Philadelphia, W. B. Saunders (1976)

56 ROWED, D. W., McLEAN, J. A. and TATOR, C. H. Somatosensory evoked potentials in acute spinal cord injury: prognostic value. *Surgical Neurology*, **9**, (3), 203–210 (1978)

57 SEDGWICK, E. M., EL-NEGAMY, E. and FRANKEL, H. Spinal cord potentials in traumatic paraplegia and quadriplegia. *Journal of Neurology, Neurosurgery and Psychiatry*, **43**, 823–830 (1980)

58 SEDGWICK, E. M., ILLIS, L. S., TALLIS, R. C, THORNTON, A. R. D., ABRAHAM, P., EL-NEGAMY, E., DOCHERTY, T., SOAR, J. S., SPENCER, S. C. and TAYLOR, F. M. Evoked potentials and contingent negative variation during treatment of multiple sclerosis with spinal cord stimulation. *Journal of Neurology, Neurosurgery and Psychiatry*, **43**, 15–24 (1980)

59 SHIMOJI, K. The P2 wave of the evoked ESG in man – an index of presynaptic inhibition. *Electroencephalography and Clinical Neurophysiology*, **42**, 140 (1977)

60 SHIMOJI, K., MATSUKI, N. and SHIMIZU, M. Wave-form characteristics and spatial distribution of evoked spinal electrogram in man. *Journal of Neurosurgery*, **46**, 304–313 (1977)

61 SHIMOJI, K., MICHIKO, M., ITO, Y., MASUKO, K., MARUYAMA, M., IWANE, T. and AIDA, S. Interactions of human cord dorsum potential. *Journal of Applied Physiology*, **40**, 79–84 (1976)

62 SHIMOJI, K., SHIMIZU, M. and MARUGAMA, Y. Origin of somatosensory evoked responses recorded from the cervical skin surface. *Journal of Neurosurgery*, **48**, 980–984 (1978)

63 SMALL, D. G., MATTHEWS, W. B. and SMALL, M. The cervical somato-sensory evoked potential (SEP) in the diagnosis of multiple sclerosis. *Journal of Neurological Sciences*, **35**, 211–224 (1978)

64 SYMON, L., HARGADINE, J., ZAWIRSKI, M. and BRANSTON, N. Central conduction time as an index of ischaemia in subarachnoid hemorrhage. *Journal of the Neurological Sciences*, **44**, 95–103 (1979)

65 WIEDERHOLT, W. and MEYER-HARDTING, E. Recovery functions of short latency somatosensory evoked potentials in man. *Electroencephalography and Clinical Neurophysiology*, **51**, 40P (1981)

66 WILSON, S. L., BROOKS, E. R. and CHIAPPA, K. H. Scalp and spinal short latency somato-sensory evoked potentials following lower extremity stimulation in normal subjects. *Electroencephalography and Clinical Neurophysiology*, **51**, 40P–41P (1981)

13

Electroencephalography and computed tomography of the brain

Edward R. Wolpow, Stefan C. Schatzki and Linda Y. Buchwald

Introduction

In an early paper dealing with the utility of computed tomographic (CT) brain scanning for patients with dementia[50] the rather restrained statement, 'It is likely that CT will reduce the use of the EEG as a screening tool for patients with neurological disorders other than seizure disorders', evoked lively correspondence and counter-correspondence. Others have continued to question the role of electroencephalography in the new world of computed tomography. Some authors have studied whether use of EEG in various centers has changed after CT became available and concluded that numbers of EEGs are presently rising[54], falling[57, 61] or staying about the same[9].

Information dealing with the medically more germane question of how best to employ both tests is beginning to appear. A few studies in full[21] and many in abstract form, compare EEG and CT when done in patient populations with different diagnoses. Twenty-two of 144 abstracts from one recent international EEG congress[45] were devoted to such comparisons.

It is perhaps less informative to highlight the concordances between CT scanning and EEG – situations in which both are positive or both negative – than to attempt to point out clinical settings in which the findings are discordant. In these situations, decision-making as to which diagnostic tests to employ is most challenging and instructive. Speculations as to the causes of such discordances may lead to new insights into brain function.

This review of selected clinical topics will attempt to emphasize circumstances with disparate CT and EEG findings, and to suggest how each test may be used in various settings.

Overview of EEG

Although electrical potential changes represent the common interactive currency for all neurons, the scalp-recorded EEG is a very restricted derivation of the electrical pattern of the billions of central nervous system (CNS) nerve cells. To begin with, to be recordable at the scalp, a high value must be placed on neuronal synchronization; asynchronous discharges from cortical neurons are silent (cancel out) at the surface of the head. It is largely for this reason that the more numerous of the two morphological varieties of cortical neuron, the *stellate* cell, makes no direct impression on the EEG. There is general agreement that normal surface EEG represents only postsynaptic potential changes in the second variety of neuron, the *pyramidal* cell (not synonymous with the cells of origin of the 'pyramidal' or corticocospinal tract), and most particularly, changes within apical dendrites. Excitatory postsynaptic potentials seem the major contributor, but inhibitory postsynaptic potentials may also play a part[11, 14]. In addition, recording of the EEG from the scalp fails to monitor activity faster than about 40 Hz, due only partly to limitations of response of the ink-writing apparatus.

The requisite pyramidal neuronal synchronization is brought about by pacemakers, presumably located in the 'non-specific' nuclei of the thalamus. Although the activity of pyramidal neurons may be modified by many subcortical and intracortical mechanisms, the normal (and probably most of the abnormal) clinical EEGs encountered are reflections purely of the electrical activity in this restricted population of neurons. It appears likely that various neuronal groups in the thalamus 'take turns' in the role of cortical pacing[3]. Theoretically, if the thalamic pacers were totally desynchronized, the scalp EEG would appear 'flat', even though all or most of the neurons of the CNS were healthy. Yet, the truly flat EEG ('electrocortical silence') reliably indicates extremely severe brain damage. In many other ways as well, the variations of the scalp EEG do reliably point to the underlying state of the brain, even though an understanding of basic mechanisms for generation of pathological EEGs is rudimentary. That clinical EEG is useful, then, is admittedly somewhat surprising, considering that it represents such a small and 'special' fraction of the brain's electrical output.

However imperfect, the EEG (along with more recently developing evoked potential techniques) stands with the clinical examination of the patient as the only two widely available measures of cerebral neurophysiology. It is this unique qualitative difference from other diagnostic modalities that retains for electroencephalography its great clinical utility and interest, even in the face of dramatic advances in technology for *in vivo* monitoring of brain structure and metabolism. It remains the pre-eminent clinical barometer for cerebral neuronal function.

Overview of CT scanning

Computed tomography is an imaging technique that combines X-rays, tomography and computers to provide radiographic transverse tomographic sections of the brain[1]. As in the case of conventional radiography, the ability to image various structures depends upon the distribution of X-ray attenuation coefficients through the part being studied. CT is an important advance over conventional X-ray chiefly because it allows definition of tissues that have very similar contrasts (densities) – ready distinction being made, for example, between brain, CSF and blood – refinements not possible with plain radiographs. These tissues can be delineated in a way that preserves detailed anatomical relationships. Further, computerized technology permits definition of intracranial contents even when surrounded by bone.

Computed tomography demonstrates thin sections of brain, from 13 mm to less than 1 mm in thickness, by calculating the relative absorption coefficients of structures in the section from multiple well-collimated beams of X-ray that pass through the section being examined from many different angles. The computer is able to reconstruct with very great precision the various anatomical structures and these may then be displayed on a cathode-ray tube.

As with any anatomical test, the CT scan has limits in the minimum size structure that can be detected (spatial discrimination) at any given difference in contrast (difference of attenuation coefficients). Spatial discrimination is rapidly improving with newer equipment.

The value of CT scanning is further extended with the use of intravenous iodinated contrast materials to visualize better both normal and abnormal structures. Knowledge that certain pathological entities enhance (increase in density) after the intravenous injection of contrast media in a different manner than normal tissue is often helpful in detecting and characterizing cerebral lesions. The phenomenon of iodinated contrast enhancement is not fully understood but the most likely mechanisms involved include:

(1) widening of the capillary tight junctions, allowing contrast to leak out, as may occur in or near brain tumors;
(2) increased density of blood pool such as in arteriovenous malformations; and
(3) temporarily increased local blood flow, as in infarcts and areas of inflammation.

CT is least accurate in those regions where there is an abrupt change in density, as where brain or CSF lies close to bone. For this reason, certain intracranial sites such as the posterior fossa, the sella, and the subfrontal and subtemporal regions pose more inherent difficulties for CT scanning, although the newer scanners reduce this problem. Another inherent limitation of CT scanning is its inability to separate two adjacent tissues which have the same density (isodense). For example, an intracerebral lesion with the same density as surrounding brain cannot be recognized unless it produces secondary changes, such as edema or distortion in the surrounding normal tissue.

Vascular disease

CT scanning has had pre-eminent success in the diagnosis of intracranial hemorrhage. Almost all acute supratentorial intracerebral hemorrhages more than about 5 to 10 mm in diameter are seen unless the patient has a very low hematocrit. Following the ictus, a hematoma eventually becomes isodense and then hypodense, and 'ring-enhancement' may occur. Results of CT scanning have given rise to a change in the traditional teaching regarding the almost uniformly poor prognosis with intracerebral hemorrhages. It is clear with scanning that small intracerebral hemorrhages, especially in hypertensive patients, are often compatible with good recovery; these hematomas communicate neither with the ventricular system nor the subarachnoid space over the convexities, so that the CSF contains no blood. Before CT scanning, these small strokes would otherwise have been considered ischemic and anticoagulation possibly recommended. Pathologically, some of these strokes conform to so-called 'subcortical slit hemorrhages'[16]. Focal EEG slowing cannot help to differentiate between a small ischemic cortical infarct and a small subcortical hemorrhage. Large supratentorial hemorrhages invariably produce profound EEG slowing and disorganization[70].

CT scanning is central to the care of patients with subarachnoid hemorrhage due to ruptured saccular aneurysm[5, 52]. In many such patients, the presence of blood in the subarachnoid space can be readily detected. The initial CT scan permits differentiation of intracerebral hematoma from subarachnoid blood and also allows assessment of the presence and extent of intraventricular blood, the presence of ischemia manifest by areas of decreased density, and often suggests the most likely location of the bleeding aneurysm, thereby helping direct subsequent angiography. The development of ischemia due to vasospasm, the appearance of hydrocephalus as well as possible rebleeding can be evaluated by CT without the potential risks of lumbar puncture or angiography. The EEG is now seldom of great importance in management of patients with subarachnoid hemorrhage, although focal slowing may indicate ischemia due to evolving vasospasm, and long-term monitoring of such patients may reveal when vasospasm is beginning. Marked paroxysmal activity may indicate need for additional anticonvulsant coverage. In the small number of patients for whom treatment of aneurysmal rupture consists of gradual surgical occlusion of the cervical carotid artery[67], the EEG is a most useful instantaneous monitor of whether or not hemispheral ischemia is occurring.

EEG assumes a much more important role relative to CT scanning in cerebral ischemia, than in intracranial hemorrhage[69, 70]. One reason for this is that the abnormalities in the EEG following hemispheral ischemia appear as early as 6 s after the insult, while even with large ischemic strokes, the CT scan may not show abnormalities for 24 hours or more. Focal disorganization of the background, as well as tall polymorphic δ-slowing are the EEG characteristics of focal cortical ischemia; sharp waves may be prominent, especially with emboli to the cortical branches of the middle cerebral artery. However, there is a tendency for the slowing to occur anteriorly and laterally so that the localization of polymorphic δ-activity does not depict the site of infarction in an absolutely reliable manner.

Ischemic cerebral injury can be due to embolism from the heart or great vessels (aorta, innominate, common or internal carotid arteries) or to thrombosis in large arteries (internal carotid, basilar) by atherosclerosis or in small penetrating end-arteries in hypertensive patients by non-atheromatous disorganization of the arterial wall (lacunar strokes)[16, 17]. In addition, low cardiac output or hypotension can result in infarction of the distal fields of various cerebral arterial territories, particularly the middle cerebral artery. Although it is clearly true that the patient's clinical presentation may strongly suggest which of these mechanisms is responsible, it is often important to collect non-invasive diagnostic information quickly, since there are several different therapeutic options for patients with cerebral ischemia of different causation, and precise diagnosis is therefore desirable.

CT scanning should, of course, be carried out in patients with acute onset of cerebrovascular symptoms, especially to rule out small deep hemorrhages or other unsuspected entities such as tumor. In ischemia in the territory of the middle cerebral artery, or in the retina, operable lesions such as stenosis or ulcerated plaques in the ipsilateral internal carotid artery must be considered. Surgery should be postponed for a period of weeks if an actual stroke, as opposed to a transient ischemic attack, has occurred, but within the first 24 hours it may not be possible to determine if an ischemic event is transient or not. A focally abnormal EEG strongly suggests structural ischemic injury (stroke) in this setting. Some clinical syndromes such as hemiparesis may occur either with large vessel (middle cerebral artery territory) disease or lacunar disease, and here EEG can be most instructive in that it is very likely to be normal with an acute lacunar infarction and very likely to be focally slow with hemispheral ischemia[7]. In cases where the clinical symptoms may be due either to lacunar or cerebral cortical damage, the combination of CT scanning and EEG has been shown to be useful in determining which mechanism is responsible[10].

In one study[6] it was noted that CT abnormalities occurred in 48 percent of patients scanned on the first day of the infarct and that the number of positive scans increased until it reached 76 percent on the 10th day, gradually declining after that. The consistent use of contrast media might have raised these figures since CT enhancement occurs in the majority of infarcts in the first to fourth weeks[55]. It was noted[6] that while brain swelling or a mass effect was seen in 25 percent of cases, sometimes as early as the day of infarct, it frequently began to decrease by the 10th day and was never seen after 25 days. This course of the mass effect is helpful in separating infarcts from tumors.

Case report

A 67-year-old man with a past history of two myocardial infarctions presented two days after he suddenly noted difficulty with word-finding. Neurological examination revealed occasional uncorrected spoken aphasic errors, poor calculations, left-right confusion, but no hemiparesis or visual field cut.

302

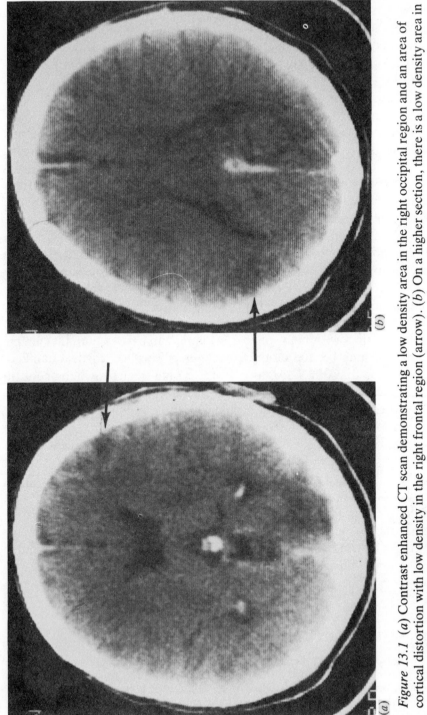

Figure 13.1 (*a*) Contrast enhanced CT scan demonstrating a low density area in the right occipital region and an area of cortical distortion with low density in the right frontal region (arrow). (*b*) On a higher section, there is a low density area in the left posterior parietal region (arrow)

CT scanning showed three low density lesions, in the right occipital lobe, in the right frontal lobe, and in the left posterior temporal region (*Figure 13.1*). Radioisotope scanning showed a single positive region of uptake in the left posterior temporal region and the EEG demonstrated a sharp-wave focus in the left anterior temporal region (*Figure 13.2*).

The presumption after these tests was that he had had multiple cerebral cortical lesions of different age, only the left posterior temporal lesion being symptomatic. The differential considerations included multiple emboli and multiple metastases.

Two months later, he was completely normal, and a repeat CT scan showed no significant changes. He was begun on warfarin sodium with a presumptive diagnosis of cardiac emboli and was neurologically normal five months after the hospitalization.

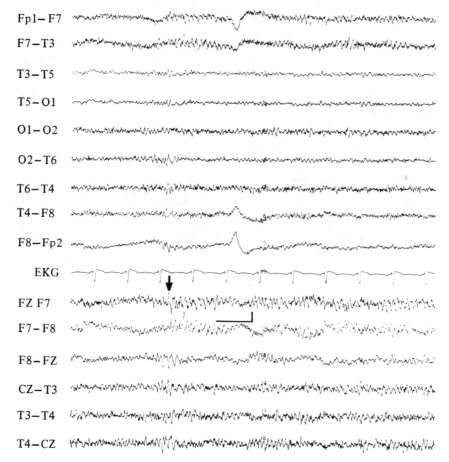

Figure 13.2 EEG showing focus of sharp waves in the left anterior temporal region (arrow). Calibration for EEG figures: 50 μV (vertical) and 1 s (horizontal). EKG: electrocardiogram

Comment

This case demonstrates that the complete evaluation of a patient with multiple cerebral lesions may require the summation of several diagnostic modalities. It is particularly interesting that the single sharp EEG focus did not correspond with positive CT or radioisotope scan lesions and probably represented a very small cortical embolism at some point in the past, which had evolved into an irritative focus.

In the chronic or later phases of infarction, as with trauma, if the EEG has returned to normal, the prognosis for further recovery of neurological deficits is poor.

There are substantial difficulties correlating diagnostic tests with clinical symptoms in vertebrobasilar disease, although there are indications of usefulness of CT[42] as well as EEG[69] in cases of brainstem infarction.

In states of low cerebral perfusion, distal field infarction occurs and the EEG is immediately abnormal. Periodic electric discharges have been observed in this setting, for example after cardiac arrest[33]. Hemispheral distal field infarction is often associated with clinical seizures and the EEG may show a variety of irritative phenomena acutely, including spiking. Once again, the CT scan may not show evidence of cortical damage for more than a day after the ischemic event.

One further important use for EEG in vascular disease is the intraoperative monitoring of electrocortical activity during carotid endarterectomies[8], especially as focal EEG changes correlate well with changes in regional cerebral blood flow[63].

Brain tumor and abscess

The EEG in supratentorial brain tumor has been studied for as long as this technique has been available. Hans Berger, the founder of human EEG, indicated that intracranial tumors effect the EEG and Walter demonstrated the usefulness of EEG in the diagnosis of brain tumor in man in 1936[72]. In the region of a cerebral hemispheral tumor is found attenuation of background rhythms and at the borders of tumor, irregular slowing in θ (4–8 Hz) and δ (less than 4 Hz) range[43]. Irregular δ-slowing is thought to be due to lesions in subcortical white matter[23]. Sharp waves and spiking may correlate with clinical epileptogenicity. In posterior fossa tumors, 'projected' runs of bifrontal slowing may appear, which may be indistinguishable from slowing produced by authentic bifrontal pathological processes, although cerebellar tumors may produce focal EEG changes as well[48, 68]. If the patient is obtunded, diffuse slowing may obscure focal EEG abnormalities. When there are multiple cerebral lesions, these may be difficult to identify individually, even when the patient is alert. Peritumoral edema appears not to have much effect on the extent of focal EEG abnormality[22]. As many as 13 percent of patients with brain tumor, however, may have normal EEGs[31] although most of this group have posterior fossa lesions. Very slow-growing tumors such as meningiomas may reach enormous size without changes in the EEG. The figure of 16 percent (8 of 50) of patients with histologically proven supratentorial brain tumors showing normal EEGs[36] seems inordinately high.

CT scanning has been consistently reported very highly likely to be positive in patients with brain tumor[2, 76]. In the first large series reported, CT scanning detected 93 percent of a large series of supratentorial and 80 percent of infratentorial tumors with all of the negative latter cases showing hydrocephalus as indirect evidence[2]. However, in a more recent study[40] CT scanning failed to identify tumor in only 8 of 2015 cases. CT scanning allows identification of the mass itself, as well as shift of midline structures, ventricular or sulcal displacement, distortion or effacement, ablation of normal tissue planes, regions of abnormal density, including intratumoral hemorrhage or calcification and edema and hydrocephalus. In addition, changes in the bony calvarium are detectable. The accuracy of CT scanning is slightly less in the detection of posterior fossa tumors. In a recent series[71], 92 percent of such tumors were detected with only 4 of 11 brain stem gliomas being missed. Further, it is occasionally difficult, even with correlation of clinical and CT changes, to differentiate an infiltrating glioma from an enhancing cerebral infarct.

Tumors may occur that are so small that they cannot be detected on routine CT scanning done with non-overlapping sections. Metastases particularly fit in this category and the CT is often performed in one of two clinical settings: (1) work-up for a focal seizure in a patient without previous neurological disease; and (2) screening a patient with known or suspected non-CNS malignancy but no neurological signs or symptoms, to determine if the spread to CNS has already occurred. Metastases to brain commonly occur at the deep layers of the cerebral cortex, where epileptigenicity is quite high, and therefore, where symptoms (focal seizures such as limb movements, abnormal sensation, aphasia) may occur when the tumor is very small. This type of

small deep cortical tumor, however, especially if causing focal seizures, may well show a sharp or slow focus on EEG. CT scanning may
also fail to detect the rare tumor that is isodense, non-contrast
enhancing, and not producing a mass effect. Low-grade infiltrating
astrocytomas best fit this category, and indeed, even histological
review of cerebral material in grade I astrocytoma may reveal little
that is abnormal.

Several studies have appeared that set out to compare EEG and CT
scanning in patients with brain tumor. In one study of 116 patients[12],
CT was positive in 90 percent and EEG in 68 percent, but only two
cases, of brainstem gliomas, were missed by both examinations. Four
patients with cerebral metastases were positive on EEG and negative
on CT scanning. In a much larger study[40] using CT alone, 1.5 percent
of patients with metastases were missed, but without pathological
confirmation of all cases, this figure would have to be considered a
minimal value. In a series of 200 patients[73] with known primary
non-CNS tumors and cerebral symptoms, all but two showed CT
findings of tumor and the remaining two, led by an abnormal EEG,
were scanned a second time, at which point the metastatic lesions were
identified.

EEG may have a particular value, then, in supplementing CT
scanning in cases where CT shows a single tumor, but EEG, showing
an abnormal focus at a different cerebral location, makes the diagnosis
of metastases (or at least, multiple lesions) likely. In such cases, a
repeat scan with the use of high-dose contrast media, including
overlapping sections in the area of suspicion, should be carried out.

Considering the highly irritating nature of cerebral abscess, it is not
surprising that most patients with this condition demonstrate concor-
dant abnormalities on EEG and CT scanning[51, 75] and there are few
false negatives. EEG slowing is usually more pronounced with an
abscess than with a neoplasm of the same size and location[51]. The use
of CT scanning has already resulted in markedly improved mortality
statistics for brain abscess[60]. It is usually possible with CT scanning to
distinguish the focal cerebritis preceding abscess formation from the
encapsulated abscess itself, and in addition, CT scanning may demonstrate multiple lesions. Neither EEG nor CT scanning, however, can
differentiate abscess from neoplasm in all cases.

In inflammatory viral invasion of the cerebral hemispheres, both
EEG and CT scanning show focal abnormalities[24, 39] but the electrical
abnormalities are detectable earlier than the anatomical ones.

Head trauma

The management of acute head injury has been revolutionized by CT scanning which has become the primary diagnostic modality[18]. In some centers, it has almost eliminated the need for cerebral angiography for acute head trauma. CT scanning is particularly valuable as it is able to depict accurately the status of the extracranial and intracranial structures as well as the calvarium. The orbits and orbital contents can be readily imaged. When a decision for surgery must be made within the first minutes or hours after head injury, EEG is seldom relevant. The acute life-threatening epidural, subdural or intracerebral hematoma is located rapidly and accurately by CT scanning[65].

Non-acute extracerebral collections, especially the subacute subdural hematoma, are diagnostically more challenging and several testing modalities may be required. The subacute subdural hematoma may fail to be detected because it is isodense, and detection may require the use of contrast media and the utilization of indirect CT signs that have recently become better understood[41]. Extracerebral collections of any age, in the posterior fossa or near the base of the skull, are particularly difficult to detect.

The EEG is approximately 90 percent likely to be abnormal (but not diagnostic) in subdural hematomas, the most common findings being slowing of rhythms over the lesion and attenuation of background rhythms as well as attenuation of drug-induced fast activity[67]. The clinician may elect to use several EEGs over months or years after head trauma in preference to multiple CT scans, since the latter involves repeated small doses of radiation.

With regard to direct cerebral damage, the presence of a traumatic intracerebral hematoma can be easily delineated on CT scanning. All intracranial hematomas undergo predictable changes in density so that by the second to fourth week, a high-density lesion may become isodense, and occasionally presents a differential diagnostic problem. In cerebral contusion-laceration, areas of low density are seen to be interspersed with focal areas of increased density, both of which may enhance. Both with contusion and intracerebral hematoma, varying degrees of associated edema may appear. At a later stage, the contused brain may present low-density areas of encephalomalacia, most commonly seen at the temporal tips and the anterior inferior frontal lobes. Cerebral concussion, with only transient loss of consciousness, may show no CT changes, although some degree of EEG slowing is not uncommon. Care of the patient with acute head trauma is optimized by using both EEG and CT scanning[53].

Focal EEG changes after acute head injury include voltage attenuation which may reflect hematoma, laceration or focal ischemia, with localized edema. However, 40 percent of tracings with focal EEG abnormality show no gross lesions[13], indicating that the EEG is often more sensitive to minor degrees of brain trauma than any of the anatomical diagnostic tests. Focal slowing is usually polymorphic and tends to occur at the temporal derivations in adults and in the occipital areas in children, as well as frontally at all ages. If slow-wave foci resolve quickly, it is likely that brain injury has been minimal. Failure of slow-wave foci to resolve in one week may indicate significant injury. Persistent foci tend with time to 'shrink down' and may migrate within the first few days or weeks of the insult[66]. The most characteristic EEG feature of traumatic lesions and disturbances, then, is their marked tendency for gradual recovery as evidenced in follow-up studies[13]. Patients with head trauma resulting in an abnormal EEG but normal CT scan tend to do well[74] and the prognostic value of EEG after head trauma has been underlined[4].

Case report

A 25-year-old passenger hit her head in an automobile accident and was comatose with right-sided hyperreflexia on arrival at the hospital. Emergency CT scanning was normal and she awoke within a few hours. High dose steroids were instituted and on the fifth day, when the examination revealed drowsiness, confusion, ataxia and four-limb hyperreflexia, the CT scan was again normal (*Figure 13.3*). The EEG showed generalized paroxysms of tall, sharp activity with a minimally slowed and disorganized background (*Figure 13.4*), although there was no clinical evidence for seizures. Three weeks after the accident, she was much less confused, with some ataxia of gait and repeat EEG showed independent sharp foci in the right and left temporal regions.

Comment

The normal CT scans in the acute phase of the injury belied the altered cerebral physiology as expressed by the neurological examination and the EEG. The EEG suggested at first generalized cortical irritability and later coup and contrecoup temporal lobe injuries and led to prophylactic use of anticonvulsants.

When clinical seizures do not develop after head injury, the EEG tends to return eventually to normal, even if damage to the brain with severe permanent deficits has occurred. It appears that abnormal slowing on the EEG depends upon ongoing injury to neurons: after a time of healing, as many cortical neurons as remain produce a normal EEG. Regarding post-traumatic seizures, if an irritative focus (sharp waves, spikes) evolves from a slow wave focus, clinical seizures occur

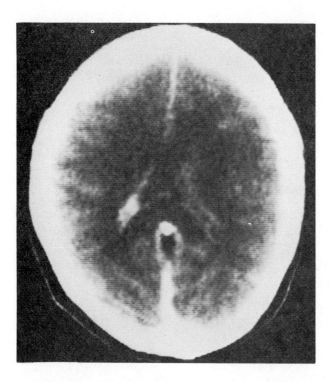

Figure 13.3 A single representative section of a normal CT scan is shown. Intravenous contrast material has been used

in about two-thirds of cases[66]. Focal non-paroxysmal irregularities are, nonetheless, found much more often in patients with post-traumatic clinical epilepsy than is paroxysmal activity. The persistence then, of a slow wave focus months or years after serious head injury is correlated with epilepsy. On the other hand, a normal EEG does not mitigate against the later development of seizure disorder as 48 percent of patients with clearly defined post-traumatic seizures developed a normal EEG[66]. A persistently slow EEG focus, long after head trauma, especially when there is clinical deficit, should lead to further evaluation, including CT scanning, since some late symptomatic, post-traumatic lesions such as chronic subdural hematoma or hygroma and porencephalic cyst are surgically treatable. In addition, sequential CT scanning may point to the development of late hydrocephalus.

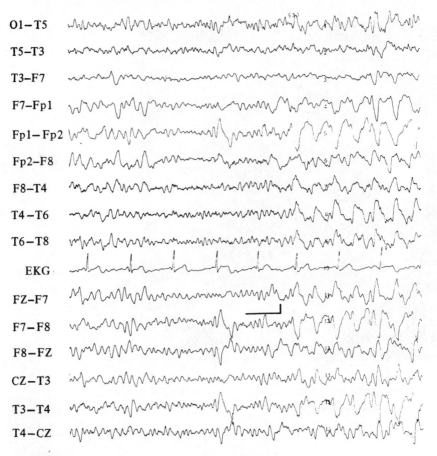

O1–T5
T5–T3
T3–F7
F7–Fp1
Fp1–Fp2
Fp2–F8
F8–T4
T4–T6
T6–T8
EKG
FZ–F7
F7–F8
F8–FZ
CZ–T3
T3–T4
T4–CZ

Figure 13.4 EEG showing bursts of tall sharp δ-activity, most prominent anteriorly, with some slowing of the background

Epilepsy

The clinician has for the last generation used EEG in patients with epilepsy in the same way the electrocardiogram is used in following the patient with heart disease. If the seizures are difficult to control and many medication changes are necessary, it is not unusual for an epileptic patient to accumulate 10 or more EEGs in his lifetime. Each test is used as a measure of the irritability of the brain at the time the tracing is carried out. The electrical abnormalities, focal and generalized, paroxysmal and persistent, and how these changes correlate with the varieties of epilepsy are well-documented and represent the most solidly defendable subdivision within clinical electro-encephalography[32].

Since the EEG is a derivation of the activity of cortical neurons and seizures are cortical events, a close correlation is not surprising. Current medical usage of the words 'seizure' and 'epilepsy' excluding, as it does, paroxysmal electrical events outside the cortex such as spinal myoclonus, helps, perhaps arbitrarily, to ensure a good correlation. CT scanning of cortex is also positive in many patients with epilepsy, the only low-likelihood group being patients with primary generalized seizures, especially absences, and a positive family history for epilepsy.

In a series of 397 patients with focal epilepsy and focal EEG changes, excluding patients with known or strongly suspected specific diagnoses[78], CT abnormalities were found in 46 percent. This comprised 12 percent with tumors, 11 percent with generalized atrophy, 5 percent with focal atrophy and a variety of other diagnoses of low frequency. CT abnormalities were most likely in children under the age of two. In the 40 percent of patients who were over the age of 35, 62 percent were positive. In a review of 1702 patients from seven centers[19], 46 percent had positive scans, but the figure was 60 percent for patients with focal seizures and only 4 percent for 'primary generalized epilepsy'. Tumors were found in 10 percent of total cases, but in 22 percent of patients with partial (focal) seizures. 'Atrophic lesions' were the most common and it is this designation which is most troublesome, since the relationship of 'atrophy' on CT scan, especially when generalized, and either clinical symptoms or pathological changes remains to be elucidated. Similarly, 'atrophy' was the major finding in another series of 400 patients that were 'subjectively selected'[34]. In a group of 401 patients seen in one center[20], 11 percent of patients with the new onset of seizures showed tumors on CT scanning. Another study found 40 percent of 150 patients with seizures to have a positive CT scan[49], but one-third of these showed 'diffuse atrophy'. In a group of 393 epileptic patients[64] the EEG was normal in 6.8 percent and the CT scan normal in 64.6 percent. Of patients with focal EEG changes, only 38.6 percent showed a focally abnormal CT scan and this most likely reflects the fact that very small scars or other cortical lesions, especially in the temporal lobe, are difficult to detect on CT scanning. Similarly, in another group of 63 patients with focal seizures and focal EEG abnormalities, 40 percent had normal CT scans[27].

The intriguing observation has been made that some interictal epileptic foci may enhance with contrast material on CT scanning[56]. It is presently unclear if such enhancement is the result of purely structural versus physiological factors. Nevertheless, it has been shown that regional cerebral blood flow in an epileptic focus may vary with the electrical activity of the focus[62], and regional hyperemia may be demonstrated angiographically[47]. It is therefore possible that enhancement patterns on CT scanning may eventually provide data pertaining to the transient physiological activity of epileptic foci, presently the sole province of EEG.

Dementia

Considering the central role in human life of higher cortical functions – personality, intellect, emotionality – dementia qualifies as the single most painful and tragic human illness. It is remarkable how little concern is devoted to this syndrome by most clinicians. This is due in part to failure to understand that 'normal aging' is only one entry in the long differential diagnosis of this syndrome and in part due to the belief that treatable causes are so rare as to render a workup of every demented individual not cost-effective. There can be little doubt that both EEG and CT scanning are under-utilized in dementia, just as other testing modalities such as measurement of thyroid function (particularly the thyroid stimulating hormone), vitamin B_{12} level and drug levels are underutilized. Most under-used is the detailed care of the clinician, especially as it is not laboratory testing but clinical skills that distinguish dementia from depression.

Renewed interest in dementia followed the observation that the syndrome could be reversed in some individuals after lowering the intraventricular pressure by shunting, even when that pressure was not higher than the traditional upper limits of normal. It is now clear that reversible idiopathic normal-pressure hydrocephalus is an uncommon, possibly a rare condition, although this same syndrome, responding well to shunting, not uncommonly follows intracranial bleeding or infection[38].

CT scanning has proved to be of some, though limited, value in the evaluation of patients with dementia. There is a progressive, increased width of the ventricular system and the superficial sulci with increasing age. When a CT scan shows ventricular or superficial sulcal dilatation that is outside the norm for that patient's age, he is considered to have atrophy. Yet not all patients with 'atrophy' on the CT scan are demented and not all demented patients show atrophy. There tends to be little statistical relationship between the degree of dementia and the size of the lateral ventricles and superficial sulci. The presence of dilated ventricles and normal superficial sulci is compatible with, but not diagnostic of, normal-pressure hydrocephalus[35].

Clearly, for the workup of dementia, CT scanning is useful in discovering patients with chronic extracerebral collections and other chronic tumors, particularly meningioma, as well as giving evidence for there having been multiple hypertensive strokes (multi-infarct dementia; lacunar state). In 'vascular' dementia the EEG is more likely to be focally slow than in 'non-vascular' types[59].

The commonest form of dementia is Alzheimer's disease and both CT and EEG[77] may either indicate substantial abnormalities or be quite normal while the patient's symptoms are severe. When the patient with Alzheimer's disease is suffering from another health problem, however, such as fever, congestive heart failure or pneumonia, there is often a striking slowing of the EEG, along with abrupt mental decompensation. Aside from the focal slowing of a tumor or subdural hematoma, various suggestive EEG patterns in demented patients include the periodic sharp wave complexes of Creutzfeldt-Jakob disease, the very low voltage pattern of Huntington's chorea, the slowing of the background without disorganization ('slow α') in hypothyroidism and the anterior excessive fast activity (β) in patients ingesting barbiturates or benzodiazepines. Diffuse slowing of the EEG, notably with δ-waves of 'triphasic' configuration, implies a 'metabolic' encephalopathy and calls for detailed search for a specific toxic or metabolic derangement. Rarely, the EEG will indicate the presence of previously unsuspected seizures, therapy of which improves the patient's mental state.

It has been noted[28] that EEG abnormalities occur with a high incidence early in a dementing process when the disease is due to a treatable cause. Thus, the value of EEG as an early screening procedure is enhanced.

Headache

Headache is close to a universal complaint. When this symptom causes a patient to seek medical care, the differential diagnosis is almost totally confined to migraine, 'tension' headache and the somatic complaints accompanying emotional illness, particularly depression. It is unfortunate that only the far less common causes of headache, such as giant cell arteritis, sinusitis and other chronic infections and tumor are likely to show positive laboratory results, either radiological or chemical. Biochemical and anatomical tests, including CT scanning, are uniformly negative in patients with migraine, tension headache and depression. EEG, however, may be very strikingly abnormal in patients with migraine and the patterns may be identical to those seen in patients with epilepsy or focal cerebral lesions. A paroxysmal EEG in a migraineur may suggest to the physician a trial of treatment with an anticonvulsant. Paroxysmal stroboscopic light activation suggests that the patient might benefit from the use of tinted glasses. However, many headache sufferers have only incomplete benefit from therapy and the long, frustrating patient–physician contact often raises the question of what other tests are appropriate to rule out other causes of headache.

CT scanning can most often be deferred if the neurological examination is normal[29] and if the headaches are not clinically uniform. Of greater concern is the migrainous patient who describes absolutely identical headaches at the same part of the head over a period of time, even if accompanied by migrainous auras and scintillations, since a rare patient with this complaint may harbor a meningioma or arteriovenous malformation at the part of the brain referable to the location of the headaches and the neurological accompaniments. When, as is often the case, migrainous pain centers in or behind the eye, a full ophthalmological examination is also appropriate. If questions of ocular or orbital pathology are raised, the CT scan may be very profitably used to study this region, as well as to visualize the paranasal sinuses.

Altered states of consciousness

Several comprehensive approaches to patients with altered states of consciousness have appeared in recent years[15, 37, 58] and these influential monographs along with new interest in such topics as 'brain death', sleep and cerebral effects of various drugs have focussed a great deal of medical attention on stupor, delerium and coma and related conditions.

Obtunded patients raise immediate questions as to the presence of structural disease of the brain versus toxic or metabolic derangements.

Much can be determined confidently by careful clinical examination, as outlined in the sources noted. Yet many different factors are commonly at play in the same patient, and the full force of diagnostic technology often needs to be brought to bear. CT scanning in its present state aids greatly in the workup of the obtunded or comatose patient. In the future, improvements will allow investigation of the finer infratentorial anatomy, especially pertaining to small hemorrhages, infacts or small displacements of the cerebellum or the brainstem itself.

In parallel with the interest in altered states of consciousness has been the sorting out of a variety of EEG patterns in obtunded or comatose patients. Some specific syndromes with EEG findings, such as dialysis encephalopathy[46] are being delineated, but a variety of other EEG abnormalities, such as 'periodic lateralized epileptiform discharges', 'burst-suppression'[44] and 'α-coma'[26] do not as yet have a single firm pathological basis; CT scanning may help to correct these deficiences.

Summary and speculations

In the past, CT scanning has been primarily an anatomical methodology. While continued improvements in scanners will allow smaller structures to be recognized at lower contrast, the greatest future progress in cranial CT appears to be in the area of dynamic scanning, which allows analysis of physiological circulatory events[30]. Dynamic scanning is at present being carried out with iodinated contrast media and with xenon.

Some of the newer scanners are able to perform several scans within a 30 s period, allowing a sophisticated analysis of the blood flow to different parts of the brain. By observation of the sequential opacification of homologous points on both sides of the brain, it is possible to compare blood flow to various brain regions. These studies have already begun to become helpful in the evaluation of patients with extracerebral vascular disease who are possible candidates for surgery.

The time–density curves that are developed after intravenous contrast media, in different kinds of tumor, infarcts and other types of intracranial pathology are now being studied with the hope that they may help in making specific diagnoses on the basis of these physiological events, rather than depending, as in the past, on changes in the anatomical CT data.

To declare EEG a test of physiology and CT scanning a test of anatomy is surely too simplistic. In a great many clinical settings, some of which were discussed, both will be required, and there seems scant prospect that this will change. In spite of the economic burdens of new and better technology, it is potentially to patients' detriment to speak of curtailing availability of EEG to help pay for CT. In fact, CT will help the science of electroencephalography to advance by improving the ability to make accurate EEG-pathological correlations.

Case report

A 56-year-old hypertensive lady developed a very severe headache along with dizziness and drowsiness, with some loss of recent memory, and sought medical attention two days later. She showed some resistance to flexion of the neck and the optic discs were slightly blurred. The neurological exam was otherwise normal.

A CT (*Figure 13.5*) showed blood filling a dilated left lateral ventricle and also some blood in the right lateral ventricle and to a lesser extent in the subarachnoid space. A bleeding site was suggested on CT scan in the region of the left caudate nucleus, close to the ventricular surface, but subsequent angiography failed to reveal any abnormalities. CSF was under raised pressure and there were 10 000 RBCs/mm^3. The EEG (*Figure 13.6*) showed bursts of tall, generalized slowing against a normal background.

She had an uneventful recovery, with both CT and EEG returning completely to normal within one month. The diagnosis was hypertensive intracerebral hemorrhage, virtually entirely intraventricular in location.

Comment

Prior to the advent of CT scanning, there would have been no way to be assured of the diagnosis of intraventricular hemorrhage, and its subsequent spontaneous resolution. Collection in parallel of clinical, radiographic and electrophysiological data in patients with intraventricular hemorrhage will allow a confident statement to be made about the EEG in this special stroke syndrome, thereby strengthening the usefulness of clinical EEG.

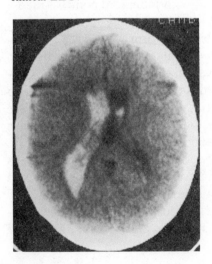

Figure 13.5 CT scan section showing blood in the body of both lateral ventricles, although more so the left. Contrast material has not been used

It is anticipated that the success of EEG in intraoperative cerebral monitoring during carotid surgery will lead to its increasing use in many other settings, both in neurosurgery and general surgery. Of particular note are prolonged cardiac, vascular or orthopedic operations in elderly patients, where minor intraoperative falls in blood pressure may give rise to cerebral ischemia due to arterial stenosis. Changes in regional cerebral oxygenation will be reflected rapidly in the EEG and prompt pharmacological elevation of the blood pressure during surgery may thereby prevent stroke.

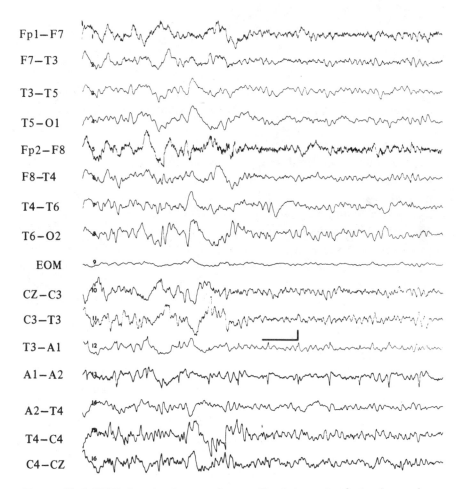

Figure 13.6 EEG showing bursts of generalized, irregular δ-slowing and a normal background. A_1: left ear reference. A_2: right ear reference. EOM: eye movement monitor

Particularly with monitoring for hours at a time, as in the operating room, computer programs which simplify the interpretation of large quantities of EEG data will be needed and are being devised. Outside of surgical uses, long-term EEG monitoring is becoming increasingly useful in certain cases of epilepsy, in the study of coma, sleep and states with unstable cerebral perfusion.

Some of the disparities between EEG and CT, notably in early stroke, in epilepsy and in metabolic disorders, may be expected to find resolution when techniques for demonstrating regional cerebral blood flow, oxygen utilization, carbon dioxide production and glucose metabolism[25] become widely available.

References

1 ABRAMS, H. L. and McNEIL, B. J. Medical implications of computed tomography ('CAT scanning') (First of two parts). *New England Journal of Medicine*, **298**, 255–261 (1978)

2 AMBROSE, J., GOODING, M. R. and RICHARDSON, A. E. An assessment of the accuracy of computerized transverse axial scanning (EMI scanner) in the diagnosis of intracranial tumour. A review of 366 patients. *Brain*, **98**, 569–582 (1975)

3 ANDERSEN, P. and ANDERSSON, S. A. *Physiological Basis of the Alpha Rhythm*, 235 pp. New York, Appleton-Century-Crofts (1968)

4 BRICOLO, A., TURAZZI, S. and FACCIOLI, F. Combined clinical and EEG examinations for assessment of severity of acute head injuries. *Acta Neurochirurgica*, Supplement **28**, 35–39 (1979)

5 BRYAN, R. N., SHAH, C. P. and HILAL, S. Evaluation of subarachnoid hemorrhage and cerebral vasospasm by computed tomography. *CT: the Journal of Computed Tomography*, **3**, 144–153 (1979)

6 CAMPBELL, J. K., HOUSER, O. W., STEVENS, J. C., WAHNER, H. W., BAKER, H. L., JR. and FOLGER, W. N. Computed tomography and radionuclide imaging in the evaluation of ischemic stroke. *Radiology*, **126**, 695–702 (1978)

7 CAPLAN, L. R. and YOUNG, R. R. EEG findings in certain lacunar stroke syndromes. *Neurology*, **22**, 403 (1972)

8 CHIAPPA, K. H., BURKE, S. R. and YOUNG, R. R. Results of electroencephalographic monitoring during 367 carotid endarterectomies. Use of a dedicated minicomputer. *Stroke*, **10**, 381–388 (1979)

9 CHIAPPA, K. H. and YOUNG, R. R. Impact of CT on EEG. *Neurology*, **29**, 421–422 (1979)

10 CHOKROVERTY, S. and RUBINO, F. A. Pure motor hemiplegia due to cerebral cortical infarction. *Archives of Neurology*, **34**, 93–95 (1977)

11 CREUTZFELDT, O. (Editor) In *Handbook of Electroencephalography and Clinical Neurophysiology*, Editor-in-Chief: A. Rémond. Volume **2**, *Electrical Activity from the Neuron to the EEG and EMG. Part C: The Neuronal Generation of the EEG*. 157 pp. Amsterdam, Elsevier Scientific Publishing Co. (1974)

12 CULEBRAS, A., HENRY, C. E. and WILLIAMS, G. H., JR. Evaluation of intracranial space-occupying lesions by computed tomography and electroencephalography. *Cleveland Clinic Quarterly*, **45**, 275–280 (1978)

13 DAWSON, R. E., WEBSTER, J. E. and GURDJIAN, E. S. Serial electroencephalography in acute head injuries. *Journal of Neurosurgery*, **8**, 613–630 (1951)

14 ELUL, R. The genesis of the EEG. *International Review of Neurobiology*, **15**, 227–272 (1972)

15 FISHER, C. M. The neurological examination of the comatose patient. *Acta Neurologica Scandinavica*, **45**, Supplementum 36, 1–56 (1969)

16 FISHER, C. M. The anatomy and pathology of the cerebral vasculature. In *Modern Concepts of Cerebrovascular Disease*, edited by J. S. Meyer, 1–41. New York, SP Division of Spectrum Publications (1975)

17 FISHER, C. M. Capsular infarcts. The underlying vascular lesions. *Archives of Neurology*, **36**, 65–73 (1979)

18 FRENCH, B. N. and DUBLIN, A. B. The value of computerized tomography in the management of 1000 consecutive head injuries. *Surgical Neurology*, **7**, 171–183 (1977)

19 GASTAUT, H. Conclusions: computerized transverse axial tomography in epilepsy. *Epilepsia*, **17**, 337–338 (1976)

20 GASTAUT, H. and GASTAUT, J. L. Computerized transverse axial tomography in epilepsy. *Epilepsia*, **17**, 325–336 (1976)

21 GASTAUT, J. L. and MICHEL, B. The impact of cranial computerized tomography on electroencephalography. *Electroencephalography and Clinical Neurophysiology*, Supplement **34**, 123–132 (1978)

22 GASTAUT, J. L., MICHEL, B., HASSAN, S. S., CERDA, M., BIANCHI, L. and GASTAUT, H. Electroencephalography in brain edema (127 cases of brain tumor investigated by cranial tomography). *Electroencephalography and Clinical Neurophysiology*, **46**, 239–255 (1979)

23 GLOOR, P., BALL, G. and SCHAUL, N. Brain lesions that produce delta waves in the EEG. *Neurology*, **27**, 326–333 (1977)

24 GO, R. T., ABU YOUSEF, M. M. and JACOBY, C. G. The role of radionuclide brain imaging and computerized tomography in the early diagnosis of Herpes simplex encephalitis. *CT: the Journal of Computed Tomography*, **3**, 286–296 (1979)

25 GOTOH, F., NAGAI, H. and TAZAKI, Y. (Editors) Cerebral blood flow and metabolism. *Acta Neurologica Scandinavica*, **60**, Supplementum 72, 1–649 (1979)

26 GRINDAL, A. B., SUTER, C. and MARTINEZ, A. J. Alpha-pattern coma: 24 cases with 9 survivors. *Annals of Neurology*, **1**, 371–377 (1977)

27 HAJNŠEK, F., GUBAREV, N., NUTRIZIO, V., IVAČIČ-BOHACEK, V. and ĆEMA-LOVIĆ-BOKO, Z. A comparative study of partial epilepsies using computerized tomography, EEG, echo and brain scanning. *Acta Medica Iugoslavica*, **32**, 323–332 (1978)

28 HARNER, R. N. EEG evaluation of the patient with dementia. In *Psychiatric Aspects of Neurological Disease*, edited by D. F. Benson and D. Blumer, 63–82. New York, Grune and Stratton (1975)

29 HAUG, G. Computer-Tomographie-Befunde bei Kopfschmerzpatienten. Überlegungen zur Indikationsstellung. *Der Nervenarzt*, **48**, 197–204 (1977)

30 HEINZ, E. R., DUBOIS, P., OSBORNE, D. DRAYER, B. and BARRETT, W. Dynamic computed tomography study of the brain. *Journal of Computer Assisted Tomography*, **3**, 641–649 (1979)

31 HESS, R. Significance of EEG-signs for location of cerebral tumours. *Electroencephalography and Clinical Neurophysiology*, Supplement **19**, 75–110 (1961)

32 HESS, R. Electroencephalography. In *Handbook of Clinical Neurology*, **15**, (*The Epilepsies*), edited by P. J. Vinken and G. W. Bruyn, 498–532. Amsterdam, North-Holland Publishing Co. (1974)

33 HOCKADAY, J. M., POTTS, F., EPSTEIN, E., BONAZZI, A. and SCHWAB, R. S. Electroencephalographic changes in acute cerebral anoxia from cardiac or respiratory arrest. *Electroencephalography and Clinical Neurophysiology*, **18**, 575–586 (1965)

34 ISHIDA, S., YAGI, K., FUJIWARA, T., SAKUMA, N., SEINO, M. and WADA, T. Cranial computed tomography on epilepsy: A correlation study with electroencephalographic findings. *Folia Psychiatrica et Neurologica Japonica*, **32**, 373–387 (1978)

35 JACOBS, L., KINKEL, W. R., PAINTER, F., MURAWSKI, J. and HEFFNER, R. R., JR. Computerized tomography in dementia with special reference to changes in size of normal ventricles during aging and normal pressure hydrocephalus. In *Alzheimer's Disease: Senile Dementia and Related Disorders* (*Aging*, **7**), edited by R. Katzman, R. D. Terry and K. L. Bick, 241–260. New York, Raven Press (1978)

36 JALLON, P., CONSTANT, P., CAILLE, J.-M. and LOISEAU, P. Encéphalo-tomographie axiale transverse et E.E.G. dans les tumeurs cérébrales. *Révue d'Electroencéphalographie et de Neurophysiologie Clinique*, **6**, 421 (1976)

37 JENNETT, W. B. and PLUM, F. The persistent vegetative state: a syndrome in search of a name. *Lancet*, **1**, 734–737 (1972)

38 KATZMAN, R. Normal pressure hydrocephalus. In *Alzheimer's Disease: Senile Dementia and Related Disorders (Aging, 7)*, edited by R. Katzman, R. D. Terry and K. L. Bick, 115–124. New York, Raven Press (1978)

39 KAUFMAN, D. M., ZIMMERMAN, R. D. and LEEDS, N. E. Computed tomography in Herpes simplex encephalitis. *Neurology*, **29**, 1392–1396 (1979)

40 KAZNER, E., GRUMME, T., LANKSCH, W. and WENDE, S. Computed tomography (CT) and the operative indications for brain tumors. A cooperative study of 3 university hospitals. *International Congress Series No. 433*, 28–36. Amsterdam, Excerpta Medica (1978)

41 KIM, K. S., HEMMATI, M. and WEINBERG, P. E. Computed tomography in isodense subdural hematoma. *Radiology*, **128**, 71–74 (1978)

42 KINGSLEY, D. P. E., RADUE, E. W. and DuBOULAY, E. P. G. H. Evaluation of computed tomography in vascular lesions of the vertebrobasilar system. *Journal of Neurology, Neurosurgery, and Psychiatry*, **43**, 193–197 (1980)

43 KRENKEL, W. The electroencephalogram in tumours of the brain. In *Handbook of Clinical Neurology*, **16** (*Tumours of the Brain and Skull. Part I*), edited by P. J. Vinken and G. W. Bruyn, 418–454. Amsterdam, North-Holland Publishing Co. (1974)

44 KUROIWA, Y. and CELESIA, G. G. Clinical significance of periodic EEG patterns. *Archives of Neurology*, **37**, 15–20 (1980)

45 LECHNER, H. and ARANIBAR, A. (Editors) *2nd European Congress of EEG and Clinical Neurophysiology*, International Congress Series No. **506**, Amsterdam, Excerpta Medica (1979)

46 LEDERMAN, R. J. and HENRY, C. E. Progressive dialysis encephalopathy. *Annals of Neurology*, **4**, 199–204 (1978)

47 LEE, S. H. and GOLDBERG, H. I. Hypervascular pattern associated with idiopathic focal status epilepticus. *Radiology*, **125**, 159–163 (1977)

48 MARTINIUS, J., MATTHES, A. and LOMBROSO, C. T. Electroencephalographic features in posterior fossa tumors in children. *Electroencephalography and Clinical Neurophysiology*, **25**, 128–139 (1968)

49 McGAHAN, J. P., DUBLIN, A. B. and HILL, R. P. The evaluation of seizure disorders by computerized tomography. *Journal of Neurosurgery*, **50**, 328–332 (1979)

50 MENZER, L., SABIN, T. and MARK, V. H. Computerized axial tomography. Use in the diagnosis of dementia. *Journal of the American Medical Association*, **234**, 754–757 (1975)

51 MICHEL, B., GASTAUT, J. L. and BIANCHI, L. Electroencephalographic cranial computerized tomographic correlations in brain abscess. *Electroencephalography and Clinical Neurophysiology*, **46**, 256–273 (1979)

52 MODESTI, L. M. and BINET, E. F. Value of computed tomography in the diagnosis and management of subarachnoid hemorrhage. *Neurosurgery*, **3**, 151–156 (1978)

53 NAU, H.-E., BONGARTZ, E. B., BOCK, W. J. and WEICHERT, C. Computerized tomography (CT), electroencephalography (EEG), and clinical symptoms in severe cranio-cerebral injuries. A comparative study. *Acta Neurochirurgica*, **45**, 209–216 (1979)

54 NEWMAN, S. E. Comparative utilization of EEG and computerized tomography: the effect of computerized tomographic scanning on EEG usage. *Clinical Electroencephalography*, **8**, 70–76 (1977)

55 NORTON, G. A., KISHORE, P. R. S. and LIN, J. CT contrast enhancement in cerebral infarction. *American Journal of Roentgenology*, **131**, 881–885 (1978)

56 OAKLEY, J., OJEMANN, G. A., OJEMANN, L. M. and CROMWELL, L. Identifying epileptic foci on contrast-enhanced computerized tomographic scans. *Archives of Neurology*, **36**, 669–671 (1979)

57 OLDENDORFF, W. H. The quest for an image of brain: A brief historical and technical review of brain imaging techniques. *Neurology*, **28**, 517–533 (1978)

58 PLUM, F. and POSNER, J. B. *Diagnosis of Stupor and Coma*, 3rd edition. *Contemporary Neurology Series*, **19**, 373 pp. Philadelphia, F. A. Davis (1980)

59 ROBERTS, M. A., McGEORGE, A. P. and CAIRD, F. I. Electroencephalography and computerised tomography in vascular and non-vascular dementia in old age. *Journal of Neurology, Neurosurgery and Psychiatry*, **41**, 903–906 (1978)

60 ROSENBLUM, M. L., HOFF, J. T., NORMAN, D., WEINSTEIN, P. R. and PITTS, L. Decreased mortality from brain abscesses since advent of computerized tomography. *Journal of Neurosurgery*, **49**, 658–668 (1978)

61 SABIN, T. D. and MARK, V. H. Computerized axial tomography and electroencephalography. *Journal of the American Medical Association*, **236**, 138 (1976)

62 SAKAI, F., MEYER, J. S., NARITOMI, H. and HSU, M.-C. Regional cerebral blood flow and EEG in patients with epilepsy. *Archives of Neurology*, **35**, 648–657 (1978)

63 SHARBROUGH, F. W., MESSICK, J. M., JR. and SUNDT, T. M., JR. Correlation of continuous electroencephalograms with cerebral blood flow measurements during carotid endarterectomy. *Stroke*, **4**, 674–683 (1973)

64 SOREL, L., RUCQUOY-PONSAR, M. and HARMANT, J. Electroencéphalogramme et tomographie assistée par calculateur dans 393 cas d'épilepsie. Étude des correspondences des localisations EEG et des localisations découvertes par la tomographie assistée par calculateur. *Acta Neurologica Belgica*, **78**, 242–252 (1978)

65 STEINER, L., BERGVALL, U. and ZWETNOW, N. Quantitative estimation of intracerebral and intraventricular hematoma by computer tomography. *Acta Radiologica*, Supplement **346**, 143–154 (1975)

66 STOCKARD, J. J., BICKFORD, R. G. and AUNG, M. H. The electroencephalogram in traumatic brain injury. In *Handbook of Clinical Neurology*, **23** (*Injuries of the Brain and Skull, Part I*), edited by P. J. Vinken and G. W. Bruyn, 317–367. Amsterdam, North-Holland Publishing Co. (1975)

67 TINDALL, G. T. and ODOM, G. L. Saccular aneurysms of the brain. Surgical treatment. In *Handbook of Clinical Neurology*, **12** (*Vascular Diseases of the Nervous System. Part II*), edited by P. J. Vinken and G. W. Bruyn, 205–226. Amsterdam, North-Holland Publishing Co. (1972)

68 VAN DER DRIFT, J. H. A. *The Significance of Electro-Encephalography for the Diagnosis and Localisation of Cerebral Tumours*. 132 pp. Leiden, H. E. Stenfert Kroese (1957)

69 VAN DER DRIFT, J. H. A. (Editor) In *Handbook of Electroencephalography and Clinical Neurophysiology*. Editor-in-Chief A. Rémond. Volume **14**, *Clinical EEG. Part A: Cardiac and Vascular Diseases*. 88 pp. Amsterdam, Elsevier Publishing Co. (1971)

70 VAN DER DRIFT, J. H. A. The EEG in cerebrovascular disease. In *Handbook of Clinical Neurology*, **11** (*Vascular Diseases of the Nervous System. Part I*), edited by P. J. Vinken and G. W. Bruyn, 267–291. Amsterdam, North-Holland Publishing Co. (1972)

71 VAN KIRK, O. C., CORNEL, S. H. and JACOBY, C. G. Posterior fossa intra-axial tumors: A comparison of computed tomography with other imaging methods. *CT: the Journal of Computed Tomography*, **3**, 31–39 (1979)

72 WALTER, W. G. The location of cerebral tumours by electroencephalography. *Lancet*, **2**, 305–308 (1936)

73 WEISBERG, L. A. Computerized tomography in intracranial metastases. *Archives of Neurology*, **36**, 630–634 (1979)

74 WEISBERG, L. A. CT and acute head trauma. *Computerized Tomography*, **3**, 15–28 (1979)

75 WEISBERG, L. A. Cerebral computerized tomography in intracranial inflammatory disorders. *Archives of Neurology*, **37**, 137–142 (1980)

76 WENDE, S., AULICH, A., KRETZSCHMAR, K., GRUMME, T., MEESE, W., LANGE, S., STEINHOFF, H., LANKSCH, W. and KAZNER, E. Die Computer-Tomographie der Hirngeschwülste. Eine Sammelstudie über 1658 Tumoren. *Radiologe*, **17**, 149–156 (1977)

77 WILSON, W. P., MUSELLA, L. and SHORT, M. J. The electroencephalogram in dementia. In *Dementia*, 2nd Edn., edited by C. E. Wells. *Contemporary Neurology Series*, 205–221. Philadelphia, F. A. Davis (1977)

78 ZIMMERMAN, R. A., GONZALEZ, C., BILANIUK, L. T. and LAFFEY, P. Computed tomography in focal epilepsy. *Computed Axial Tomography*, **1**, 83–91 (1977)

14
On the need to collect EEG data from so-called normal individuals

K. G. Ingemar Petersén and Ulla Selldén

Introduction

When electroencephalograms came into clinical use, criteria for normality evolved and it was long customary to give details of these normal EEGs and of the incidence of normal EEGs in various patient populations. These criteria were sometimes arbitrary and referred to the EEG of adult individuals, especially the α-dominated EEG, but also to an EEG in which, besides the α-activity, there was, for example, less than 10 per cent θ-activity. A small degree of asymmetry was allowed. Certain norms were also promulgated for EEG during childhood and adolescence.

In the late 1950s, at the Department of Clinical Neurophysiology in Göteborg the question was asked: 'What does the EEG look like in individuals who satisfy well-defined criteria which provide a reasonable guarantee that the individual's central nervous system has not been exposed to injury, disease or other detrimental effects?' In 1958, Petersén began to collect such material from children and adults, work which has continued ever since. It is no longer sufficient to describe the incidence of normal EEGs. Instead, attention should be focussed on finding out more about EEG in normal individuals who may be characterized as healthy and without damage to the CNS. The term 'normal' is used primarily because it is short; it is difficult to say what is 'normal' but subjects were selected according to the following criteria[37].

(1) An uneventful prenatal (i.e. gestational age not less than 37 weeks, birth weight above 2500 g) and neonatal period.

(2) No disorders of consciousness.

(3) No head injury with cerebral symptoms.

(4) No history of central nervous system disease.

(5) No obvious somatic diseases which may have a secondary effect on the central nervous system.

(6) No convulsions of a febrile or other nature (including so-called emotional ones).

(7) No family history of convulsive disorders other than those secondary to acquired cerebral damage.

(8) No paroxysmal headaches or abdominal pains.

(9) No enuresis or encopresis after the fourth birthday.

(10) No tics, stuttering, pavor nocturnus or excessive nailbiting.

(11) No obvious mental disease, e.g. psychosis, depression or obsessive or compulsive symptoms.

(12) No conduct disorders; e.g. delinquency, criminality.

(13) No deviation with regard to mental and physical development.

These criteria were relatively uniform for all groups of individuals investigated though certain exceptions were made because of age. For example, in Göteborg it was possible in nearly 100 per cent of the childhood and adolescent subjects to establish the particulars of their delivery with respect to possible complications by studying hospital delivery files and through information from parents and others. For the material from adults it was more difficult. In all groups, EEG investigations were combined with a thorough somatic examination, including blood pressure measurement and establishment of neurological status including ophthalmoscopy.

Individuals from a wide cross-section of the community were invited to take part in the investigations. Children were collected from child welfare centres, children's homes, nursery schools and schools. The 'normal case' criteria were sent out to maternity clinics, child welfare centres, school health centres etc. and children who preliminarily satisfied the criteria came along with their parents to the Department of Clinical Neurophysiology. Further selection took place at the laboratory after interviewing the children and parents and after the children had undergone a thorough clinical examination by doctors with paediatric and neurological qualifications. In the case of children and adolescents, final selection did not take place before information from delivery files and other hospital case-records had been obtained where relevant. Clinical neurophysiologists, paediatricians and neurologists took part in these investigations. In a large number of cases, siblings of normal volunteers were also investigated, with a view to performing certain genetic analyses.

EEG signals from this extensive and representative sample were tape-recorded for subsequent analyses by different methods. The studies included: 29 children (18 girls and 11 boys) from birth to 1 year[16]; 743 children (389 girls and 354 boys) aged 1–15 years[37, 42]; 185 adolescents (94 girls and 91 boys) aged 16–21 years[10]; and 220 adults (106 females, 114 males) aged 22–80 years[39].

Special attention was paid to puberty, birth order, handedness and social data such as social group and parental marital status.

In the literature there are a considerable number of studies of EEG in so-called normal individuals. However, in many of these investigations no statement about the criteria for normality is made. Others do not include both sexes, or are only concerned with resting EEG. The authors, therefore, will chiefly restrict themselves to their own experiences and in particular, aim to demonstrate the importance of obtaining normative values for different EEG parameters.

The visual assessment of EEG records comprises the following.

(1) Resting EEG

  (a) Background activity:
     (i) α- and β-activity;
    (ii) subjectively assessed amount of low frequency activity under the main headings: normal amount of low frequency activity, slight increase of low frequency activity (SIL) and moderate increase of low frequency activity (MIL) (*Figure 14.1*).

  (b) Special rhythmic patterns:
     (i) slow α-variant;
    (ii) polyphasic potentials, mainly in the temporo-occipital derivations, blocked by opening the eyes and accentuated by hyperventilation;
   (iii) slow posterior rhythm (SPR), 2.5–4.5 Hz activity in posterior derivations, blocked by eye-opening, often increased by hyperventilation;
   (iv) diffuse 3–5 Hz activity in drowsiness, blocked by alerting stimuli. This pattern may appear in lower age groups with posterior accentuation;
    (v) rhythmic 6–7 Hz activity in occipital derivation;
   (vi) rhythmic 6–7 Hz activity in anterior derivations;
  (vii) μ-rhythm.

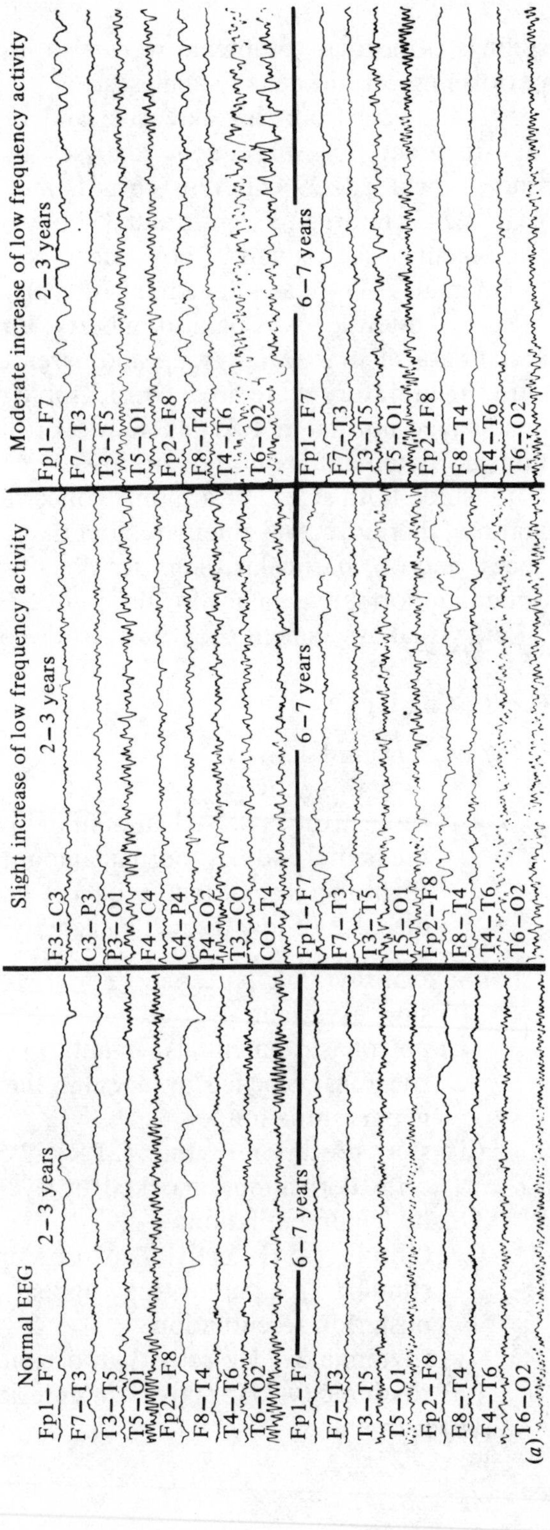

Normal EEG   2–3 years

Fp1–F7
F7–T3
T3–T5
T5–O1
Fp2–F8
F8–T4
T4–T6
T6–O2

Fp1–F7 —————— 6–7 years
F7–T3
T3–T5
T5–O1
Fp2–F8
F8–T4
T4–T6
T6–O2

Slight increase of low frequency activity   2–3 years

F3–C3
C3–P3
P3–O1
F4–C4
C4–P4
P4–O2
T3–CO
CO–T4

Fp1–F7 —————— 6–7 years
F7–T3
T3–T5
T5–O1
Fp2–F8
F8–T4
T4–T6
T6–O2

Moderate increase of low frequency activity   2–3 years

Fp1–F7
F7–T3
T3–T5
T5–O1
Fp2–F8
F8–T4
T4–T6
T6–O2

Fp1–F7 —————— 6–7 years
F7–T3
T3–T5
T5–O1
Fp2–F8
F8–T4
T4–T6
T6–O2

(a)

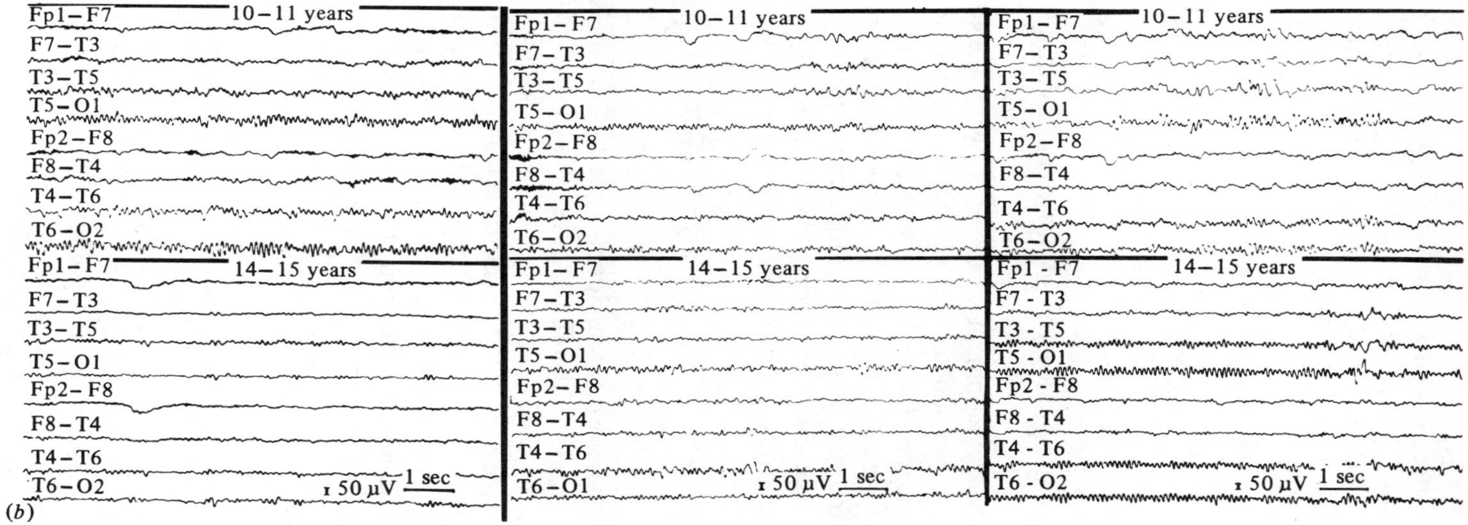

Figure 14.1 Normal EEG, slight (SIL) and moderate (MIL) increase of low frequency activity in normal children. Age (*a*) 2–3 and 6–7 years; (*b*) 10–11 and 14–15 years. (From Petersén and Eeg-Olofsson[37], courtesy of the Editor and publisher, *Neuropädiatrie*)

(c) Paroxysmal activities: spikes, sharp waves, paroxysmal slow waves, special paroxysmal patterns such as the psychomotor variant pattern, 14-6 Hz positive spike pattern, 6 Hz spike and wave pattern or 6 Hz phantom spike waves.
(2) Response to hyperventilation.
(3) Response to intermittent photic stimulation.
(4) Response to sleep.

Results

Development of the electroencephalogram in normal individuals

One goal was to ascertain the development of the EEG with age in male and female individuals. A detailed account will not be given here of all the patterns studied in normal individuals from birth to 80 years of age, but rather the development illustrated by some variables of special interest including α-frequency, slight to moderate increase in the amount of low frequency activity in resting EEGs, paroxysmal activity whilst awake, 14-6 Hz positive spikes, 6 Hz spike wave activity and psychomotor variant pattern.

α-Activity
The frequency of α-activity in all normal individuals aged 1–80 years is shown in *Figure 14.2*. Previous publications have shown that α-frequency increases successively during childhood and adolescence[10, 27, 29, 30], and that in old people[32, 35, 49, 51], even in selected healthy individuals, a lower α-frequency is found than in selected healthy young adults. In order to determine more closely at what age these frequency changes take place, a linear regression analysis was made of the data after dividing them into three different age intervals, with varying age limits. The method of 'least squares' was used to ascertain the age division at which the obtained regression line best expressed the actual conditions.

The analysis showed that α-activity reached a maximum frequency at 17 years of age. It was less easy to pin-point the age when α-frequency started to decrease but it occurred within the age interval 40–60 years. Finally, the age groups 0–17 years, 18–49 years and 50 years or over were chosen. A statistically significant increase ($P <$ 0.01) in the frequency of α-activity up to the age of 17 could be

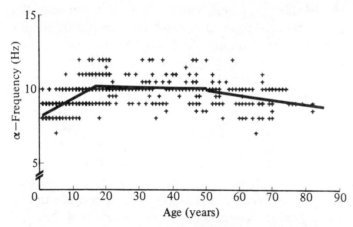

Figure 14.2 α-Frequency in relation to age. Regression lines are based on observations between the ages 1–17 years, 18–49 years and ⩾ 50 years respectively

distinguished; between the ages of 18–40, the slope of the regression line did not significantly vary from 0; after 50 years of age there was a statistically significant decrease $(P < 0.01)$.

In previously published data[47] on normal adults between the ages of 26 and 55 years, females exhibited an α-activity of 11 Hz or greater significantly more often and an α-activity of 9 Hz or less, significantly less often than males $(P < 0.05)$. When the data were divided into males and females of under and over 40 years of age respectively, an α-activity of 9 Hz or less was found in significantly more men than women $(P < 0.05)$. The same tendency, but without statistical significance, can be found if the age limit is set at 60 years.

Increase of low frequency activity

Conventional visual assessment shows that SIL and MIL occur to a certain extent in all age groups. However, the number of individuals with SIL or MIL varies unsystematically in the different age groups. In children and adolescents, investigated annually, the percentage varies from 2–3 to 25 per cent; in the adult material, analyzed per decade, there is a variation of between 7.5 and 24 per cent. Focal localization is unusual and only occurs in a few individuals over the age of 50. Throughout the whole age spectrum from 14 years onwards, there is a higher frequency of SIL and MIL in females than in males. A statistically significant difference only occurs, however, between the ages of 14 and 22 ($P < 0.05$). In the adult material, a higher frequency of SIL and MIL was registered in individuals over 50 years of age than under (12.6 per cent against 5.6 per cent). The difference is not significant overall, but a significantly higher MIL frequency was noted in females over 50 than in those under 50 ($P < 0.05$). In boys and adolescents of both sexes, a significant correlation between SIL–MIL and low α-frequency was found ($P < 0.05$), but not even a tendency in this direction has been found in adults.

These various findings in different age groups emphasize the difficulty in drawing conclusions from the SIL and MIL content respectively. It is possible that these findings have different importance in different age groups; longitudinal studies of normal material are presently being undertaken to ascertain whether those EEG patterns may also serve as indices of cerebral lesions or not.

Paroxysmal activity in resting EEGs. This occurs in all age groups but to a very minor extent and without a significant age correlation. There is a significantly higher incidence in women than in men ($P < 0.05$). The incidence in children was 2.7 per cent, in adolescents 1.6 per cent and in the adult material 3.3 per cent. This paroxysmal activity usually consisted of focal sharp waves which appeared more distinctly in children. The significance of these paroxysmal changes in normal subjects is at present unclear and longitudinal studies are required in order to determine their significance.

14-6 Hz positive spikes. A pronounced correlation is found with age; they successively increase in frequency from 2 up to 13 years of age, after which a level of approximately 25 per cent is maintained up to, and including, 15 years of age. Thereafter a decline is noted between 16 and 21 years of age to 14.6 per cent. In the adult material, there is a considerable and rapid decrease to 7.3 per cent between the ages of 20 and 23 and to 2.6 per cent between the ages of 30 and 39. In older age groups, 14-6 Hz positive spike activity does not occur (*Figure 14.3*).

6 Hz spike-wave activity. This also occurs extremely rarely, i.e. in one boy of 14 years, 7 adolescents and 6 adults. 14-6 Hz positive spikes have a more distinctive configuration in children and adolescents than in adults. 6 Hz spike-wave activity is almost non-existent in children and appears later in life, when 14-6 Hz positive spikes, if present, are less well-defined. Silverman[48] found that 14-6 Hz positive spikes and

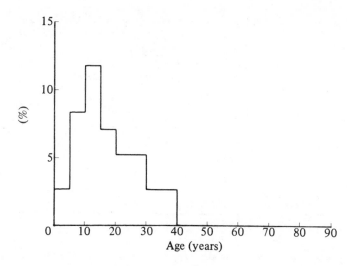

Figure 14.3 Percentage distribution of 14-6 Hz positive spike activity in relation to age

6 Hz spike waves often coincide in the same patient and therefore suggested that both phenomena might be of the same origin. Age may play a role in the configuration these activities show. Neither of them showed any systematic variation between the sexes.

The strikingly high frequency of these findings at puberty with their noticeable decrease in later years may be a sign that they reflect factors in physiological development. Positive correlations between 14-6 Hz positive spikes and certain behavioural disturbances have been demonstrated, however[7].

The psychomotor variant pattern. This pattern occurred in 6 children between the ages of 6 and 14, in two 18-year-olds and in six adults[15] (*Figure 14.4*).

An especially interesting finding is the difference between sexes, both for α-frequencies in certain age groups and several of the EEG patterns observed. Women show a higher α-frequency and a more frequent occurrence of different kinds of EEG patterns mentioned above. Even when statistical significance does not emerge, there is a consistent tendency for a higher incidence in women[47]. This relationship applies also to different kinds of activation effects. The threshold for appearance of EEG changes provoked by, for example, hyperventilation, photic stimulation and administration of Megimide

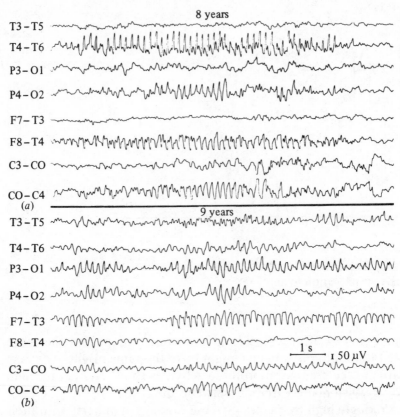

Figure 14.4 Psychomotor variant patterns. (*a*) Saw-toothed waves; (*b*) flat-topped waves

(bemegride) is lower for women than for men. The difference between the sexes should be taken into consideration when evaluating different EEG patterns and effects of activation clinically.

Psychiatric assessment of healthy children with various EEG patterns

EEGs from normal children[37] contained a number of deviations from what has customarily been called normal in everyday clinical EEG. If these EEGs had been recorded from patients with certain symptoms, such EEG findings might have been used to suggest the presence of disease.

The possibility of proving, with current psychiatric diagnostic methods, any clinical or other correlations with various EEG patterns was investigated in children who, as far as it was known, had not been exposed to cerebral damage of any kind or who were judged to be healthy according to general paediatric norms[7]. A total of 222 normal children (112 girls and 110 boys), aged between 5 and 16 years were randomly chosen from the sample for examination by a child-psychiatrist. Their EEG findings appear in the following categories.

(1) Normal EEG, at rest and on provocation.
(2) Normal resting EEG, with 14-6 Hz positive spikes during sleep.
(3) Normal resting EEG, paroxysmal activity on activation (without 14 and 6 Hz positive spikes).
(4) Slight increase of low frequency activity or moderate increase of low frequency activity.
(5) Paroxysmal activity in resting EEG.
(6) Psychomotor variant pattern.

Each EEG was taken recently and each child had again undergone paediatric examination to ascertain whether he or she still, after several years, satisfied the criteria for normality. The child-psychiatrist and assistants had no information about the EEG investigation when they made their examinations. Besides a medical examination, the investigation included an interview with the parents by a social worker and determination of the IQ in accordance with the Wechsler Intelligence Scale for children[52], as well as two tests of organicity[1, 2].

Particular attention was paid to 13 so-called 'suspected lesion symptoms', i.e. increased fatiguability, irritability, hypersensitivity to sound and light, emotional instability, proneness to cry, poor concentration, circumstantiality, obstinacy, stubbornness, perseveration tendency, paroxysmal traits and hyperactivity (restlessness, motor deviations and abnormal interests in detail). Each symptom was rated on a 3-point scale: 0 = negative findings, 1 = slight symptoms, 2 = more pronounced symptoms. If the total points for any child was six or more, it was listed under the subjective heading 'suspected lesion syndrome'.

Because of the criteria for normality, children with mental deviations and behavioural disorders had been excluded as far as possible. In the psychiatric assessment, however, individual children were found who initially were considered 'normal' but now could be described as having behavioural disorders. Previous behavioural disorders were considered present if the parents had consulted a doctor on the child's behalf because of behavioural symptoms, (13 per cent). Current behavioural disorders were judged to be present if, at the psychiatric examination, the case history and mental status gave evidence for them (3 per cent), even though the parents did not regard the child as deviant or troublesome. Isolated symptoms were classified as 'other clinical symptoms', i.e. aggressiveness, anxiety, abdominal pains, headaches, food problems, sleep disturbance, head-banging, tics, disturbed peer relationship, school problems, vagrancy, pilfering, thumb-sucking and nail-biting. Amongst the results[7], those which appeared in the correlation studies are particularly remarkable. The findings of a *'normal EEG at rest and on activation' were negatively correlated (P < 0.05 at least) with those clinical variables listed above. Furthermore, it was found that other, different EEG patterns were positively correlated with some of the different psychiatric variables.*

The 'suspected lesion syndrome', observed in 30 children, was in all cases positively correlated ($P < 0.05$) with paroxysmal activity in the resting EEG. In a few subgroups of the total material, there were even positive correlations between the 'suspected lesion syndrome' and the EEG pattern 'SIL and MIL', as well as with 'normal resting EEG, paroxysmal activity on provocation'. The most common EEG pattern in children with previous behavioural disorders or other clinical symptoms was normal resting EEG 14-6 Hz positive spikes in sleep, after which came 'normal resting EEG, paroxysmal activity on provocation'. For 'abdominal pain' a correlation was found with 'paroxysmal findings in resting EEG' and 'normal resting EEG, paroxysmal activity on provocation'. The EEG pattern 'psychomotor variant pattern' (saw-tooth pattern) gave no clinically relevant correlation.

The results of a special investigation[5], devoted to the relationship between psychological test results and EEG patterns in normal children, are summarized: 'the high frequency of defective scores in the Bender and Benton tests in this selected material of healthy children means that these tests cannot be used in clinical work for diagnosing brain injury in individual children. Nor can they be used to throw light on the clinical significance of the different EEG variables studied'.

Attention was also paid to possible correlations between psychiatric findings and EEG variables in a non-selected population of 138 of the 222 normal children where, for purposes of statistical comparison, the

EEG signal was quantified by automatic frequency analysis[6]. Clinical and EEG signs of brain immaturity failed to correlate significantly. On the other hand, children with slight symptoms of cerebral dysfunction exhibited significant deviations in their EEG frequency pattern, which could be interpreted as EEG signs of delayed maturation, i.e. increased quantity of θ-activity, prevalence of slow components within the α-band and lower values of 'age' as calculated from EEG values. There was only a doubtful relationship between IQ values and increased θ-activity in parieto-occipital derivations.

Methods for automatic diagnosis in clinical EEG based on EEG from normal individuals

While collecting EEGs from normal individuals, special methods for their automatic analysis were also developed[11, 12, 13, 24, 31, 38]. The method for automatic diagnosis is founded on the experience that brain damage caused by a tumour or a haemorrhage, for example, focally produces EEG parameters representative of normal individuals of a lower age, the more pronounced the damage the lower the age. For automatic diagnosis using background EEG activity, a mathematical method was based on tape recorded EEGs from 562 normal children and adolescents aged 1–21 years. EEGs were subjected to frequency analysis to obtain reference data on amplitudes of EEG activity in different frequency bands. Data concerning these amplitudes, as well as various amplitude ratios, were entered into the computer and processed by estimating parameters to produce a mathematical model. The model obtained could then be applied to any other EEG record in order to compare it with the normal material. This processing thus results in a single output value for each derivation relating the actual EEG to what should be normal for age. The ideal value is 100 per cent and a lower value indicates a deviation from normal. The lower the value, the more severe is the abnormality. The final results are expressed in conventional terms used in clinical electroencephalography, such as 'a normal EEG, slight, moderate or marked nonspecific abnormality, and diffuse, lateralized or focal abnormality'. Processing 1 min of EEG recording takes about 3 min in the authors' PDP 15 computer, but this can be speeded up with a more powerful computer. *Figure 14.5* shows an example of automatic clinical EEG diagnosis based on this method.

EEG Examination 1976–09–17   Patient 41–01–15

⌂

(	3	72	)
(	25	70	)
(	27	74	)
(	86	84	)

α-Activity with a frequency of 10–11 Hz and with an amplitude of about 40 μV is dominant. Rather high amount of δ-activity which is more pronounced fronto-temporally and centrally on the left side. Very small amount of β-activity diffusely. Artefacts are suspected over the fronto-temporal areas.
Conclusion: very severe abnormality in the fronto-temporal and central region on the left side.

Figure 14.5 An example of automatic evaluation of an EEG record. The figure shows a schematically depicted head with symbols indicating different grades of abnormality in various regions. The exact degree is indicated by numbers, lower values corresponding to more pronounced abnormality

In about 80 per cent of EEGs at the authors' department, these computerized diagnoses are exactly the same as ones made by an EEG expert. Exceptions are mainly due to the presence of artefacts and of components in the EEG associated with drowsiness.

This method means that routine work with clinical EEG can be reduced. For example, preliminary studies showed that normal EEGs – corresponding to about one-third of all routine EEGs at the authors' department – can be assessed automatically, with only a superficial review by an electroencephalographer. This method is also objective, thus increasing the usefulness of the EEG in recurrent examinations in longitudinal studies of separate individuals or groups of individuals.

EEG diagnosis and characteristics using EEGs from normal individuals as reference material

This EEG material from normal individuals has also been used as reference material for EEGs in patients who clinically satisfy the criteria for normal except for one symptom or disease. Idiopathic scoliosis may appear together with various neurological disorders involving different levels in the CNS. As part of a larger study of idiopathic scoliosis[45] an EEG study was therefore undertaken[43]. Of 57 children aged 10–16 years with idiopathic scoliosis, 37 were treated (brace or surgery), and 20 were observed. Controls were normal children aged 10–16 years. Thirty-four of the scoliotics met the above mentioned criteria of normality. The following EEG patterns were considered: normal EEG, slight or moderate increase of low frequency activity in resting EEG, 14-6 Hz positive spikes and/or 6 Hz spike and wave activity.

Among the results, it was interesting to note that paroxysmal abnormalities in resting EEG appeared to be statistically ($P < 0.01$) much more frequent in the scoliosis cases than in normal controls. Paroxysmal abnormalities in the scoliosis cases were, to a large extent, of a bilateral synchronous type considered to be generated subcortically, a region of special interest in discussions about the aetiology of idiopathic scoliosis.

EEG examinations using the same methods are presently being carried out on workers who have been exposed to industrial solvents for a lengthy period and on children with 'minimal brain dysfunction'.

Genetic findings

Appearing during light sleep, 14-6 Hz positive spikes[14] are most common in children and adolescents and, in the group of normal adults studied[39], not later than the 40th year. Gibbs[14] suggested that this bilateral pattern was generated in the thalamus and hypothalamus and clinical correlations with behaviour disorders and autonomic dysfunction have been described[15, 26]. Other complexes often appear, together with 14-6 Hz positive spikes or independently, which resemble abortive or questionable 14-6 Hz positive spikes. Using a reverse correlation method, an autocorrelation technique for continuous analysis of frequency interrelations in nonstationary time series[22], it was shown that typical 14-6 Hz positive spikes and the questionable 14-6 Hz positive spikes in the EEGs of normal children essentially belong to the same group of signal events[23].

A study[40] of the role played by genetic factors in the 14-6 Hz positive spikes in the EEGs of normal children showed that these spike phenomena were significantly over-represented among siblings of children with 14-6 Hz positive spikes. The same was true for the questionable cases. This material does not permit a conclusion about the way in which 14-6 Hz positive spikes are genetically transmitted; findings point to dominant autosomal inheritance, but do not exclude other means of transmission.

Certain unexpected results from work with EEG in normal individuals

An exceptionally interesting by-product of the investigation of EEG in normal children was discovered when a relationship was sought between the IQ of the children and their social group. Previously, extensive Swedish studies of relationships between social class and intelligence had shown that IQ was greater in higher social classes[3, 4, 8, 9, 17–21, 28, 34, 46, 50, 53]. Two of these investigations[4, 17] were of schoolchildren, while the others dealt with young men registered for military service. Later investigations also showed a correlation between IQ and social class[3, 9, 12, 20, 21, 34, 46, 50, 53].

The authors' study[41] included 222 children, aged 4.5–16.5 years, who were found to be normal by strict somatoneurological criteria, and were investigated by EEG and psychiatric methods. Intelligence tests were performed according to the Wechsler Intelligence Scale. The mean intelligence quotient amounted to 116.3 ± 12.4 in boys and 116.6 ± 14.1 in girls. There was no relationship of significance between IQ and social group. No relevent relationship was found between IQ and psychiatric variables, nor between IQ and EEG findings. The absence of the normal fixed relationship between IQ and social group is a notable finding as is the high average IQ. The strict criteria for normality may have contributed to the exclusion of individuals with lesions and thus diminished factors having an inhibitory effect on the development of intelligence. Such lesions may be explained by the fact that children in lower social groups run a greater risk of physical damage to the cerebral structures of importance for intelligence, including IQ, than is the case with children belonging to higher social groups. The authors look upon their results rather as a challenge: new investigations ought to be undertaken in line with them. If their results prove to be correct this should lead to important political consequences, not least in view of the fact that the results obtained are probably very similar in other countries and particularly in countries where there is a lower degree of social equality.

Discussion

As emphasized in the introduction, the word 'normal' is not a good term to denote a single individual or group of individuals[25,33]. EEGs were studied from individuals who fulfil a series of well-defined criteria, which indicate that they have not been exposed to any injuries or diseases which, directly or indirectly, can have a negative effect on the CNS. In this way, the development of EEG with age in males and females was studied which permits the use of EEG together with other methods for analysis of the development of the brain.

EEG from normal individuals provides reference data from which something new can be learnt about the diagnostic possibilities and limitations of EEG. Knowledge regarding EEGs in normal individuals is presently not sufficient to establish what constitutes a normal EEG. For this purpose, longitudinal studies are needed to look for connections between development of the individual and EEG patterns – do normal children with, for example, paroxysmal EEGs run a greater risk of epilepsy, headache or behavioural disturbances than normal children without paroxysmal EEGs? Preliminary results of one such longitudinal study show that individuals who fulfilled the criteria for normal at the time of EEG examination and who later repeatedly committed larceny of a defined type exhibited a higher α-amplitude, more paroxysmal EEG findings during sleep and different hyperventilation effects than comparable individuals in the study who have not committed larceny. This study was performed in collaboration with the Social Science Research Institute, University of Southern California.

Amongst the deficiencies of the data is the fact that, during a sleep EEG, only the appearance of paroxysmal phenomena such as spikes, sharp waves, 14-6 Hz positive spikes etc. were noted. Neither a systematic study of the development of different sleep types, nor a description of evoked potentials, has been performed on the data.

On the basis of personal experience, recommendations to other research units as to how continued investigations should be undertaken in order to gain increased knowledge of EEG in normal individuals are difficult to make. One recommendation can be made without hesitation, however. From the very first, a multi-disciplinary research project was planned with clinical neurophysiology, neurology, child neurology, psychiatry, child psychiatry, psychology, genetics, epidemiology and medical techniques to find answers to problems in the field of sociology. This involves a retroactive analysis of the social conditions which have left their mark. Any future investigation might also include an extensive analysis of the social structure of the normal material. Such a procedure could, perhaps, increase the possibility of analyzing the causes of the previously mentioned findings that normal individuals with certain abnormal EEG patterns more often commit criminal acts than normal individuals without such EEG findings. An important issue arises here: can social pressures, such as those found in members of the authors' study, be the cause, not only of changes in social behaviour, but also of changes in EEG?

The authors' results are representative for parts of Europe, North America, Canada and some other areas. Special investigations are possibly necessary for countries with a tropical or arctic climate, for population groups living at high altitude and for population groups with special nutritional characteristics, etc. etc.

Knowledge of human normative data is an important prerequisite for research into preventive medicine. Demand for normative data regarding EEG increases in proportion to the risks of toxic and other damaging influences to which human beings today, more rapidly than at any time previously, are increasingly exposed. Finally, it is emphasized that the need for increased knowledge about normative EEG data must not be confined to the experience collected from protected research laboratories. The influence of the working environment on the EEG of normal individuals is of vital importance. Based on normal data, EEG results can, far better than before, contribute to revealing the effects of toxic influences on the CNS. Normative data is also essential to studies of circadian variations of EEG and how these are affected by shift-work and other stress factors at work[44]. These activities create the basis of occupational EEG[36].

References

1 BENDER, L. *A Visual Motor Gestalt Test and its Clinical Use*, 176. New York, Orthopsychiatric Association (1938)

2 BENTON, A. *The Revised Visual Retention Test*, 74. Dubuque, Iowa, W. M. C. Brown Co. Inc. (1963)

3 BIRCH, H. and GUSSOW, J. *Disadvantaged Children: Health, Nutrition and School Failure*, 322. New York, Harcourt, Brace and World (1970)

4 BOALT, G. *Skolutbildning och Skolresultat för Barn ur Olika Samhällsgrupper i Stockholm*, 149. Stockholm, Nordstedt and Söners Förlag (1947)

5 BOSAEUS, E. The relationship between psychological test results and EEG patterns in healthy children. *Scandinavian Journal of Psychology*, **19**, 181–191 (1978)

6 BOSAEUS, E., MATOUSEC, M. and PETERSÉN, I. Correlation between paedopsychiatric findings and EEG-variables in well-functioning children of ages 5 of 16 years. An EEG frequency analysis study. *Scandinavian Journal of Psychology*, **18**, 140–147 (1977)

7 BOSAEUS, E. and SELLDÉN, U. Psychiatric assessment of healthy children with various EEG patterns. *Acta Psychiatrica Scandinavica*, **59**, 180–210 (1979)

8 DAHLQUIST, R. Prestationer i svenska krigsmaktens inskrivningsprov i Göteborg år 1945 med särskild hänsyn till den regionala fördelningen. *Folkskolan*, **1**, 87–98 (1947)

9 DEUTSCH, M., KATZ, J. and JENSEN, A. *Social Class, Race and Psychological Development*. New York, Rinehart and Winston (1968)

10 EEG-OLOFSSON, O. The development of the electroencephalogram in normal adolescents from the age of 16 through 21 years. *Neuropädatrie*, **3**, 11–45 (1971)

11 FRIBERG, S. *A Program System for Automatic Evaluation of the Background Activity in the Human Electroencephalogram*. Technical Report **3:80**, 53. Research Laboratory of Medical Electronics, Chalmers University of Technology, Göteborg (1980)

12 FRIBERG, S., MAGNUSSON, R., MATOUSEK, M. and PETERSÉN, I. Automatic EEG diagnosis by means of digital signal processing. In *Quantitative Analytic Studies in Epilepsy*, edited by P. Kellaway and I. Petersén, 289–307, New York, Raven Press (1976)

13 FRIBERG, S., MATOUSEK, M. and PETERSÉN, I. *A Mathematical Model for the Age Development of the Background Activity in the Human Electroencephalogram*. Technical Report **2:80**, 45. Research Laboratory of Medical Electronics, Chalmers University of Technology, Göteborg (1980)

14 GIBBS, E. L. and GIBBS, F. A. Electroencephalographic evidence of thalamic and hypothalamic epilepsy. *Neurology*, **1**, 136–144 (1951)

15 GIBBS, F. A. and GIBBS, E. L. *Atlas of Electroencephalography*, **2**, 422, Cambridge, Mass., Addison-Wesley (1952)

16 HAGNE, I. Development of the EEG in normal infants during the first year of life. In *Clinical Electroencephalography of Children*, edited by P. Kellaway and I. Petersén, 97–118. Stockholm, Almqvist and Wiksell (1968)

17 HALLGREN, S. Intelligens och social miljö. Några resultat från en undersökning vid Malmö folkskolor och privata skolor. *Studia Psychologica et Pedagogica*, **115**, 126–146 (1946)

18 HUSÉN, T. *Begåvning och Miljö. Studier i Begåvningsutvecklingens och Begåvningsurvalets Psykologiskpedagogiska och Sociala Problem*, 196. Stockholm, Hugo Gebers Förlag (1948)

19 HÅRNQVIST, K. Relative changes in intelligence from 13 to 18 years. *Scandinavian Journal of Psychology*, **9**, 50–65 (1968)

20 JENSEN, A. How much can we boost IQ and scholastic achievement? *Harvard Educational Revue*, **29**, 1–23 (1969)

21 JONSSON, G. and KÄLVESTEN, A. L. *222 Stockholmspojkar*, 684. Stockholm, Almqvist and Wiksell (1964)

22 KAISER, E. and PETERSÉN, I. Automatic analysis in EEG, reverse correlation. *Acta Neurologica Scandinavica*, Supplementum **22**, 20–31 (1966)

23 KAISER, E. and PETERSÉN, I. Reverse correlation of 14 and 6 per second positive spikes. In *Clinical Electroencephalography of Children*, edited by P. Kellaway and I. Petersén, 155–166. Stockholm, Almqvist and Wiksell (1968)

24 KAISER, E., PETERSÉN, I., SELLDÉN, U. and KAGAWA, N. EEG data representation in broad band frequency analysis. *Electroencephalography and Clinical Neurophysiology*, **17**, 76–80 (1964)

25 KARLBERG, P. Assessment of health in studies of child development. *Modern Problems in Pediatrics*, **7**, 208–218 (1962)

26 KELLAWAY, P., CRAWLEY, J. W. and KAGAWA, N. A. A specific electroencephalographic correlate of convulsive equivalent disorders in children. *Journal of Pediatrics*, **55**, 582–592 (1959)

27 KELLAWAY, P. An orderly approach to visual analysis: Parameters of the normal EEG in adults and children. In *Current Practice of Clinical Electroencephalography*, edited by D. W. Klass and D. D. Daly, 147 (1978)

28 KLACKENBERG-LARSSON, I. and STENSSON, J. The development of children in a Swedish urban community. A prospective longitudinal study. IV. Data on mental development during the first five years. *Acta Paediatrica Scandinavica*, Supplementum **187**, 67–93 (1968)

29 KNOTT, J. R. and GIBBS, F. A. A Fourier transform of the electroencephalogram from one to eighteen years. *Psychological Bulletin*, **36**, 512–513 (1939)

30 LINDSLEY, D. B. A longitudinal study of occipital alpha rhythm in normal children: Frequency and amplitude standards. *Journal of Psychology*, **55**, 197–213 (1939)

31 MATOUSEK, M. and PETERSÉN, I. Automatic evaluation of EEG background activity by means of age-dependent EEG quotients. *Electroencephalography and Clinical Neurophysiology*, **35**, 603–612 (1973)

32 OBRIST, W. D. The electroencephalogram of normal aged adults. *Electroencephalography and Clinical Neurophysiology*, **6**, 235–244 (1954)

33 OFFER, O. and SABSHIN, M. *Normality. Theoretical and Clinical Concepts of Mental Health*, 253. New York, Basic Books (1960)

34 OLIVE, H. The relationship of divergent thinking to intelligence, social class, and achievement in high-school students. *Journal of Genetic Psychology*, **186**, 121–179 (1972)

35 OTOMO, E. Electroencephalography in old age: dominant alpha pattern. *Electroencephalography and Clinical Neurophysiology*, **21**, 489–491 (1966)

36 PERSSON, J. and PETERSÉN, I. Occupational EEG. In *Proceedings of the 2nd International Industrial and Environmental Neurology Congress* (Prague, Czechoslovakia) 94–101 (1976)

37 PETERSÉN, I. and EEG-OLOFSSON, O. The development of the electroencephalogram in normal children from the age of 1 through 15 years. Non-paroxysmal activity. *Neuropädiatrie*, **2**, 247–305 (1971)

38 PETERSÉN, I. und MATOUSEK, M. EEG-Breitbandfrequenz-analyse bei normalen Kindern und Jugendlichen. *EEG-EMG*, **3**, 134–138 (1972)

39 PETERSÉN, I. and SELLDÉN, U. (unpublished observations)

40 PETERSÉN, I. and ÅKESSON, H-O. EEG studies of siblings of children showing 14 and 6 per second positive spikes. *Acta Genetica*, **18**, 163–169 (1968)

41 PETERSÉN, I., SELLDÉN, U. and BOSAEUS, E. The relationship between IQ, social class and EEG findings in healthy children investigated by child-psychiatric methods. *Scandinavian Journal of Psychology*, **17**, 189–197 (1976)

42 PETERSÉN, I., SELLDÉN, U. and EEG-OLOFSSON, O. The evolution of the EEG in normal children and adolescents from 1 to 21 years. In *Handbook of Electroencephalography and Clinical Neurophysiology*, **6**, Part B, edited by C. G. Lairy, 30–68. Amsterdam, Elsevier (1975)

43 PETERSÉN, I., SELLDÉN, U. and SAHLSTRAND, T. Electroencephalographic investigation of patients with adolescent idiopathic scoliosis. *Acta Ortopaedica Scandinavica*, **50**, 283–293 (1979)

44 PETERSÉN, I., HERBERTS, P., KADEFORS, R., PERSSON, J., RAGNARSSON, K. and TENGROTH, B. The measurement evaluation and importance of electroencephalography and electromyography in arduous industrial work. In *Society, Stress and Disease, 1974*, edited by L. Levi, Oxford, Oxford University Press (in press)

45 SAHLSTRAND, T. Equilibrium factors in adolescent idiopathic scoliosis. A clinical study including stabilometry, electroencephalography and electronystagmography. *Thesis*, 34. Göteborg, Uno Lundgren Tryckeri AB (1977)

46 SCARR-SALAPTEK, S. Race, social class and IQ. *Science*, **174**, 1285–1295 (1971)

47 SELLDÉN, U. Electroencephalographic activation with Megimide in normal subjects. *Acta Neurologica Scandinavica*, Supplementum **12**, 69 (1964)

48 SILVERMAN, D. Phantom spike-waves and fourteen and six per second positive spike pattern. A consideration of their relationship. *Electroencephalography and Clinical Neurophysiology*, **23**, 207–213 (1967)

49 SILVERMAN, A. J., BUSSE, E. W. and BARNES, R. H. Studies in the process of aging: Electroencephalographic findings in 400 elderly subjects. *Electroencephalography and Clinical Neurophysiology*, **7**, 67–74 (1955)

50 SVENSSON, A. Hembakgrund och prestationsnivå. *Rapporter från Pedagogiska Institutionen, Göteborgs Universitet*, **73**, 1–40 (1972)

51 WANG, H. S., OBRIST, W. D. and BUSSE, E. W. Neurophysiological function of elderly persons living in the community. *American Journal of Psychiatry*, **126**, 1205–1212 (1970)

52 WECHSLER, D. Wechsler Intelligence Scale for Children. *Manual*, 114. New York, Psychological Corporation (1949)

53 WILLERMAN, L., BENMAN, S. and FIEDLER, M. Infant development, preschool IQ, and social class. *Child Development*, **41**, 69–77 (1970)

15
Electroencephalography in cerebral monitoring: coma, cerebral ischaemia and epilepsy

Pamela Prior

Introduction

In the last decade the introduction of a number of new methods for assessing the function and structure of the brain has given an opportunity to reconsider the place of electroencephalography. As a diagnostic technique it remains a necessary complement to the other main non-invasive procedure, the computerised transaxial tomogram or CT scan (*see* Chapter 13). Whilst the scan provides a static picture primarily concerned with details of structure, the electroencephalogram (EEG) is the objective (i.e. non-clinical) source *par excellence* of information about brain function. It is this characteristic that enables us to consider a different emphasis and broader scope for clinical neurophysiology, that of cerebral monitoring.

Substantial pioneering experience with EEG monitoring has already been gained in the operating theatre and intensive care unit. Both physiological and pathological correlates of the EEG and optimal methods of monitoring have been explored extensively, often using large laboratory computer installations. Recent technological advances enable the EEG to be processed to give practical, small, relevant and relatively cheap monitoring devices. These range from miniature cassette recorders or radiotransmitters attached to the patient, to small versatile pre-programmed or programmable bedside monitors. They enable precise and objective measurements to be recorded automatically and have been successfully applied to gross phenomena like seizures or subtle unobtrusive ones such as cerebral responses in comatose patients. These developments have exciting implications in the care of individual patients and also in improving our general understanding of the mechanisms and therapeutic possibilities in many disorders of brain function.

Clinical relevance

Modern neurophysiological monitoring techniques have much to offer. Well tested applications[6, 7, 53, 68, 86] of interest to the neurologist and neurosurgeon include the following:

(1) severe disorders affecting the brain, e.g. coma of traumatic or toxic origin, acute encephalitides and encephalopathies, status epilepticus.
(2) Patterns of seizure discharge in epilepsy, e.g. petit mal status versus temporal lobe epilepsy, often studied by ambulatory monitoring, and quantification of their modification by treatments of both medical and surgical type.
(3) Behavioural studies, sleep patterns and other biological cycles in relation to precipitation or patterns of occurrence of disease, e.g. narcolepsy, epilepsy, drug effects (*see* Chapter 16).
(4) Prevention or minimization of ischaemic brain damage during elective surgical or anaesthetic procedures where the brain may be at risk, e.g. cardiopulmonary bypass, carotid artery surgery and hypotensive anaesthesia.
(5) Intrapartum fetal monitoring and detection of perinatal brain hypoxia and ischaemia; also behavioural cycles in the newborn as an indicator of maturity and state.

Feasibility of clinical monitoring

It is one thing to record biological variables from a carefully prepared sleeping subject and analyze the resulting data by computer in the controlled situation of a research laboratory. It is quite another to monitor several patients simultaneously for days at a time in a busy neurological-neurosurgical intensive care unit – much simpler, sturdier and more flexible routines are required with unambiguous display of significant data without delay for processing. Such methods can incorporate automatic alarms to obviate the need for nurse or clinician to watch the writeout continuously. Modern EEG data acquisition and monitoring equipment have permitted study of brain function in exceptionally difficult environments where orthodox methods of recording would have been impossible. Sleep was monitored in men working at a survey base in Antarctica where loss of 24 hour light/dark patterns reduced the proportion of slow wave sleep[64]. Soldiers from an infantry company underwent ambulatory monitoring during a 9-day exercise in harsh climate and terrain. With increasing sleep deprivation, sleep occurred during 'wake' periods with a decline in efficiency in cognitive tasks and, interestingly, in one soldier paroxysmal discharge was activated *de novo*[1]. Polygraphic ambulatory monitoring of aircrew during 20-hour flights from Buenos Aires to London emphasied the need for methods and data relevant to real-life problems[17]. Similar considerations apply to extrapolation of techniques and results derived from young healthy animals in a quiet laboratory to diseased or ageing humans in the stressful environment of a hospital ward.

General techniques

Essentially, the EEG represents the only biological activity suitable for *continuous* non-invasive monitoring of brain function. Serial assessment of evoked potentials can provide intermittent surveillance of the integrity of specific pathways (*see* Chapter 11). However the procedures are somewhat cumbersome and specialized and are used more for diagnosis than as widely applicable monitoring methods. In contrast, clinical experience with continuous monitoring by EEG is now considerable and its benefits well established. The main question is how best to refine it and extract the useful features without becoming submerged in extraneous data. The reader is referred to more general reviews for details of the many available methods[6, 7, 38, 46, 47, 49a, 53, 68, 69, 86, 87]

The requirements for collection, processing and display of information vary substantially according to the clinical reason for cerebral monitoring. The choice of an appropriate system depends on factors such as whether information is required instantaneously or delays for processing are acceptable, whether any degree of restraint of patient or modification of medical or nursing procedures is permissible, whether to have a permanent recording or a transient display, whether detection of gross trends or quantification of transient events is required, whether an automatic alarm when certain features occur is desirable, whether combined assessment of several biological variables and their interaction is advantageous, whether display of 'pictorial' (analog signal), graphical or alpha-numeric form is preferred, and finally, whether analysis and statistical treatment such as detection of significant trends, decision-making procedures or even feedback systems, e.g. to aid control of drug administration, are required.

It is noteworthy that many technologically perfect, computer-based monitoring systems incorporating EEG have fallen into disuse because they are too complex for user acceptability in the clinical setting[40,71]. However, with the simplification of equipment in recent years there is much more widespread use of monitoring as part of routine patient care. The specific limitations of many of the methods used must be clearly understood[19] and the place of monitoring as a supplement to more comprehensive EEG studies emphasized.

The general groups of commercially available EEG monitoring methods are classified in *Table 15.1*. Examples of their use are given in the remainder of the chapter.

For monitoring where immediate display of data is required, two essentially different types of system are widely available. Both show long-term trends far better than conventional EEG. The more elaborate, the compressed spectral array (CSA), is based on Fourier analysis of short (about 4 s) periods of EEG and sequential plots of power at various frequencies are written out[7]. Each plot summarizes the events of the period of time analyzed, thus brief events such as single spikes or short isoelectric periods (in burst suppression activity) will not be seen. CSAs have an intensely detailed pictorial quality and changing frequency patterns or interhemispheric asymmetries are easily recognised. They can be difficult to interpret and measure however and the inexperienced may not be able to utilize all the information they contain. Protagonists find that this method of presenting data renders it readily intelligible to all operating theatre and intensive care staff, creating enthusiasm and confidence in use of EEG monitoring and raising standards of care[12,20]. Such comments also apply to the simpler cerebral function monitor (CFM)[52] which provides a *continuous* compressed display of EEG amplitude variation somewhat resembling an intra-arterial blood pressure recording. The EEG is processed to minimize artefacts and the state of electrode contact is recorded simultaneously on a second channel with indication of any remaining artefacts and of muscle potentials from the vicinity of the scalp electrodes. The recording pen follows, via a 0.5 s time constant, the amplitude fluctuation of the EEG waves after weighting

Table 15.1 Techniques for EEG monitoring

Method (and references)	Useful for	Advantages	Disadvantages
Conventional EEG (4, 6, 38, 46, 87)	Short term study of seizure discharges, sleep, coma, status epilepticus, anaesthesia and cardiovascular surgery.	Detailed information about EEG patterns and regional features.	Expensive (*5–15), voluminous paper trace, hard to see trends, needs skilled personnel and/or computer analysis.
Compressed spectral array (Berg Fourier analyzer†) (7, 12)	Longer term monitoring in surgery, anaesthesia, intensive care and sleep.	Convenient immediate display of 2-channel frequency spectra, trends easily seen.	Relatively expensive (*9.5–12.7), brief events not detectable (depends on epoch length), needs experience to interpret, artefacts may confuse.
Cerebral function monitor (Par-Medex Ltd§) (53, 68, 69)	Long term monitoring in surgery anaesthesia, intensive care, sleep, epilepsy, intrapartum fetal monitoring.	Convenient, small, cheap (*2) Immediate display, no skilled operator needed, easy to recognise trend and brief events, artefacts eliminated or indicated. Trace easily measured and continuous.	No frequency information, unsuitable for detecting asymmetries (both will be available on modified instrument (51)).
Telemetry: often combined with closed circuit TV and video tape (several systems available) (66, 67, 88)	Clinical and EEG correlates of epilepsy or undiagnosed attacks.	Allows patients freedom within range of telemetry and camera. Multichannel transmission possible. Helpful format for teaching.	Very expensive (*6.5–40), needs skilled personnel and playback for visual or automatic analysis of EEG recordings.
Miniature cassette recorders (Oxford Medical Systems 'Medilog'**) (43, 82)	24-h recording for identification, quantification and timing of seizure discharges, also collection of polygraphic data.	Relatively cheap (*3–7.5). No attention required during recording, pocket-sized recorder suitable for ambulatory monitoring, subjects not restricted.	Limited to 4 channels of information. Only delayed playback possible. Needs skilled interpreter or program for automatic analysis.

*Approximate 1980 price ranges are given in units of £1000 for comparison.
†O.T.E. Biomedica SPA, 15 via di Caciolle, 50100 Florence, Italy or S.L.E. Ltd., 15 Campbell Road, Croydon, Surrey, CRO 2SQ, UK.
§Par Medex Ltd., 16 Leyden Road, Stevenage, Herts, SG1 2BP, UK.
**Oxford Medical Systems, Nuffield Way, Ashville Industrial Park, Abingdon, Oxon, OX14 1BZ, UK or Oxford Medilog Inc., 9130/H, Redbranch Road, Colombia, Maryland 21045, USA.

by a filter and logarithmic amplitude compression. Thus if α-rhythm increased suddenly from 10 up to 100 μV peak to peak the CFM pen would move from half to full scale with a time constant of 0.5 s. Precise measurements can be made of the lower and upper margins of the trace (minimum and maximum peak to peak voltages) and the band width (voltage range at any one moment). The semilogarithmic scale is designed to give a close approximation to a normal Gaussian distribution of amplitude measurements, taken in millimetres on the CFM chart. It also obviates the need for gain control and emphasizes the character of low voltage, e.g. burst suppression or tracé alternant activity. Although the expert neurophysiologist may feel deprived of frequency information the recognition of trends, simple patterns and drug or stimulus responses is eased for the non-specialist.

The other techniques listed in *Table 15.1* relate to investigations where data is analyzed at some later stage after recording. These are mostly used in the investigation of seizure disorders and are discussed later in this chapter (*see* pp. 367–373).

Monitoring in comatose patients

Reasons for monitoring

Cerebral monitoring in unconscious patients is concerned with obtaining continuous information to help in the following:

(1) assessing the adequacy of internal and external life-support systems in perfusing the brain with oxygenated blood in order to prevent secondary hypoxic-ischaemic brain damage (*see* p. 362)
(2) Recording an objective measure of the functional state of the brain to indicate depth of coma and both general and specific EEG responses to external stimuli.
(3) Recognizing changes in state, whether short-lived events or longer term trends, in order to indicate the need for or effect of treatment.
(4) Detection of developing localized abnormalities such as mass lesions.
(5) Making a prognosis by identifying normal features, signs of reversible depression of function or of irreparable damage to the brain.

The aetiological factors of the comatose state require little mention in this regard. Depression of neuronal function is the nonspecific effect of a wide range of processes. The clinical and neurophysiological signs have many features that are related more to the depth of coma than its cause. With the exception of evidence of space-occupying lesions such signs can be of general value in management and prognosis whatever the underlying cause of coma.

Depth of coma and cerebral responses to stimuli

The careful observation of key neurological signs[30, 65] at regular intervals is the cornerstone for understanding the comatose patient. For precision in recognizing change and in recording the state of the patient, structured coma scales[5, 45, 94] are imperative. However, the use of such methods is very labour intensive and only some form of continuous monitoring will detect all changes of functional state. Automatic EEG monitoring systems can give a permanently recorded, objective, quantifiable measure which is not subject to observer error. Furthermore EEG monitors, by direct recording of neuronal activity, are not affected by the pharmacological (e.g. muscle relaxant or mydriatic drugs) and physical (e.g. cerebrospinal fluid or blood leaking from the ear, orbital injuries or limbs in plaster) factors which may restrict neurological examination.

Long term trends in EEG of comatose patients are particularly well seen in monitor tracings because of the data reduction and time compression. Increasing depth of coma is reflected in the EEG by initial slowing of frequency and increase in voltage with loss of variability and response to stimulation. This is followed by increasing periods of reduction of activity until electrical silence occurs. The recovery sequence reverses that order. These alterations are well exemplified in barbiturate coma[37].

Global EEG responses to alerting stimuli are a useful index of the functional state of the brain in comatose patients. These are much simpler to record than the computer-averaged cortical or brainstem evoked potentials to specific stimuli mentioned earlier. In the awake or drowsy subject arousal produces 'blocking' or attenuation (decrease in voltage and amount) of EEG rhythms, via the brainstem reticular activating system. In sleep or light coma short-lived (1–2 s) high voltage arousal responses occur. In patients with brainstem injuries or dysfunction, responses are of prolonged (5 s to several minutes), widespread, high-voltage slow waves[83], accompanied by increases in cardiac and respiratory rate[28] and other autonomic phenomena. All three forms of EEG arousal response are clearly seen on CFM traces and may be evident on CSA displays depending on their duration.

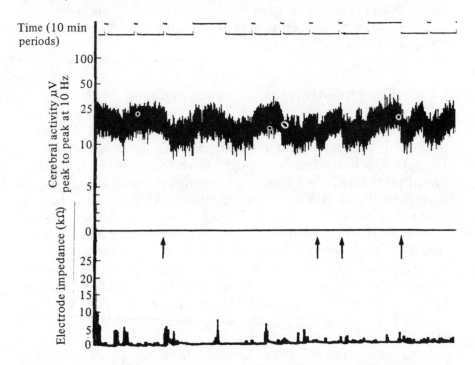

Figure 15.1 Reactivity in post-traumatic coma: CFM recording (biparietal electrodes, P3–P4) in a 30-year-old woman 12 days after head injury. She was lightly unconscious for a further month; some residual spasticity, ataxia and intellectual slowing were noted at follow-up 5 months later. The thick band in the upper part of the figure records the continually varying voltage of cerebral electrical (EEG) activity. The lower margin indicates the minimum peak to peak voltages in the filtered EEG at any one moment and the upper margin is related to the maximum voltages. The lowest trace monitors electrode contact continuously and also indicates scalp muscle potentials and electrode movements. The arrows indicate observed stimuli. Notice how the trace shows frequent changes in level indicating a variable, and relatively normal, pattern of EEG activity over the 2 hour sample. With nursing attention (first arrow) and the patient's mother calling her (remaining arrows) the level drops abruptly suggesting an attenuation or 'blocking' of EEG activity. This response is accompanied by scalp muscle potentials on the electrode impedance trace confirming a greater degree of arousal. (Patient of R. Campbell Conolly, unpublished data)

Patients emerging from coma may show a gradual change from the prolonged high voltage response to the normal 'blocking' response (*Figure 15.1*) in advance of actual waking.

The finding of prominent EEG responses, particularly to familiar stimuli (*Figure 15.2*) in monitor traces is helpful in recognition of

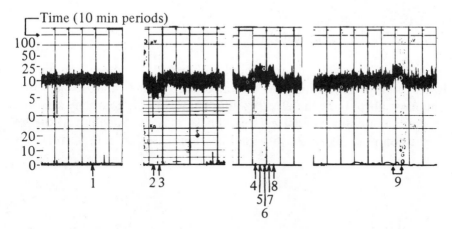

Figure 15.2 Reactivity in 'locked-in' syndrome: samples of CFM recording (electrodes P3–P4) in a 48-year-old man 6 weeks after onset of 'coma' with flaccid quadriplegia. (Vertical calibration as for *Figure 15.1*). Vertical eye movements (to command) preserved. EEG showed plentiful 7–9 Hz, intermittently responsive, α-rhythm. Paradoxical δ-responses to stimuli[83], especially when familiar, were accompanied by tachycardia. The first sample shows initial monotonous trace with no alteration when patient is spoken to. The second sample shows considerable variation in the trace at the time of auditory and painful stimuli. The third and fourth samples show abrupt increases in voltage in response to relatives, equivalent to the high voltage δ-bursts seen in the EEG. The patient died 10 weeks later and neuropathological examination revealed gross arteriosclerosis of vertebrobasilar and carotid arterial systems with major stenosis of basilar artery. Cerebral hemispheres were normal. A cystic infarct in the brainstem extended from the cerebral peduncles to the lower border of the pons and also from the floor of the aquaduct and IVth ventricle to the ventral aspect of the brainstem. (Patient of M. Bozza Marrubini; neuropathologist: A. Allegranza, unpublished data.)

Key to events:

1 Doctor speaking	6 Brother leaves room
2 Doctor speaking	7 Brother returns and speaks
3 Painful stimuli	8 Brother leaves room
4 Brother in visual field	9 Wife speaking
5 Brother speaking	

patients with the 'locked-in' syndrome[39, 62]. In these coma is mimicked by total paralysis of all motor function except vertical eye movements and the patient may be awake but suffering from a de-efferented state[65] due to a ventral pontine lesion.

Seizure discharges and status epilepticus

In addition to responses to stimuli, other sudden alterations in the EEG monitor recording may be encountered in comatose patients. The most abrupt are the electrical discharges that accompany seizures or status epilepticus (*Figure 15.3*). These may be 'subclinical' or the motor components of the fits may be suppressed by muscle relaxant

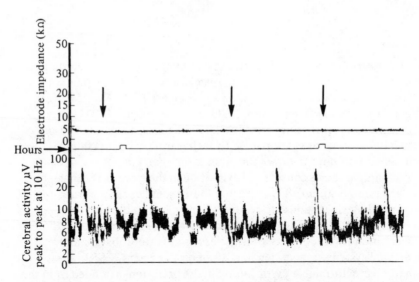

Figure 15.3 Status epilepticus: CFM recording (left temporal electrodes F7–T3) in a man in his forties deeply unconscious after head injury and evacuation of left subdural haematoma. Seizures were not controlled by intravenous diazepam or by thiopentone with muscle relaxants and controlled ventilation. The cerebral activity (lower trace) shows abrupt high voltage peaks followed by a gradual decline to below the previous level. Each peak coincides with a minor right facial twitch and a spreading focal seizure discharge originating in the left temporal region in the EEG. Intravenous paraldehyde 2 ml at each arrow reduces the discharge rate. (Patient of T. T. King, unpublished data)

drugs and the discharges unsuspected. Their successful control, necessary even when the motor accompaniments have been suppressed, is an important factor in preventing additional brain damage[55] and here EEG monitoring can guide anticonvulsant therapy[63].

Intracranial pressure

Somewhat similar but slightly less dramatic changes in EEG monitor traces may coincide with the various waves of intraventricular pressure described by Lundberg[50]. Accompanying 'cerebellar', 'mesencephalic' or 'decerebrate seizures' are associated with minor EEG alterations unlike those in epilepsy and typical of abnormal arousal patterns. Polygraphic recording[22] has defined relationships between EEG, intracranial pressure fluctuations and other variables during sleep. Higher amplitude EEG, tachycardia, periodic respiration, decreased cortical blood flow and oxygen availability are evident during waves of higher pressure.

These fluctuations in intraventricular pressure, whether spontaneous or induced by introduction of fluid or gas into the ventricular system, are considered evidence of an untoward state with alternating decompensatory and compensatory mechanisms. Their recognition is, therefore, an important warning sign of impending pressure problems. Processing the EEG with the cerebral function monitor has shown up the alterations associated with intracranial pressure waves much more clearly than in conventional EEG recording (*Figure 15.4*). This finding suggests that such non-invasive cerebral monitoring methods may well have a larger part to play in the neurological-neurosurgical intensive care unit than heretofore.

Localized abnormalities

Lateralised or localised features will only be evident with monitoring systems comprising more than one channel of recording and with appropriate electrode placement. Clearly, for their diagnosis other methods are generally more appropriate. However, the development of, for instance, an haematoma after head injury, or of hemispheric infarction after carotid occlusion, may be detected in comatose or anaesthetised patients by suitable monitoring. Lateralized lesions are indicated by asymmetries such as that in *Figure 15.5*.

358

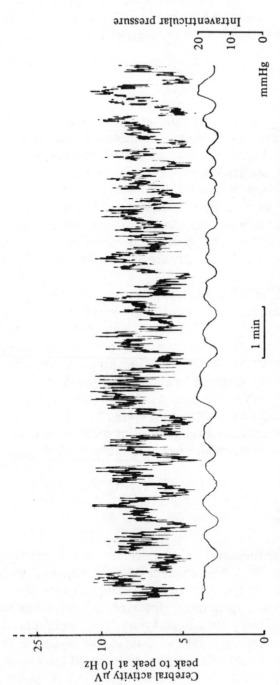

Figure 15.4 Intraventricular pressure (IVP) waves: simultaneous CFM (upper thick trace) and IVP (lower linear trace) recording (time runs from right to left) during preparation for postoperative carotid angiogram in a 45-year-old man who was confused 1 week after clipping of a right internal carotid artery aneurysm. He subsequently made a full recovery. Note the parallel courses of CFM and IVP traces during transient run of 'one-per-minute' intraventricular pressure waves occurring at a relatively low CSF pressure. The method of signal processing in the CFM accentuates the pattern of episodes of increasing EEG slow waves. This suggests that the non-invasive CFM recording may well be able to indicate when periodic fluctuations are occurring in IVP. $PaCO_2$ falling from 5.95 to 4.41 kPa (44.6–33.1 mmHg); rCBF[init.] and rCBF[10] at site of parietal CFM electrode both 53 ml · (100 g)$^{-1}$ · min^{-1}; $CMRO_2$ = 2.25 ml · (100 g)$^{-1}$ · min^{-1}; A-V oxygen content difference = 4.41 ml · (100 ml)$^{-1}$ (Patient of J. Overgaard and T. Rosendal, unpublished data)

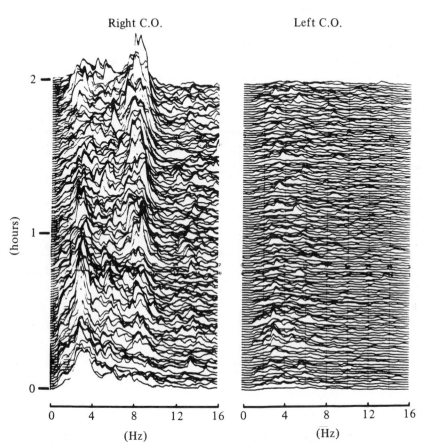

Right C.O.   Left C.O.

Figure 15.5 Lateralized lesion: CSA recording from right and left centro-occipital regions showing inter-hemispheric asymmetry. Comatose patient, 75 years old, four days after head injury with equal and reactive pupils and severe right hemiparesis; spontaneous breathing. Skull X-rays: no fractures. CT scan: left temporal lobe contusion with hemispheric oedema and brain shift to the right. The patient survived with severe disturbance of mental state and right hemiparesis. Note the relative lack of activity from the left hemisphere recording compared with the large waves over a relatively wide frequency range on the right. The persistent reduction of left-sided activity suggests that contusion has led to some permanent left hemisphere damage. (Unpublished data of A. Bricolo and S. Turazzi)

Prognostic signs

Appearance of normal EEG features such as sleep patterns[18, 74] (*Figures 15.6 and 15.7a*) and other cyclical changes gives evidence of recovering brain function in a comatose patient. These can be recognized with simple bedside monitors and do not require the whole apparatus of the sleep laboratory. They may occur in the absence of obvious clinical change. In contrast, monotonous, unreactive tracings (*Figure 15.7b*) suggest major impairment of brain function. In drug-induced coma this may be reversible providing adequate and early cardiorespiratory support is given[37].

The extreme abnormality of electrical silence may be suspected from one or two channel monitor tracings but these are quite inadequate for its proper confirmation. When clinical signs of brain-stem function[21] are absent and a full EEG recording is required, it must be carried out according to prescribed guidelines[2], and if isoelectric will support the diagnosis of brain death[19, 48, 93].

In an extensive study of the use of EEG monitoring techniques in patients with head injury Bricolo, Faccioli and Turazzi[11] and Bricolo *et al.*[12] have categorized the main patterns found in 1600 comatose

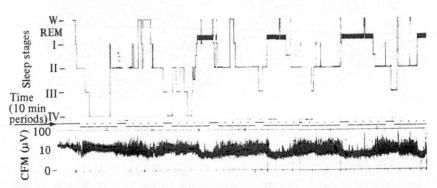

Figure 15.6 Physiological sleep: sleep scores[74] derived from assessment of polygraphic overnight sleep recording (EEG, EKG, electro-oculogram, submental electromyogram and respiration) in upper part of illustration. Shaded areas indicate paradoxical (rapid eye movement) sleep; W, waking periods and I, II, III, IV, the stages of orthodox (slow wave) sleep. Below the time marker the simultaneous CFM trace documents the paradoxical and orthodox stages of sleep offering a simple and automatic method of recording them. (From Romano *et al.*[77], courtesy of the Editor and publisher, *Annales de l'Anésthesiologie Française*)

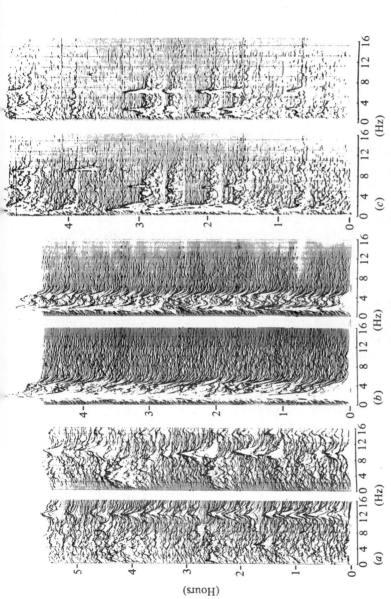

Figure 15.7 Changeable and monotonous pattern CSAs: from 3 patients, in each case recordings derived from right and then left centro-occipital regions. (*a*) 'Changeable sleep-like' spectrogram recorded 14 hours after head injury in a 25-year-old patient who was comatose with equal and reactive pupils and normal motor responses to stimuli on both sides. Skull X-rays: no fractures. CT scan: no expanding lesion. The patient survived without neurological sequelae. Note features of normal sleep including 13 Hz spindles. (*b*) 'Slow monotonous' spectrogram recorded 5 days after head injury in a 14-year-old deeply comatose patient. Left pupil fixed and dilated, extensor rigidity, assisted ventilation. Surgical intervention for bilateral depressed fractures at the vertex and superior longitudinal sinus laceration. The patient survived with severe physical and mental sequelae. Note relatively unchanging band of activity between 0.5 and 5 Hz. (*c*) 'Changeable diphasic' spectrogram 8 hours after head injury in an 18-year-old comatose patient. Pupils equal, spontaneous breathing, normal movements of right arm and weakness of left. Skull X-rays showed left temporal fracture. CT scan: no expanding lesions. The patient survived with slight left hemiparesis. This spectrogram shows intermittent bursts of high voltage slow waves separated by periods of low voltage activity. (Unpublished data of A. Bricolo and S. Turazzi)

patients (with 9658 conventional EEGs and 250 CSAs). 'Changeable' tracings were relatively common and carried a much better prognosis than the less usual unreactive, unvarying tracings (*Figure 15.7*). 'Changeable sleep-like' records (*Figure 15.7a*) were associated with 13 per cent mortality (8 per cent if non-cerebral deaths excluded). The 'changeable diphasic' records (*Figure 15.7c*) (41 per cent mortality) showed high-voltage bursts of slow waves accompanied by variations in heart and respiratory rate and in muscle tone[28, 83]. Presumably these may be related to intracranial pressure waves of the type illustrated in *Figure 15.4*. 'Borderline' records (66 per cent mortality) showed unreactive activity at 7–8 Hz, i.e. near the normal waking range and inappropriate for coma. These were quite rare (up to 10 per cent of patients) and were associated with brainstem lesions at or below the ponto-mesencephalic junction. 'Slow monotonous' records (*Figure 15.7b*) were unaltered by external stimuli and carried an 86 per cent mortality, whilst in totally silent traces this was 100 per cent.

Thus, recognition of relatively simple patterns in prolonged conventional EEG or monitor traces taken over the first 48 hours gives a considerable amount of prognostic information in patients unconscious after head injury. With both CSA and CFM it becomes a practical matter to monitor in spite of the extreme technical difficulties with both the patient and the environment, as well as the vast volume of paper tracing to assess, that would generally preclude prolonged recording with conventional EEG.

Monitoring and cerebral ischaemia

Reasons for monitoring

(1) Prevention or minimization of brain damage by identification in individual patients in coma or during elective procedures of situations where cerebral perfusion may be compromised either locally or globally.
(2) Prediction of outcome and assistance in management of patients who have suffered ischaemic insults to the brain.

Prevention of hypoxic-ischaemic brain damage

The anaesthetist can be given much help by the clinical neurophysiologist both when managing the intensive care of the comatose patient and during elective procedures in the operating theatre.

Recognition of cerebral ischaemia is an aspect of monitoring the unconscious that deserves careful consideration since inadequate oxygen delivery to neurons may impair the chances of recovery from the primary condition.

Patients with head injury

Secondary ischaemic damage may be avoidable[16, 57, 75] providing there is awareness of failing brain perfusion or oxygenation. Cerebral monitoring from early in the resuscitation period provides an effective means of assessing both the adequacy of systemic factors in supporting the brain and also detecting ischaemia due to rising intracranial pressure. The EEG as a 'final common denominator' of cerebral perfusion and oxygenation continuously reflects changes in cortical function within seconds as opposed to measurements such as intracranial pressure, systemic blood pressure, arterial blood gases or end-expired PCO_2 whose relationships to cerebral function are more indirect, less immediate and less all-encompassing[20]. Arterial hypotension, hypoxia and raised intracranial pressure may all respond to urgent treatment before secondary brain damage is sustained.

Prevention or limitation of ischaemic brain damage by reducing neuronal metabolic requirements and by lowering intracranial pressure is the aim of the somewhat controversial use of large doses of barbiturates in coma[56, 76, 90]. Further experimental studies in appropriate animal models and clinical trials are required to establish the value of this approach. In both, adequate EEG monitoring of brain function is important to assess and standardize the degree of drug-induced neuronal depression. The additional use of serial multi-modality averaged evoked potential examinations[34, 35, 36, 42], particularly of brainstem type, during this period allows monitoring of the integrity of functional pathways. The brainstem potentials appear to be unaffected by the drug whilst the EEG is isoelectric or shows burst suppression activity and cortical evoked potentials are degraded or absent.

Monitoring of patients during elective procedures

Where there is risk of global or focal brain ischaemia, specific techniques are fully described elsewhere,[6, 10, 20, 53, 60, 68, 84, 91] and here more general comment will be made on the rationale.

Neurons are damaged by critical reduction in the supply of oxygen for oxidative metabolism. In clinical practice combinations of ischaemia or oligaemia and hypoxia are more common than single factors[29]. The resulting patterns of selective neuronal necrosis[13] reflect differing cellular sensitivities to oxygen lack due to differing metabolic demands and local blood-flow factors. These latter determine the typical arterial boundary zone distribution in cerebrum and cerebellum of ischaemic lesions due to reduced cerebral perfusion seen in a wide range of clinical situations[33]. The EEG fails when cerebral blood flow and hence oxygen supply fall below a critical threshold[3, 58, 92, 95]. This depression of neuronal electrical activity is reversible. However, a second threshold beyond which neurons are irreversibly damaged will be reached, at least in subhuman primates, following continuing or increasing ischaemia[15, 58, 59]. The existence of these two thresholds provides the basis for preventive monitoring. If the initial phase of decline and extinction of the EEG activity can be recognized it will give a warning period of several minutes in which to take corrective action before neuronal damage is inevitable. Automatic trend alarms that indicate when the slope of the monitor trace changes rather than waiting for the level itself to reach some theoretical threshold are equally applicable to blood flow (R. R. Young, personal communication) and to CFM monitoring[51].

Monitoring during carotid artery surgery in man[9, 20, 23, 60, 91] confirms the unique capacity of the EEG to reveal when neurons are actually in jeopardy due to inadequate perfusion. Although related data on 'critical' carotid stump pressures and regional cerebral blood flows exist[54] the range associated with EEG failure is wide suggesting considerable inter-individual differences[95]. These may depend on local intracranial factors such as anomalies of the circle of Willis or vascular disease.

Certain groups of patient are at particular risk when cerebral perfusion is reduced[9]. In hypertensives the lower limit for autoregulation can be 'reset' at a higher level[31]. Subjects with extra- or intracranial vascular disease may have occlusions which not only are unsuspected but can only be compensated for when collateral flow is at adequate pressure[20, 78, 79, 96] and their intracranial vessels may be too sclerotic to permit autoregulation. Similarly, vasoparalysis may be encountered in diseased or injured brains and lead to pressure passive flow[49].

The warning signs of impending cerebral ischaemia are similar to those of deepening coma, i.e. decrease in frequency with associated increase in amplitude of EEG followed by activity becoming increasingly broken up by periods of silence until the tracing becomes isoelectric. The rate of change can be rapid with electrical silence within a few seconds of onset of severe ischaemia. Three such episodes are illustrated in *Figure 15.8*.

The effect of resuscitatory procedures in also evident from the rate of recovery of the monitor trace. The duration of EEG depression together with the rate and degree of its recovery forms the basis for predictions of the severity of ischaemic brain damage[15, 84].

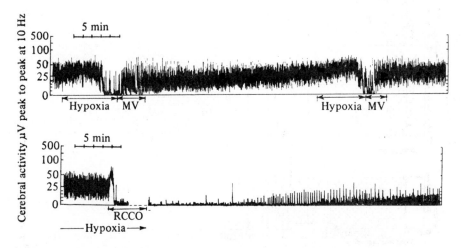

Figure 15.8 Cerebral hypoxia and ischaemia: samples from CFM recording (cortical electrodes C3–C4) in a spontaneously breathing baboon (light Althesin anaesthesia) exposed to profound hypoxia. In the upper sample two periods of hypoxia lead to apnoea necessitating mechanical ventilation (MV). With each the lower margin of the CFM trace falls to zero as hypoxia produces cardiac failure. The trace recovers more rapidly following the second episode, and the conventional EEG became normal. In the lower sample, right common carotid artery occlusion (RCCO) during hypoxia ($PaO_2 = 3.95$ kPa, 29.6 mmHg) leads to a higher voltage narrower trace due to hypoxic activation of the EEG, which is mediated via carotid and/or brainstem chemoreceptors and the reticular activating system[26, 41]. This is followed by abrupt fall in level to zero (7 min omitted). Slow and very incomplete recovery begins over the next 80 min. Subsequent neurological deficit (asymmetrical bilateral paresis); neuropathological demonstration of congenitally small left internal carotid artery, severe bilateral arterial boundary zone ischaemic infarcts maximal in the parietal areas. (Unpublished data of J. B. Brierley and P. F. Prior)

Prediction of outcome after ischaemia

Experimental studies with animal models have indicated the range of periods for both total brain ischaemia and for oligaemia which can be followed by recovery and also those associated with various degrees of brain damage[14, 15, 44, 61, 89, 90]. Before seeking to apply the results to clinical practice such studies must, however, be critically evaluated.

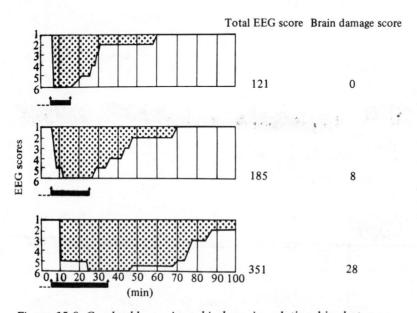

Figure 15.9 Cerebral hypoxia and ischaemia: relationships between quantified EEG and brain damage in three baboons. Under light Althesin anaesthesia spontaneously breathing animals were exposed to hypoxia ($PaO_2 = 2.67$–3.33 kPa, 20–25 mmHg) followed by bilateral common carotid artery occlusion (black bars). Plots show minute by minute EEG scores (1 = continuous activity, 2–5 = increasing burst suppression, 6 = isoelectric trace), total EEG scores (minute by minute scores summed when below baseline anaesthetic level) and total brain damage scores (histological evidence assessed in 16 regions on a 0–3 point scale, maximum possible score being 48). Note variation in time taken for EEG to become isoelectric (score 6) after carotid occlusion occlusion and in rate and degree of EEG recovery. The animal in the top plot was neurologically normal, that in the middle plot was hyperactive and clumsy with flailing limbs, that in the bottom plot was decerebrate with repetitive myoclonic jerks. (After J. B. Brierley *et al.*[15])

They need to be appropriate in terms of species, type of insult and pattern and reproducibility of brain damage produced. Survival must be sufficient for functional recovery to be recognizable, i.e. a period without anaesthesia or muscle relaxants is necessary. The criteria for recovery should be adequate. Brain damage must be confirmed neurologically and eventually with optimal neuropathological techniques which can exclude as well as identify lesions. These cautions are equally pertinent, of course, to clinical investigations about factors affecting brain damage.

The relationship between quantified EEG features at the time of ischaemia and subsequent neurological and neuropathological assessment of brain damage is close[15]. In man 83 per cent accuracy in the prediction of neurological outcome was possible on the basis of intra-operative CFM records in 100 patients undergoing cardiopulmonary bypass[84]. In the baboon typical arterial boundary zone ischaemic lesions were produced in the cerebral hemispheres in 18 animals by a combination of hypoxia and ischaemia from bilateral common carotid occlusion[15]. EEGs were assessed visually and by computer[70] and also monitored simultaneously with the CFM (*Figure 15.8*). Brain damage only occurred when there had been EEG silence during hypoxia and ischaemia lasting at least 8 min. The total EEG scores during ischaemia and recovery showed a near linear relationship[15] with quantified histological scoring of severity of brain damage (*Figure 15.9*).

Monitoring in epilepsy

Reasons for monitoring

EEG monitoring can contribute information otherwise unobtainable that allows objectivity and measurement techniques to be applied to epilepsy.

(1) Acute problems, such as status epilepticus or seizures complicating coma, requiring immediate monitoring displays to guide treatment: these have already been discussed (*see* p. 356 and *Figure 15.3*).
(2) Diagnosis of attacks of uncertain origin, i.e. whether some form of epilepsy, syncope, hysteria etc.

(3) Type of discharge in epilepsy, i.e. whether focal or generalized, to assist in choice of appropriate treatment whether medical or surgical.
(4) Frequency of attacks or discharges in relation to natural history, precipitants, behaviour and biological cycles such as sleeping/waking.
(5) Obtaining evidence about the effect of treatment, i.e. in relation to pharmacological studies, surgical extirpation, lesions or stimulators, other new forms of therapy.

In many of the applications the main requirement is for prolonged recording with or without related clinical surveillance. Although this end may be achieved with conventional EEG and experienced observers it makes almost insurmountable demands on all but the most well-staffed specialist units. It is also incompatible with the need for ambulatory monitoring. Thus, a number of sophisticated systems have been developed for use in epilepsy. Delayed processing of data can often be used rather than real-time displays necessary for the acute uses described earlier (*see* p. 350).

The techniques used for monitoring in epilepsy are summarized in *Table 15.1*.

Video systems and telemetry

Closed circuit television and videotape systems[8, 24, 66, 67, 88] have largely replaced cine-film recording of the clinical features of seizures. They have been used extensively for prolonged observations by day and by night, using infrared lighting, and can be monitored visually throughout or stored for future examination. Particular value may accrue to information about the mode of onset of seizures as well as their EEG correlates. Combined EEG and video displays on split screens or with superimposition allow close comparison of clinical and electrical features.

Systems for transmitting the EEG by radio or light-weight cable to recorders at a distance from the patient give relative freedom of activity during prolonged recording. To reduce artefact from lead movement small pre-amplifiers are incorporated near the scalp electrodes[72]. Radio transmitter packs are carried on shoulder or belt and typically have ranges of the order of 30–50 m. Radio systems are more expensive and artefact-prone but allow greater freedom of movement than cable transmission; in many national regulations govern permissible transmitter power and frequency. The recordings can be written out on an EEG machine or stored on tape; various automatic analysis programs are available. Although mainly applied to seizure disorders the techniques have also been used to study pilots, parachutists, astronauts, footballers, divers, free-ranging animals and the states of narcolepsy and sleep[67].

Miniature cassette recorders

Prolonged, e.g. during sleep, or ambulatory monitoring away from the hospital in the patients own environment may conveniently employ small portable tape recorders[24, 43, 82]. These use domestic 120 min cassettes to record four channels of information at slow speed (2 mm/ min) for 24 hours. They are played back at fast speeds (up to × 60) for analysis. Pre-amplifiers near electrodes reduce artefacts[72] but these and any faults will be undetectable until replay. Playback uses video display to view the EEG page by page and can also incorporate automatic analysis programs to count paroxysmal features. Activity from scalp, sphenoidal or depth electrodes can be recorded as well as other biological variables such as EOG, EMG and EKG. This allows relationships between paroxysmal discharges and sleep phases to be explored and cardiogenic attacks identified.

Analysis of EEG monitor recordings

Automation has an important place in the recognition and quantification of stereotyped repetitive patterns such as paroxysmal discharges in the EEG of patients with epilepsy. It is applicable to tape recordings from miniature cassette recorders. The pattern recognition procedures are complex, for instance it is necessary to be able to detect generalized spike and wave or focal spike discharges and to differentiate them from the many physiological artefacts of similar morphology. This may present a substantial problem when prolonged monitoring includes events like eating. Implementation of these objectives has generally necessitated computers although small programmable microprocessor systems for specific purposes are becoming available. In most instances adjustment of recognition parameters is necessary for each individual patient according to the exact morphology of their discharges. Furthermore changing patterns may occur with development of drowsiness or sleep and automatic scoring of associated EEG stages may be required. Various analysis systems have been utilized to evaluate a patient's suitability for neurosurgical treatment, to test the effects of anticonvulsants and to assess the behavioural correlates of paroxysmal discharges[8, 24,32, 73].

Clinical value of monitoring in epilepsy

Cost-benefit analysis of these elaborate monitoring techniques has to be made. The clinician rightly requires to know whether and when they are justified by improvement in diagnosis or treatment. The place for monitoring in the preparation of patients for neurosurgical treatment of epilepsy has been established by the Montreal and Paris schools. In neurological practice the most frequent reason for monitoring appears to be the diagnosis of the nature of attacks of uncertain origin i.e. whether they are epileptic or not. Differentiation of psychogenic seizures from those arising in the temporal lobe, or of cardiogenic attacks from epilepsy, may often be aided by actually observing and recording an attack: indeed this has been considered a reasonable goal in the investigation of most patients with epilepsy. Other clinical applications include study of seizure frequency, particularly in petit mal where assessment of performance during EEG discharges is also needed if it is suspected that they may be affecting schooling or work.

Binnie *et al.*[8] have reviewed 181 telemetric EEG and video monitor recordings taken over 18 months in an institute for epilepsy. Details are shown in *Table 15.2*. The overall success rate in answering the questions of the referring clinician was 60–70 per cent, similar to that in the survey of Stålberg[88]. The particular areas where the technique was most successful are evident. The most common diagnosis, in 50 per cent of patients, was partial epilepsy, most frequently of temporal lobe type, and primary or secondarily generalized epilepsies were present in another 25 per cent of patients. Interestingly 'no epilepsy' was the final diagnosis in 12 per cent and in 30 instances it was concluded that observed episodes were psychogenic. Self-induced and other reflex epilepsies were also very successfully investigated by this method and appeared not to be great rarities.

Cull *et al.*[24] make the point that many seizure problems can be investigated during the 8-hour working day and that nocturnal recording is not always required. The need for pleasant and relaxing surroundings with facilities such as books, card games or television is emphasized. In their experience prolonged closed circuit television and EEG observation doubled the incidence of paroxysmal discharges

Table15.2 Evaluation of EEG monitoring in epilepsy

Clinical question	Total patients*	Total recordings	Attacks with EEG discharge	Attacks without EEG discharge	Question answered	
Are attacks epileptic?						
Self-reported attacks	17	18	6	6	10	
Myoclonic jerks	6	6	2	4	5	
Other diurnal attacks	47	55	13	19	30	(57%)
Unusual nocturnal motor activity	12	14	4	4	8	
Nocturnal enuresis	6	6	ND	3	3	
EEG correlates of known epileptic seizures	20	23	9	1	9	(39%)
Seizure frequency determination	16	31	23	2	31	(100%)
Sensory-precipitated seizures?						
Self-induction	10	12	9	ND	12	(95%)
Other precipitating factors	6	7	4	ND	6	
Are EEG discharges accompanied by cognitive impairment?	6	6	2	ND	5	(83%)
Miscellaneous	3	3	0	ND	3	(100%)
Total	149	181	72	39	122	(67%)

From Binnie *et al*[8], courtesy of the Editor and publisher, *Neurology*.
*10 patients are listed in two categories.
ND = No data.

recorded compared with standard 30-minute routine EEGs and increased the yield of clinical attacks 3–5-fold. Economies in technician and medical time are made by telemetry and cassette monitoring systems compared with prolonged EEGs but the capital cost is quite high. However, recording is automatic once set up and playback for visual or automatic analysis is rapid.

Relationships between sleep and epilepsy

The complexity of the relationship between seizures and circadian cycles and especially with the different phases of sleep is often emphasized[25, 81] (*see also* Chapter 16). Reports of the value of EEG monitoring indicate the utility of a period of drowsiness or sleep in increasing the yield of paroxysmal discharges. It is well known that seizures arising in the temporal lobe are activated in this way. The generalized epilepsies also show relationships with sleep and arousal, e.g. the typical early morning exacerbation of myoclonus epilepsy. Automatic methods are generally required to quantify the relationships between various types of discharge and the character of EEG background activity.

Pharmacodynamics and epilepsy

The practice of sampling to ascertain whether serum levels of anticonvulsant drugs are within the therapeutic range is one of the major advances in the care of patients with epilepsy in recent years.

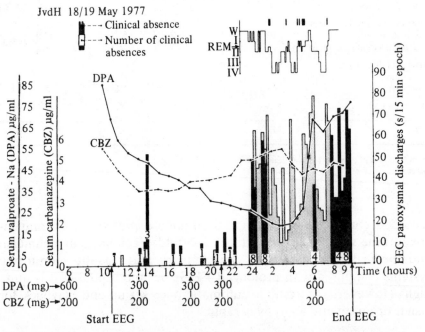

Figure 15.10 EEG and pharmacodynamics in epilepsy: baseline study of a 53-year-old woman with absence attacks. Black bars: duration of one or more seizures with 3/s generalized spike-wave discharges; stippled bars: duration of interictal spike-waves during wakefulness and slow spike-waves or poly-spike-waves during sleep. Sleep scores[74] from 2300–0800 hours shown top right: note nocturnal increase of discharges and absence attacks. Total of 67 seizures. Sodium valproate (DPA) total dose of 1500 mg administered in enteric coated form. Peak DPA concentration at 0930 (85 µg/ml) with steady decline to minimum at 0300 (18 µg/ml). (From Rowan *et al.*[80], courtesy of the Editor and publisher, *Neurology*)

Considerable improvement in seizure control may be achieved when the drug is at optimal levels throughout the 24 hours. What is optimal at what time of night or day will vary according to the natural propensity for different types of seizure to occur preferentially at different times in the circadian cycle[25]. Many are activated nocturnally or around the time of waking when levels of shorter-acting drugs may be lowest. Combined monitoring of paroxysmal discharges and clinical attacks together with pharmacodynamic studies has proved a valuable tool in investigation of patients with refractory seizures[80]. Altering the distribution and not increasing the amount of the total daily dose may change the pattern of clinical seizures and paroxysmal EEG discharges for the better (*Figure 15.10* and *15.11*).

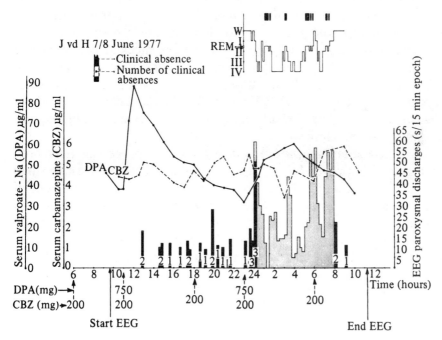

Figure 15.11 EEG and pharymacodynamics in epilepsy: second study in patient illustrated in *Figure 15.10*. DPA total dose (plain tablets) unchanged but given in two divided doses 12 hours apart. Total seizures reduced to 28. Note relationship between discharges and REM sleep. Peak DPA concentrations at 1200 (88 µg/ml) and 0400 (60 µg/ml). (From Rowan *et al.*[80], courtesy of the Editor and publisher, *Neurology*)

Future trends in EEG monitoring

Increasing clinical interest in recording and measurement of cerebral events has been matched by rapid technological advances. Investigations and service commitments that were unthinkable with conventional EEG recording are becoming commonplace with purpose-built cerebral monitoring systems. Apart from their precision and objectivity the prime attractions of the neurophysiological monitoring techiques are their ability to replace some invasive methods and also to derive previously unavailable information.

One may summarize by citing the care of a patient with traumatic coma as an example of the extent to which monitoring techniques can be applied. Initially, monitoring is used to confirm the adequacy of brain perfusion and oxygenation (*Figure 15.8*). Later, detection of variations in intracranial pressure (*Figure 15.4*) becomes important and can only be made by continuous recording methods, whereas the course of white matter swelling can be observed by repeated measurements of central somatosensory conduction time[42]. Control of early post-traumatic seizures (*Figure 15.3*) can be checked or lateralized lesions (*Figure 15.6*) detected. Depth of coma and the nature of reactivity to stimuli can be monitored (*Figure 15.1* and *15.2*) and early prognostic predictions made (*Figure 15.7*). All these can be carried out non-invasively at the bedside and to a large extent evaluated immediately by the clinician.

Recording equipment for monitoring and data processing have both been greatly improved by microprocessors and these are making small versatile apparatus available. This may allow bedside assessment of combinations of variables by multivariate analysis with indication of significant trends. Such integrated approaches are very attractive in the neurosciences where the overall functional state of the nervous system requires mapping[27] preferably on a continuous basis. Different aspects of function may be assessed most advantageously by different methods and the results combined to give an overall statement e.g. as in coma scoring systems employing both neurological and neurophysiological variables[85].

Most of the widely used clinical neurophysiological monitoring techniques simplify data. By reducing it, compared with conventional EEG, to essentials pertinent to a particular purpose, clarity is given. Then all staff can gain useful insight into the functional state of the brain and the effects upon it of their actions. This leads to the more efficient and responsible care of the individual patient which is the prime aim of cerebral monitoring.

Acknowledgements

The author would like to thank colleagues who have kindly given illustrations for this chapter.

References

1 ABRAHAM, P., DOCHERTY, T. B. and HASLAM, D. R. Ambulatory EEG recording for extended periods under adverse conditions. In *ISAM 1977. Proceedings of the Second International Symposium on Ambulatory Monitoring*, edited by F. D. Scott, E. B. Raftery, P. Sleight and L. Goulding, 85–90. London, Academic Press (1978)

2 AMERICAN EEG SOCIETY. Guidelines in EEG: Minimum technical standards for EEG recording in suspected cerebral death. (1976) Reprinted in *Current Practice of Clinical Electroencephalography*, edited by D. W. Klass and D. D. Daly, 492–496. New York, Raven Press (1979)

3 ASTRUP, J., SYMON, L., BRANSTON, N. M. and LASSEN, N. A. Cortical evoked potential and extracellular K^+ and H^+ at critical levels of brain ischaemia. *Stroke*, **8**, 51–57 (1977)

4 BARLOW, J. S. and DUBINSKY, J. Some computer approaches to continuous automatic EEG monitoring. In *Quantitative Analytic Studies in Epilepsy*, edited by P. Kellaway and I. Petersén, 309–327. New York, Raven Press (1976)

5 BATES, D., CARONNA, J. J., CARTLIDGE, N. E. F., KNILL-JONES, R. P., LEVY, D. E., SHAW, D. A. and PLUM, F. A prospective study of non-traumatic coma; methods and results in 310 patients. *Annals of Neurology*, **2**, 211–220 (1977)

6 BICKFORD, R. Computer analysis of background activity. In *EEG Informatics. A Didactic Review of Methods and Applications of EEG Data Processing*, edited by A. Rémond, 215–232. Amsterdam, Elsevier/North Holland Biomedical Press (1977)

7 BICKFORD, R. G., BRIMM, J., BERGER, L. and AUNG, M. Application of compressed spectral array in clinical EEG. In *Automation of Clinical Electroencephalography*, edited by P. Kellaway and I. Petersén, 55–64. New York, Raven Press (1973)

8 BINNIE, C. D., ROWAN, A. J., OVERWEG, J., MEINARDI, H., WISMAN, T., KAMP, A. and LOPEZ DA SILVA, F. A clinical evaluation of telemetric EEG and video monitoring in epilepsy. *Neurology* (in press)

9 BOYSEN, G., ENGELL, H. C., PISTOLESE, G. R., FIORANI, P., AGOLI, A. and LASSEN, N. A. On the critical lower level of cerebral blood flow in man with particular reference to carotid surgery. *Circulation*, **49,** 1023 –1025 (1974)

10 BRANTHWAITE, M. A. Prevention of neurological damage during open heart surgery. *Thorax*, **30,** 258–261 (1975)

11 BRICOLO, A., FACCIOLI, F. and TURAZZI, S. L'EEG dans le coma traumatique aigu valeur diagnostique et pronostique. *Revue d'électroencéphalographie et de neurophysiologie clinique*, **9,** 116– 130 (1979)

12 BRICOLO, A., TURAZZI, F., FACCIOLI, F., ODORIZZI, F., SCIARRETTA, G. and ERCULIANI, P. Clinical applications of compressed spectral array in long-term EEG monitoring of comatose patients. *Electroencephalography and Clinical Neurophysiology*, **45,** 211–225 (1978)

13 BRIERLEY, J. B. Cerebral hypoxia. In *Greenfield's Neuropathology*, 3rd Edn,, edited by W. Blackwood and J. A. N. Corsellis, 43–85. London, Arnold (1976)

14 BRIERLEY, J. B., BROWN, A. W., EXCELL, B. J. and MELDRUM, B. S. Brain damage in the Rhesus monkey resulting from profound arterial hypotension. 1. Nature, distribution and general physiological characteristics. *Brain Research (Amsterdam)*, **13,** 68–100 (1969) ·

15 BRIERLEY, J. B., PRIOR P. F., CALVERLEY, J., JACKSON, S. J. and BROWN, A. W. Pathogenesis of ischaemic neuronal damage along the cerebral arterial boundary zones in *Papio anubis*. *Brain*, **103,** 929–965 (1980)

16 BRUCE, D. A., GENNARELLI, T. A. and LANGFITT, T. W. Resuscitation from coma due to head injury. *Critical Care Medicine*, **6,** 254–269 (1978)

17 CARRUTHERS, M., COOKE, E. and FREWIN, P. Ambulatory monitoring of aircrew. In *ISAM 1977. Proceedings of the Second International Symposium on Ambulatory Monitoring*, edited by F. D. Scott, E. B. Raftery, P. Sleight and L. Goulding, 23–27, London, Academic Press, (1978)

18 CHATRIAN, G. E. Electrographic and behavioural signs of sleep in comatose states. In *Handbook of Electroencephalography and Clinical Neurophysiology*, **12,** edited by A. Rémond, R. Harner and R. Naquet, 63–77. Amsterdam, Elsevier (1975)

19 CHATRIAN, G. E. Electrographic evaluation of brain death. In *Electrodiagnosis in Clinical Neurology*, edited by M. J. Aminoff, 553–560. New York, Churchill Livingstone (1980)

20 CHIAPPA, K. H., BURKE, S. R. and YOUNG, R. R. Results of electroencephalographic monitoring during 367 carotid endarterectomies. *Stroke*, **10,** 381–388 (1979)

21 CONFERENCE OF MEDICAL ROYAL COLLEGES AND FACULTIES IN THE U.K. Diagnosis of brain death. *Lancet*, **2**, 1069–1070 (1976)

22 COOPER, R. and HULME, A. Changes of the EEG, intracranial pressure and other variables during sleep in patients with intracranial lesions. *Electroencephalography and Clinical Neurophysiology*, **27**, 12–22 (1969)

23 CUCCHIARA, R., SHARBROUGH, F., MESSICK, J. and TINKER, J. An electro-encephalographic filter-processor as an indicator of cerebral ischaemia during carotid endarterectomy. *Anesthesiology*, **51**, 77–79 (1979)

24 CULL, R. E., GILLIATT, R. W., QUY, R. J. and WILLISON, R. G. Prolonged observation and EEG monitoring of epileptics. In *Textbook of Epilepsy*, 2nd Edn., edited by J. Laidlaw and A. Richens, Edinburgh, Churchill Livingstone (in press)

25 DALY, D. D. Circadian cycles and seizures. In *Epilepsy: its Phenomena in Man*, edited by M. A. B. Brazier, UCLA Forum in Medical Sciences No. **17**, 215–233, New York, Academic Press (1973)

26 DELL, P., BONVALLET, M. and HUGELIN, G. Effects of hypoxia on the reticulo-cortico-reticular system and on motor excitability. In *Cerebral Anoxia and the Electroencephalogram*, edited by H. Gastaut and J. S. Meyer, 46–58. Springfield, Illinois, Charles Thomas (1961)

27 DUFFY, F. H., BURCHFIEL, J. J. and LOMBROSO, C. T. Brain electrical activity mapping (BEAM): a method for extending the clinical utility of EEG and evoked potential data. *Annals of Neurology*, **5**, 309–321 (1979)

28 EVANS, B. M. Patterns of arousal in comatose patients. *Journal of Neurology, Neurosurgery and Psychiatry*, **39**, 392–402 (1976)

29 FAHN, S., DAVIS, J. N., ROWLAND, L. P. (Editors) *Cerebral Hypoxia and its Consequences. Advances in Neurology*, **26**, 1–350. New York, Raven Press (1979)

30 FISHER, C. M. The Neurological Examination of the Comatose Patient. *Acta Neurologica Scandinavica*, **45**, Supplementum 36, 1–56 (1969)

31 FITCH, W., JONES, J. V., GRAHAM, D. I., McKENZIE, E. T and HARPER, A. M. Effects of hypotension induced by halothane on the cerebral circulation in baboons with experimental renovascular hypertension. *British Journal of Anaesthesia*, **50**, 119–125 (1978)

32 GOTMAN, J., IVES, S. R. and GLOOR, P. Automatic recognition of interictal epileptic activity in prolonged EEG recordings. *Electroencephalography and Clinical Neurophysiology*, **46**, 510–520 (1979)

33 GRAHAM, D. I. Pathology of hypoxic damage in man. In *Hypoxia and Ischaemia*, edited by B. C. Morson, *Journal of Clinical Pathology*, **30**, Supplement 11, 170–180 (1977)

34 GREENBERG, R. P., MILLER, J. D. and BECKER, D. P. Early prognosis after severe human head injury utilizing multi-modality evoked potentials. *Acta Neurochirurgia (Vienna)*, Supplement **28**, 50 (1979)

35 GREENBERG, R. P., MAYER, D. J., BECKER, D. P. and MILLER, J. D. Evaluation of brain function in severe human head trauma with multimodality evoked potentials. Part 1: evoked brain-injury potentials, methods and analysis. *Journal of Neurosurgery*, **47**, 150–162 (1977)

36 GREENBERG, R. P., BECKER, D. P., MILLER, J. D. and MAYER, D. J. Evaluation of brain function in severe head trauma with multimodality evoked potentials. Part 2: localisation of brain dysfunction and correlation with post-traumatic neurological conditions. *Journal of Neurosurgery*, **47**, 163–177 (1977)

37 HAIDER, I., MATTHEW, H. and OSWALD, I. Electroencephalographic change in acute drug poisoning. *Electroencephalography and Clinical Neurophysiology*, **30**, 23–31 (1971)

38 *Handbook of Electroencephalography and Clinical Neurophysiology*, Editor-in-chief A. Rémond. **4** Part B: Digital Processing of Bioelectric Phenomena, edited by D. O. Walter, 1–64 (1972); and **5** Part A: Frequency and correlation methods of analysis, edited by M. Matoušek, 1–137. Amsterdam, Elsevier Scientific Publishing Company (1973)

39 HAWKES, C. H. and BRYAN-SMYTH, L. The electroencephalogram in the 'locked-in' syndrome. *Neurology*, **24**, 1015–1018 (1974)

40 HEMEL, N. M. VAN and PRONK, R. A. F. *Monitoring of the Seriously Ill*. European Travelling Fellowship Report M–1973–3, 1–45. Utrecht, Medisch fysisch instituut TNO (1977)

41 HUGELIN, A., BONVALLET, M. and DELL, P. Activation réticulare et corticale d'origine chémoceptive au cours de l'hypoxie. *Electroencephalography and Clinical Neurophysiology*, **11**, 325–340 (1959)

42 HUME, A. L., CANT, B. R. and SHAW, N. A. Central somatosensory conduction time in comatose patients. *Annals of Neurology*, **5**, 379–384 (1979)

43 IVES, J. R. and WOODS, J. F. 4-channel 24 hour cassette recorder for long term EEG monitoring in clinical electroencephalography. *Electroencephalography and Clinical Neurophysiology*, **39**, 88–92 (1975)

44 JACKSON, D. L. and DOLE, W. P. Total cerebral ischemia: a new model system for the study of post-cardiac arrest brain damage. *Stroke*, **10**, 38–43 (1979)

45 JENNETT, B. and TEASDALE, G. Aspects of coma after severe head injury. *Lancet*, **1,** 878–881 (1977)

46 KELLAWAY, P. and PETERSÉN, I. (Editors) *Automation of Clinical Electroencephalography*. New York, Raven Press (1973)

47 KELLAWAY, P. and PETERSÉN, I. (Editors) *Quantitative Analytic Studies in Epilepsy*. New York, Raven Press (1976)

48 KOREIN, J. (Editor) Brain death: interrelated medical and social issues. *Annals of the New York Academy of Sciences*, **315,** 1–454 (1978)

49 LASSEN, N. A. and TWEED, W. A. Anaesthesia and cerebral blood flow. In *A Basis and Practice of Neuroanaesthesia*, edited by E. Gordon, 113–133. Amsterdam, Excerpta Medica (1975)

49a LEVY, W. J., SHAPIRO, H. M., MARUCHAK, G. and MEATHE, E. Automated EEG processing for intraoperative monitoring: a comparison of techniques. *Anesthesiology*, **53,** 223–236 (1980)

50 LUNDBERG, N. Continuous recording and control of ventricular fluid pressure in neurological practice. *Acta Psychiatrica et Neurologica Scandinavica*, Supplement **149,** 1–193 (1960)

51 MAYNARD, D. E. Development of the CFM: the cerebral function analysing monitor (CFAM) *Annales de l'Anesthésiologie Française*, **20,** 253–255 (1979)

52 MAYNARD, D., PRIOR, P. F. and SCOTT, D. F. Device for continuous monitoring of cerebral activity in resuscitated patients. *British Medical Journal*, **4,** 545–546 (1969)

53 McDOWALL, D. G. Monitoring the brain. *Anesthesiology*, **45,** 117–134 (1976)

54 McKAY, R. D., SUNDT, T. M., JR., MICHENFELDER, J. D., GRONERT, G. A., MESSICK, J. M., SHARBOROUGH, F. W., PEIPGRAS, D. G. Internal carotid artery stump pressure and cerebral blood flow during carotid endarterectomy: modification by halothane, enflurane, and Innovar. *Anesthesiology*, **45,** 390–399 (1976)

55 MELDRUM, B. S., VIGOUROUX, R. A. and BRIERLEY, J. B. Systemic factors and epileptic brain damage. *Archives of Neurology (Chicago)*, **29,** 82–87 (1973)

56 MILLER, J. D. Barbiturates and raised intracranial pressure. *Annals of Neurology*, **6,** 189–193 (1979)

57 MILLER, J. D., SWEET, R. C., NARAYAN, R. and BECKER, D. P. Early insults to the injured brain. *Journal of the American Medical Association*, **240,** 439–442 (1978)

58 MORAWETZ, R. B., CROWELL, R. H., DeGIROLAMI, U., MARCOUX, F. W., JONES, T. H. and HALSEY, J. H. Regional cerebral blood flow thresholds during cerebral ischemia. *Federation Proceedings*, **38**, 2493–2494 (1979)

59 MORAWETZ, R. B., DeGIROLAMI, U., OJEMANN, R. G., MARCOUX, F. W. and CROWELL, R. M. Cerebral blood flow determined by hydrogen clearance during middle cerebral artery occlusion in unanesthetized monkeys. *Stroke*, **9**, 143–149 (1978)

60 MYERS, R. R., STOCKARD, J. J. and SAIDMAN, L. J. Monitoring of cerebral perfusion during anesthesia by time-compressed Fourier analysis of the electroencephalogram. *Stroke*, **8**, 331–337 (1977)

61 NEMOTO, E. M., BLEYAERT, A. L., STEZOSKI, S. W., MOOSY, J., RAO, G. R. and SAFAR, P. Global brain ischemia: a reproducible monkey model. *Stroke*, **8**, 558–564 (1977)

62 NORDGREN, R. E., MARKESBERY, W. R., FUKUDA, K. and REEVES, A. G. Seven cases of cerebromedullospinal disconnection: The 'locked-in' syndrome. *Neurology*, **21**, 1140–1148 (1971)

63 PAMPIGLIONE, G. and DA COSTA, A. A. Intravenous therapy and EEG monitoring in prolonged seizures. *Journal of Neurology, Neurosurgery and Psychiatry*, **38**, 371–377 (1975)

64 PATERSON, R. A. H. Seasonal reduction of slow-wave sleep at an antarctic coastal station. *Lancet*, **1**, 408–409 (1975)

65 PLUM, F. and POSNER, J. B. *The Diagnosis of Stupor and Coma*, 3rd Edn., *Contemporary Neurology Series* No. **19**, 1–373. Philadelphia, Davis (1980)

66 PORTER, R. J., PENRY, J. K. and WOLF, A. A. JR. Simultaneous documentation of clinical and electroencephalographic manifestations of epileptic seizures. In *Quantitative Analytic Studies in Epilepsy*, edited by P. Kellaway and I. Petersén, 253–268. New York, Raven Press (1976)

67 PORTER, R. J., WOLF, A. A. JR. and PENRY, J. K. Human electroencephalographic telemetry. A review of systems and their applications and a new receiving system. *American Journal of EEG Technology*, **11**, 145–159 (1971)

68 PRIOR, P. F. *Monitoring Cerebral Function*, 1–366. Amsterdam, Elsevier/North Holland (1979)

69 PRIOR, P. F. Noninvasive monitoring of cerebral function. *British Journal of Clinical Equipment*, **5**, 54–63 (1980)

70 PRIOR, P. F., MAYNARD, D. E. and BRIERLEY, J. B. EEG monitoring for control of anaesthesia produced by Althesin infusion in primates. *British Journal of Anaesthesia*, **50**, 993–1001 (1978)

71 PRONK, R.A.F. *Peri- and Postoperative Computer-assisted Patient Monitoring.* WHO Travelling Fellowship Report **M–1978–1,** 1–49. Utrecht, Medisch fysisch instituut TNO (1978)

72 QUY, R. J. A miniature preamplifier for ambulatory monitoring of the electroencephalogram. *Journal of Physiology,* **284,** 23–24 (1978)

73 QUY, R. J., FITCH, P. and WILLISON, R. G. High-speed automatic analysis of EEG spike and wave activity using and detection and micro-computer plotting system. *Electroencephalography and Clinical Neurophysiology,* **49,** 187–189 (1980)

74 RECHTSCHAFFEN, A. and KALES, A. (Editors.) *A Manual of Standardised Terminology, Techniques and Scoring Systems for Sleep Stages in Human Subjects.* National Institute of Health Publication **204,** Washington, DC, US Government Printing Office (1968) (Reprinted 1977, Brain Information Service, University of California, Los Angeles)

75 REILLY, P. L., ADAMS, J. H., GRAHAM, D. I. and JENNETT, B. Patients who talk and die. *Lancet,* **2,** 375–377 (1975)

76 ROCKOFF, M. A. and SHAPIRO, H. M. Barbiturates following cardiac arrest: Possible benefit or Pandora's Box. *Anesthesiology,* **49,** 385–387 (1978)

77 ROMANO, PH., GOLDENBERG, F., MARGENET, A., CABEN, M. C. and LABORIT, G. Utilisation du moniteur de fonction cérébrale dans l'étude du sommeil physiologique. *Annales de l'Anésthesiologie Française,* **30,** 249–252 (1979)

78 ROMANUL, F. C. A. and ABRAMOWICZ, A. Changes in brain and pial vessels in arterial border zones. *Archives of Neurology,* **11,** 40–65 (1964)

79 ROSS RUSSELL, R. W. and BHARUCHA, N. The recognition and prevention of border zone cerebral ischaemia during cardiac surgery. *Quarterly Journal of Medicine,* **47,** 303–323 (1978)

80 ROWAN, A. J., BINNIE, C. D., DE BEER-PAWLIKOWSKI, N. K. B., GOEDHART, D. M., GUTTER, T., VAN DER GEEST, P., MEINARDI, H. and MEIJER, J. W. A. Sodium valproate: serial monitoring of EEG and serum levels. *Neurology,* **29,** 1450–1459 (1979)

81 SATO, S., DREIFUSS, F. E. and PENRY, J. K. The effect of sleep on spike-wave discharges in absence seizures. *Neurology,* **23,** 1335–1345 (1973)

82 SATO, S., PENRY, J. K. and DREIFUSS, F. E. Electroencephalographic monitoring of generalised spike-wave paroxysms in the hospital and at home. In *Quantitative Analytic Studies in Epilepsy,* edited by P. Kellaway and I. Petersén, 237–252. New York, Raven Press (1976)

83 SCHWARTZ, M. S. and SCOTT, D. F. Pathological stimulus-related slow wave arousal responses in the EEG. *Acta Neurologica Scandinavica*, **57**, 300–304 (1978)

84 SCHWARTZ, M. S., COLVIN, M. P., PRIOR, P. F., STRUNIN, L., SIMPSON, B. R., WEAVER, E. J. M. and SCOTT, D. F. The cerebral function monitor. Its value in predicting the neurological outcome in patients undergoing cardiopulmonary by-pass. *Anaesthesia*, **28**, 611–618 (1973)

85 SHAKHNOVICH, A. R., THOMAS, J. G., DUBOVA, S. B., MILANOVA, L. S., KASUMOVA, S. YU., KUZNETSOV, P. S. and LALAYANTS, I. E. A study of the mechanisms of comatose states. *Seara Medica Neurocirurgica* (*São Paulo*), **8**, 269–299 (1979)

86 SHAPIRO, H. M. Monitoring in neurosurgical anesthesia. In *Monitoring in Anesthesia*, edited by L. J. Saidman and N. Ty Smith, 171–204. New York, Wiley (1978)

87 SMITH, N. T. Computers in anesthesia, In *Monitoring in Anesthesia*, edited by L. J. Saidman and N. Ty Smith, 283–329. New York, Wiley (1978)

88 STÅLBERG, E. Experiences with long term telemetry in routine diagnostic work. In *Quantitative Analytic Studies in Epilepsy*, edited by P. Kellaway and I. Petersén, 269–278. New York, Raven Press (1976)

89 STEEN, P. A., MICHENFELDER, J. D. and MILDE, J. H. Incomplete versus complete cerebral ischemia: improved outcome with a minimal blood flow. *Annals of Neurology*, **6**, 389–398 (1979)

90 STEEN, P. A., MILDE, J. H. and MICHENFELDER, J. D. No barbiturate protection in a dog model of complete cerebral ischemia. *Annals of Neurology*, **5**, 343–349 (1979)

91 SUNDT, T. M. JR., HOUSE, O. W., SHARBOROUGH, F. W. and MESSICK, J. M. JR. Carotid endarterectomy: results, complications and monitoring techniques. In *Advances in Neurology*, **16**, edited by R. H. Thompson and J. R. Green, 97–119. New York, Raven Press (1977)

92 SUNDT, T. M. JR., SHARBOROUGH, F. W., ANDERSON, R. E. and MICHENFELDER, J. D. Cerebral blood flow measurements and electroencephalograms during carotid endarterectomy. *Journal of Neurosurgery*, **41**, 310–320 (1974)

93 SWEET, W. H. Brain death. (Editorial) *New England Journal of Medicine*, **299**, 410–412, (1978)

94 TEASDALE, G. and JENNETT, B. Assessment of coma and impaired consciousness. A practical scale. *Lancet*, **2**, 81–84 (1974)

95 TROJABORG, W. and BOYSEN, G. Relation between EEG, regional cerebral blood flow and internal carotid artery pressure during

carotid endarterectomy. *Electroencephalography and Clinical Neurophysiology*, **34,** 61–69 (1973)

96 YATES, P. O. and HUTCHINSON, E. C. Cerebral infarction: the role of stenosis of the extracranial cerebral arteries. *Medical Research Council Special Report* Series No. **300,** 1–95 (1961)

16
Sleep states, polysomnography and chronomedicine
Christian Guilleminault

Introduction

Sleep is a behavior which occurs at regular intervals during a 24 hour period; although why we sleep, what triggers sleep, and how sleep is maintained are still essentially unknown. Further, the basic neuro-chemical and pharmacological events responsible for sleep are not well understood. However, there is no doubt that profound physiological changes occur during sleep and multiple central nervous system control-behaviors are different during sleep when compared to wakefulness.

Sleep and sleep states

Since 1953, and the landmark report by Aserinsky and Kleitman[2], it has been clearly established that sleep is not a unitary phenomenon and should be divided into two different states. Rapid eye movement (REM) and non-rapid eye movement (NREM) sleep are the most common terms used to describe these two physiological states of alertness. Terms such as *desychronized sleep*, *paradoxical sleep*, *active sleep*, or *dream sleep* are frequently used in the literature as synonyms for REM sleep. Similarly, *synchronized sleep*, *slow-wave sleep*, and *quiet sleep* are commonly used as synonyms for NREM sleep.

These two very different states (NREM and REM sleep) have been found in all mammals, although we have yet to clearly differentiate sleep and waking states from mere quiescence and activity in amphibians and lower species. Interestingly enough, most reptiles appear to have NREM sleep but do not show REM sleep, while birds have very well-developed NREM sleep and show occasional, very brief (approximately 1 s) episodes of what appears to be an evolutionary forerunner of REM sleep. The opossum, one of the most primitive of mammals, presents well-formed, easily recognizable REM sleep.

Sleep and sleep states are defined in humans and other mammals by the simultaneous analysis of several variables, monitored polygraphically. In the late '60s and early '70s, two international manuals were published [11, 27] outlining the minimum criteria necessary to define unambiguously sleep states (REM and NREM) and sleep stages in adults and newborns.

The electroencephalogram (EEG), chin digastric electromyogram (EMG), and electro-oculogram (EOG) are the three basic variables which must be monitored to define sleep states, and sleep stages in the young adult, which is usually taken as the frame of reference. Monitoring respiration by abdominal and thoracic strain gauges and body movements is highly recommended to score sleep in the neonatal period.

Interestingly enough, as an infant matures past the perinatal period, definitions of sleep, sleep states, and sleep stages in infancy and early childhood have not been specified internationally. This is probably because very few large-scale studies of post-perinatal infants have been performed, and profound maturational changes in sleep occur between 6 weeks and 6 months of age so that criteria must be adapted to the gestational age of the infant. Recently, the author has tried to develop a scoring system which integrates the accepted international criteria used in adult subjects with extensive 24 hour polygraphic studies performed on infants during their first year of life[16].

Sleep scoring does not require the performance of a routine sleep EEG. In fact, a one channel EEG is sufficient to allow appropriate scoring of sleep states and sleep stages. During an all-night polygraphic study, the use of two EEG derivations is usually recommended because one does not want to be at the mercy of a bad electrode during the course of a study; however, sleep states and stages are scored by the analysis of only one channel of EEG. The electrode placements must be appropriately selected and sleep researchers have agreed that the two central leads (C_3 and C_4 of the 10–20 international system) comprise the international standard. The classical derivations are C_3/A_2 and C_4/A_1. Criteria and procedures for recording sleep parameters are fully described in the *Manual of Standardized Terminology,*

Techniques and Scoring Systems for Sleep States of Human Subjects[27]. The polygraph paper speed is never under 10 mm/s; in the Americas, the usual paper speed is 10 mm/s, while in Europe it is 15 mm/s. Sleep stages and states are scored by analysis of an 'epoch', which is usually 30 s in the Americas and 20 s in Europe. These differences are a reflection of equipment differences rather than ideological ones. Often, Europeans involved in sleep research were initially electroencephalographers with standard EEG machines. Most North Amercan sleep researchers were neurophysiologists or neuropsychiatrists interested in neurophysiological phenomena, and thus used different polygraphs.

NREM sleep in the young adult has been subdivided into four stages:

Stage 1 is characterized by decrease and progressive disappearance of the α-rhythm (8–12 Hz) which is replaced by a slower alpha and, finally, by low amplitude mixed frequencies at 2–7 Hz.

Stage 2 is classically defined by the appearance of sleep or σ-spindles at 12–16 Hz and vertex sharp waves.

Stages 3 and 4, which together represent 'slow wave sleep', are characterized by the presence of large, high amplitude, slow (δ) waves of 0.5–2 Hz. The distinction between stages 3 and 4 is based upon the amount of δ-waves per 'epoch' (stage 3 = 20–50 percent; stage 4 is above 50 percent).

REM sleep can only be defined unambiguously if chin EMG and EOG are simultaneously monitored because the EEG tracing may be very similar to that of stage 1 NREM. Absence of vertex waves and presence of saw-tooth waves are the most significant EEG findings, but the association of a low amplitude, fast (desynchronized) EEG with disappearance of muscle tone in anti-gravity muscles (recorded from chin muscles) and presence of bursts of horizontal and vertical rapid eye movements permit clear identification of the REM state. REM sleep has been subdivided into tonic and phasic REM sleep, based upon the presence or absence of phasic events in the recording, such as rapid eye movements, twitches, irregular respiration, etc. This dissociation into two substates has received great attention recently with the development of clinical polysomnography. REM sleep in mammals, particularly the cat, is associated with phasic neurophysiological events[20] which include the pontine-geniculo-occipital (PGO) waves, which may appear independently or in bursts. During REM sleep in the cat, rapid eye movements are always associated with a burst of PGO waves. However, PGO waves can be seen without eye movement. In man, where PGO waves cannot be monitored, phasic events have been defined as rapid eye movements, bursts of middle ear muscle activity (MEMA), phasic integrated potentials (PIP)*, twitches, etc. 'Tonic REM sleep' is therefore a substate defined by presence of low voltage, fast activity EEG, absent muscle tone, and absence of any peripheral indices of PGO activity. Depending on which variable or variables are monitored, phasic events will be more or less numerous and tonic REM sleep may be of variable duration. Recently, respiratory physiologists have become quite interested in sleep and REM sleep phenomena[25]. They defined phasic REM sleep in terms of the presence or absence of rapid eye movements. In animal studies, this incorrect definition can be avoided by direct recording of PGO waves; in man, 'REM sleep with rapid eye movements' is a more correct term.

Sleep, sleep states, and sleep stages vary in duration at different ages. Also a function of age is the temporal organization of sleep states and stages. In a young adult, sleep follows a regular pattern during the night. Nocturnal sleep can be divided into cycles: wakefulness (W) is normally followed by NREM sleep with progressive appearance of the different sleep stages from 1 to 4 with the first REM period appearing, on the average, 90 min after sleep onset. Therefore, the combination of NREM and REM sleep represents a sleep cycle. For example, a young adult has a mean of four sleep cycles per night. As night progresses, each sleep cycle will differ slightly from the previous one, with the last sleep cycle being longer than the first. The organization of sleep stages will also vary during the night, with stages 3 and 4 essentially being seen during the first two sleep cycles and REM sleep being progressively longer in duration during the last two sleep cycles. Time spent in slow-wave sleep and REM sleep evolves in opposite directions from the beginning to the end of the night: δ-sleep is most

---

*Phasic integrated potentials (PIP) are monitored from the periorbital region. EMG activity is recorded with integrating couplers that convert phasic activity to 'spikes'. These 'spikes' have been shown to correlate with PGO waves in cats[23]. Periorbital 'spikes' obtained from extra-ocular muscles in humans (E-PIP) are excellent indicators of PGO activity during REM sleep and, to a lesser extent, during the sleep period just preceding REM sleep. During NREM sleep and sleep onset, E-PIP are related to a nonspecific generator[26].

prominent during the first third of nocturnal sleep and REM sleep most prominent during the last third of the night. In an adult, NREM sleep represents approximately 80 percent of total sleep time with stage 1 representing 1–5 percent; stage 2, 55–65 percent; stages 3 and 4, 20 percent; and REM sleep, 20–22 percent. Sleep patterns do vary with age; in the neonate, active (REM) sleep usually represents 50 percent of total sleep time. Before puberty, this percentage rapidly declines, stabilizing around 20 percent until old age. Although usually maximum during childhood, stages 3–4 NREM sleep progressively decline in duration during adulthood and reach fairly low levels past 50–55 years of age. Although several studies of sleep changes during ageing have been performed, normative data are still relatively few and there are a number of 'grey areas' to be explored.

Sleep cycles also change with age. The greatest change probably can be seen during the first year of life. In neonates, the sleep cycle is much shorter (40–50 min) but progressive variations of cycle length with age represent, once again, a fairly unexplored zone. Interestingly, in the neonatal period, infants usually fall asleep directly into REM sleep, presenting a sleep-onset REM period. This phenomenon is not experienced in young adults monitored under normal conditions. The progressive switch from sleep-onset REM sleep to the typical adult NREM/REM sleep cycle pattern is currently under investigation, but large amounts of normative data have not yet been published.

Sleep is obviously a recurrent phenomenon during any 24-hour period. In neonates, sleep and wakefulness are scattered around the clock but, progressively, sleep is 'consolidated' into a 'block' or a maximum of two to three blocks during a 24-hour period. This consolidation into long periods of sleep and wakefulness is under the control of multiple influences, including strong sociocultural factors. At the same time, it must be emphasized that a certain number of biological rhythms are linked to the sleep-wake cycle, so sleep studies must necessarily imply an understanding of chronobiology.

In the recent past, changes occurring with, or secondary to, sleep or different sleep states have attracted the attention of physicians. Sleep may sometimes give a special texture to a given disease; at other times, a disease may be revealed by, or only be associated with, sleep or a given sleep state. In North America, recognition that sleep and sleep states may have a drastic impact on patients' well-being has led to the development of a special clinical department – the Sleep Disorders Clinic. These departments have formed an association which tries to disseminate knowledge widely and educate young specialists. Thus, a new specialist, the clinical polysomnographer, has been recognized in North America; techniques are sanctioned by a special board that also sponsors a qualifying examination. Polysomnogram and polysomnographer are unfortunate terms, not so much because of the combination of Greek and Latin roots, as because they do not emphasize clearly the fact that the new specialty is *chronomedicine*, in which studies undertaken during sleep and various sleep states are interpreted with regard to time during the 24-cycle.

Chronomedicine and polysomnography

During the last 30 years, description and classification of physiological phenomena which occur during sleep, and recognition of various rhythms associated with multiple variables during the sleep-wake cycle, have progressed considerably. In free-moving, unanesthetized animals (essentially mammals) motoneurons, preganglionic autonomic nerve cells, and neurosecretory neurons have been investigated, as has the integrated activity of the effectors (visceral organs, endocrine glands, muscles, etc.). Circadian variations in circulation, respiration, digestion, excretion, thermoregulation, and metabolism have been monitored in control volunteers ranging from infancy to old age. While these investigations are far from complete, they have revealed many of the studied variables to be state-dependent, in that they are dependent not only on the state of wakefulness versus sleep but, in some cases, also on the state of REM sleep versus NREM sleep.

As already mentioned, several of the variables are linked to the 24-hour cycle but are independent of the sleep-wake cycle. Chronomedicine is aimed at deciphering pathological phenomena which may be aggravated by a specific state of alertness. Such pathology may arise from disturbances which occur at specific times during the 24-hour cycle or in relation to specific states of alertness. An undiagnosed illness may slowly progress during sleep until a crisis is seen during wakefulness; this masked process could also result in sudden, unexpected death. For example, Baust and Bonhert in 1969[3] indicated that during sleep in the adult cat there is a progressive increase in parasympathetic tone associated with a partial withdrawal of sympathetic tone. During REM sleep there is a further increase in parasympathetic activity. These changes may have a dramatic impact on the diurnal variation of heart rate and may, in some specific pathological conditions, eventually precipitate a life-threatening cardiac crisis. Clinics for sleep disorders and departments of chronomedicine have been involved in studies of some of these abnormal events using a standardized test – the polysomnogram. The following paragraphs will focus on this test and some of its clinical applications.

Standard polysomnographic procedures

Because polysomnography involves the assessment of physiological functions during the sleep-wake cycle, it must take place under conditions conducive to natural sleep. As already mentioned, the goal of polysomnography is not to obtain an EEG during sleep, which can easily be performed in any well-equipped laboratory; it is directed at the analysis of temporal variations of one, or several, physiological parameters over time and their relationship to the state of alertness.

Recording apparatus must be positioned away from the patient in a separate room. Accordingly, the desired setting is a tastefully decorated, private, sound-attenuated bedroom that can be completely darkened and from which time cues can be removed at will, depending on the test performed.

A standard polysomnogram will aways include monitoring of the state of alertness. On a polygraph, for an adult, this monitoring will require a minimum of three channels: one channel devoted to monitoring a central EEG lead (C_3/A_2) (C_4/A_1) with chin electromyogram

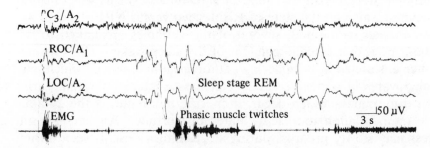

Figure 16.1 Tracing obtained during REM sleep in a 35-year-old man. From top to bottom – channel 1: recording of EEG, derivation C_3/A_2 from the 10–20 international placement system; channel 2 and channel 3: right and left electro-oculogram; channel 4: digastric electromyogram. Note the bursts of rapid eye movements, and the muscle inhibition, interrupted by phasic twitches. These phasic events are characteristic of REM sleep

and electro-oculogram being monitored on channels 2 and 3. Beckman bipotential electrodes, 7.5 mm in diameter, are taped to the forehead (ground), left and right outer canthi (eye movements), left and right mastoid (so-called 'neutral' references which are used in place of ear lobes – the true A_1 and A_2 placements), and chin. Grass gold-plated cup electrodes (R < 10 kΩ) are attached to the scalp in C_3 and C_4. The other channels will monitor different variables depending on the patient's clinical problems (*see Figure 16.1*).

Specific clinical applications of clinical polysomnography

Breathing and sleep-wake cycles

In 1965, Gastaut, Tassinari and Duron[11] opened a new era when, in massively obese (Pickwickian type) patients, they reported apneic events during sleep. Since this pioneer observation, much work has been performed, experimentally as well as clinically, to understand the delicate interaction between different states of alertness and central control of ventilation. These studies have led to the description of sleep apnea syndromes[14] and to important investigations in infants to help understand the sudden infant death syndrome.

Two major findings must be emphasized: during REM sleep, intercostal and accessory respiratory muscles are suddenly inhibited, similar to other anti-gravity muscles. This sudden inhibition has an immediate impact on the rigidity of the rib cage in infants[34] and has recently been demonstrated to be responsible, in part, for abrupt worsening of blood oxygenation in multiple respiratory syndromes in adults. Patient with severe kyphoscoliosis, thoracic deformations[15], neurological and muscle disorders involving the rib cage[6, 12], as well as patients with chronic obstructive pulmonary diseases, for example[4, 13], whose ventilation is already compromised or borderline-normal while awake, will experience an abrupt worsening of their condition during REM sleep due to simple withdrawal of activity of accessory respiratory muscles or increased deformation of the rib cage secondary to the loss of intercostal muscle activity[7, 8] (*see also* p. 81).

Secondly, sleep is characterized by a 'deafferentation', i.e. a decrease of afferent input which impinges on the neuronal network included in the mesencephalic (excitatory) reticular formation. Some of the excitatory inputs are re-entrant during wakefulness into the mesencephalic neuronal network involved in control of ventilation, reinforcing its activity. During sleep, this reinforcing excitatory input is lacking. Arousal from sleep brings this excitatory input back immediately. Arousal then appears as a major respiratory stimulant when ventilation, for any reason, is impaired during sleep. But recent studies have demonstrated that factors as simple as sleep deprivation, alcohol, or central nervous system depressant drug intake may impair this ventilatory stimulus by raising the arousal threshold during sleep.

In addition, the control of ventilation may be different during W, NREM and REM sleep. This issue is currently a controversial one but, in dogs at least, in association with bursts of rapid eye movements (called 'phasic REM' by Sullivan *et al.*[32]), the chemical control of ventilation[20], i.e. the effect of hypoxemia, hypercapnia and pH changes, would no longer be in charge – a 'REM specific system' would supercede it.

This 'REM system' involved in the central control of ventilation has been clearly demonstrated in dogs but may not play as large a role in man. Undoubtedly, in both man and other mammals, neurophysiological events associated with bursts of rapid eye movements during REM sleep induce abrupt diaphragmatic inhibition which is associated with apneic events (diaphragmatic type) of various duration, easily reaching 40–60 s. Loss of wakefulness as a respiratory stimulus may lead to progressive hypoxemia during sleep in patients with already compromised ventilation, particularly if several factors such as obesity and/or ageing are involved. In addition, bursts of rapid eye movements during REM sleep may be associated with abrupt oxygen desaturation with long apneic events in subjects who have ventilatory difficulties.

These two factors may have an impact on multiple disease entities and a simple variable such as age may increase the chance of respiratory problems during sleep. It has been shown that arterial oxygen pressure (PaO_2) decreases with age in a supine position (0.42 mmHg per year after age 14)[25]. Thus, a 70-year-old subject would be expected to have a normal resting supine PaO_2 of about 22 mmHg lower than a 20-year-old subject. The occurrence of an apneic event may additively lead to much greater oxygen desaturation in an old person than in a younger subject. Sudden hypoxemia may have an abrupt impact on the cardiovascular system and may lead to cardiac arrythmias during sleep (*see Figure 16.2*).

But sleep, for unknown reasons, may have other consequences upon respiration. It may lead to respiratory mismatch, where the upper airway suddenly occludes during inspiration: this is the classical obstructive sleep apnea syndrome[14]. It will be associated with important concomitant cardiovascular changes during sleep secondary to

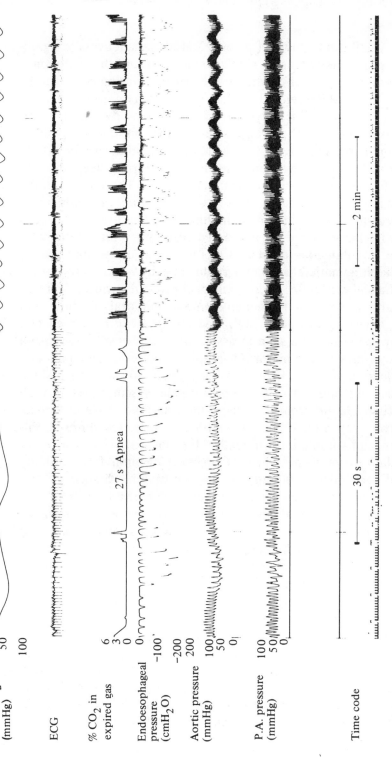

Aortic pO₂ (mmHg)

ECG

% CO₂ in expired gas

Endoesophageal pressure (cmH₂O)

Aortic pressure (mmHg)

P.A. pressure (mmHg)

Time code

Figure 16.2 Polysomnogram performed on an 18-year-old adolescent with monstrous obesity and a severe obstructive sleep apnea syndrome. From top to bottom – channel 1: continuous recording of arterial oxygen level by means of an intra-arterial electrode; channel 2: electrocardiogram (lead II); channel 3: monitoring of percent CO_2 in expired air by means of a small catheter placed in front of the nostril; channel 4: measurement of endoesophageal pressure by means of an endoesophageal balloon; channel 5: continuous tracing of arterial pressure by means of an intra-arterial catheter; channel 6: continuous recording of pulmonary arterial pressure by means of a Swan-Gantz catheter placed through the femoral vein into the pulmonary artery; channel 7: Time code (if two polygraphs are run simultaneously the time code is monitored on both machines)

repetitive Mueller maneuvres ('inverse Valsalva maneuvers'), significant hypoxemia and drastic changes imposed on the autonomic nervous system control of the heart. Obstruction during sleep can be incomplete. The sleep-related partial obstruction of the airway or 'obstructive hypopnea'[21] is polygraphically identified by decreased air flow at nose and mouth, progressive increase in endoesophageal pressure, increased intercostal muscle activity, and decrease in oxygen saturation. Obstructive hypopnea leads to nocturnal sleep disturbances but to a lesser degree than complete apnea. The impact on the cardiovascular system includes increase in systemic and pulmonary arterial pressures and cardiac arrhythmias[22]. Sleep-related central hypopnea is characterized by decreased respiratory muscle activity, marked by simultaneous decreases in intercostal electromyographic activity, diaphragmatic electromyographic activity – monitored by an endoesophageal electrode, endoesophageal pressure swings, decrease in chest and abdominal movements, nasal and oral air flow and measured oxygen saturation. Both sleep-related central apnea and central hypopnea may be seen in association with obstructive apnea syndromes or may be the major polygraphic feature in some patients. Central sleep apnea or hypopnea also leads to nocturnal sleep disturbances but both have less impact on the vascular system than their obstructive counterparts[13]. Sleep states may also have an impact on genetically determined hypoxic and hypercapnic responses. Complete absence of stimulation will lead to the classical primary alveolar hypoventilation syndrome which is, in its congenital form, usually discovered very early in infants. At times it may be dissociated and exist only during one sleep state, particularly NREM sleep[30].

Finally, abnormal breathing patterns may be associated with, or lead to, abnormal sleep-wake cycles with complete fragmentation and destructuring of sleep culminating in abnormal states of alertness and sleep-wake pathology. In these patients, the polysomnogram would be oriented toward study of respiration and ventilation which have secondary impact on the cardiovascular system. Several 24-hour monitorings are necessary if all the variables outlined above need to be studied. Depending upon the clinical protocol, the techniques used will be more or less invasive. However, *breathing problems during sleep cannot be appropriately studied with a 'nap polysomnogram' because REM sleep will probably be missing.* Long REM sleep periods with bursts of rapid eye movements are seen, in an adult with a normal day/night schedule, in the early morning hours between 0300 and 0600.

Other factors such as time spent in supine position, which may produce a progressive worsening of hypoxemia, if present, cannot be evaluated well during a nap. Technically, thoracic and abdominal strain gauges and nasal and oral thermistors will indicate the presence and type of apnea but will not help evaluate the presence of hypopnea, nor give direct information about ventilatory variables. Measurement of intraesophageal pressure by means of an endoesophageal balloon or catheter-tip pressure-transducer will provide more information about apnea, hypopnea, and similar types of events; it will also allow quantification of negative pressure efforts during obstructive events. A transducer for non-invasive monitoring of respiration (Respitrace, Ambulatory Monitoring, Inc., New York, USA) has been developed which allows calibration during wakefulness and subsequent measurement of ventilatory parameters during sleep. It also affords a good indication of the type of respiratory events involved, including an adequate definition of hypopnea. EMG recordings of intercostal, respiratory accessory, and oropharyngeal muscles, particulary the genioglossal muscle, and diaphragmatic EMGs obtained by endoesophageal recording or peripheral recording can be performed. Such varied recordings can provide different information and will disturb sleep more or less, depending on how invasive the technique is.

Abnormalities of breathing have direct impact on oxygen saturation and CO_2. Recently, a fairly accurate ear oximeter, with accurate readings down to 35 percent oxygen saturation, has been made available (Hewlett Packard A 47201). Percent expired CO_2, registered by a catheter positioned beneath the nostrils or below the mouth, can be recorded by a Beckman LB2 CO_2 analyzer. Transcutaneous O_2 electrodes, useful in infants, have not provided valid information from older children and adults. (Transcutaneous CO_2 electrodes average for several minutes and are still experimental.) Placement of arterial lines may be necessary in some cases. They permit direct measurement of blood gases and may also allow one to appreciate the impact of abnormal breathing patterns during sleep upon the cardiovascular system. Systemic and pulmonary arterial pressure, wedge pressures, and cardiac output can be monitored during the night or for 24 hours. Continuous monitoring of the electrocardiogram, a far less invasive procedure, can be performed with 24-hour Holter ECG monitoring, analysis of the tapes being performed by computer. Specific procedures such as hypoxic, hyperoxic, or hypercapnic responses during different sleep states will give very specific information but require more sophisticated monitoring equipment.

Cardiac and hemodynamic studies and sleep-wake cycles

Cardiovascular variables can be monitored using invasive techniques, as already noted (*Figure 16.3*). Placement of Swan-Gantz catheters allows measurement of right ventricular pulmonary arterial and wedge

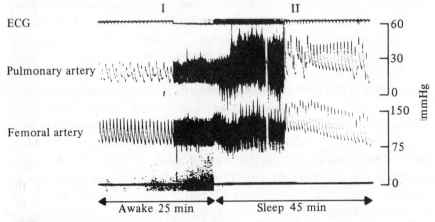

Figure 16.3 Example of changes of systemic arterial and pulmonary arterial pressures during sleep (45 min of sleep) in a sleep apneic patient

pressures without great difficulty. Systemic arterial lines permit monitoring of systemic pressure using any of the standard pressure transducers (e.g., model MP–15, Micron Instrument, Los Angeles, California, USA) coupled to electrically isolated polygraph preamplifiers (Model 8805C pressure amplifiers, Hewlett Packard, Waltham, Massachusetts, USA). These studies have been helpful in following the circadian appearance of some types of angina pectoris, particularly Prinzmetal's angina. Development of better non-invasive blood pressure recorders has permitted the performance of long-term studies of blood pressure involving usage of Doppler systems in normal and hypertensive subjects combined with analysis of hormonal secretions during the sleep-wake cycle. Significant hemodynamic changes occur during sleep in normal volunteers; there is, for example, a general decrease in systemic arterial pressure at the beginning of the night. Recent studies (*see* review[14]) indicate that a direct relationship between sleep stages and arterial pressure changes exists. The lowest systolic and diastolic values were always noted in stages 3 and 4 NREM sleep. During REM sleep, a variability of systemic arterial pressure is noted which does not correlate with changes in heart rate or arterial tone[5]. Systemic arterial pressure during REM sleep may present sudden, abrupt increases in association with bursts of rapid eye movements.

A recent study, performed on normal volunteers, indicated that the progressive drop in systemic pressure during slow wave sleep could be blocked by a bolus intravenous injection of naloxone – a specific opioid inhibitor – at sleep onset[28]. The maximum effect was seen 180 min after the injection. Interestingly, a similar intravenous bolus blocked prolactin secretion, inducing a statistical decrease when compared to placebo. This had a similar time course to the blood pressure effect in the same normal volunteers[29]. Regulation of blood pressure during sleep, and its relation to sleep states, is still not understood very well. This study is the first to implicate a peptide as one of the mediating agents involved in sleep-wake regulation of blood pressure.

There have been lengthy speculations on the diurnal variations of heart rate observed in normal volunteers and patients with heart diseases. Although the overall trend is for ventricular arrhythmias to decrease during sleep, some patients may consistently demonstrate an increase in ventricular irritability during sleep. The increase in parasympathetic tone and partial withdrawal of sympathetic tone during sleep, more marked during REM sleep, reported by Baust and Bonhert[3] in the cat, are postulated to be part of a neurophysiologic trigger which can also alter the occurrence of ventricular ectopic beats. While it seems fairly certain, based on animal work and studies in man, that the autonomic nervous system directly regulates much of the minute-to-minute and beat-to-beat variations in heart rate that occur during REM sleep, several recent observations suggest that sleep-induced changes in cardiac parasympathetic tone are not the major determinants of circadian variation in heart rate in man. Tzivoni and Stern[35] concluded after a careful study that, except for bradycardia, there were no electrocardiographic changes characteristic of increased vagal tone during sleep in either normal subjects or patients with ischemic heart disease. A study performed at Stanford involving cardiac transplantation recipients supports the results of Tzivoni and Stern. Cardiac transplant patients with completely denervated hearts experience a diurnal variation in heart rate which has the same magnitude and time course as that seen in non-transplant patients. This observation suggests that the major determinants of diurnal variation of cardiac rate are not direct changes in cardiac parasympathetic and sympathetic tone but are factors external to the heart. These could include circadian variations in body temperature, serum potassium or circulatory catecholamines; the effects of positive alterations in cardiac work load; or intrinsic cardiac responses to changes in peripheral vascular tone. To understand diurnal variations in heart rate and ventricular irritability occurring in patients with ischemic heart disease, it becomes important to study several circadian rhythm factors and to associate such studies with the polysomnogram. The development of ambulatory monitoring systems which allow continuous monitoring over several days of body (rectal) temperature, activity/non-activity cycle, heart rate, etc. are combined with the use of microprocessors and have greatly improved the performance of appropriate chronomedical studies.

Other examples: impotence and organic disorders

The polysomnogram permits the appreciation of organic causes for impotence, and may help determine the underlying cause. This is based on recording physiological REM sleep-related erections. Direct study at the peak of the reflex REM-related erection allows simultaneous evaluation of the 'buckling pressure'[36] and direct examination of the penis which may permit appropriate diagnostic and therapeutic recommendations. This involves recording penile tumescence at both tip and base of the penis with commercially available recording devices (American Medical Systems, Inc., New York, USA). Appropriate recording devices can also be easily constructed. Measurement of 'buckling pressure' must be performed on a different night than the basic penile tumescence monitoring. It allows appreciation of early deficiency with persistence of some degree of erection but objective signs of impaired function. Continuous measurement of systemic blood pressure may give clues about the etiology of the problem. Evaluation of systemic arterial pressure at the penile dorsal midline with a Doppler system may give valuable information (presence or absence of localized atheromatous plaque) particularly with diabetes or vascular disorders. Associated with evaluation of penile tumescence, continuous 24-hour samples of blood for prolactin and testosterone release and their relationship to the sleep-wake and REM/NREM cycles are frequently performed.

Polysomnography is frequently performed in conjunction with serial sampling of venous blood aimed at evaluation of hormonal changes in relation with the sleep/wake cycle or REM/NREM cycle. These studies have led to a distinction between the circadian secretion pattern of hormones, such as cortisol or corticotropin (ACTH)[10], and the sleep-related secretory pattern of growth hormone[33] or prolactin[24].

Recent studies have also explored 24-hour patterns of neurotransmitters and peptides, such as endorphin. Plasma endorphin appears to have a 24-hour cyclical pattern independent from the sleep-wake and REM/NREM cycles.

Studies of gastrointestinal juice secretions

Studies of secretion of gastrointestinal juice and its relation to the REM/NREM cycle in normal volunteers and patients have also been systematically performed frequently in association with evaluation of sphincter pressure leading to a diagnosis of abnormal reflux. The most commonly performed sphincter and reflux studies involved the gastroesophageal or gastroduodenal junctions (*see Figure 16.4*).

Sleep-related gastroesophageal reflux has been implicated in the sudden infant death syndrome[17, 18] and sudden appearance of sleep-related laryngospasm in adults. The 'Tuttle Test'[9], i.e. continuous monitoring of esophageal pH during 24 hours or during nocturnal sleep, is associated with monitoring of heart and respiration and has been a helpful technique to determine the frequency and duration of reflux episodes in sleep and their impact on cardiorespiratory variables. This test necessitates placement under fluoroscopy of a pH probe (Beckman Instrument Co.) in the esophagus 5 cm above the esophageogastric junction (cardia). Reflux presence is documented by a drop in pH below 4.0. A relationship between REM sleep and esophageal reflux in 'at risk' infants recently described by an Australian group[19] has not yet been supported by the author's own data.

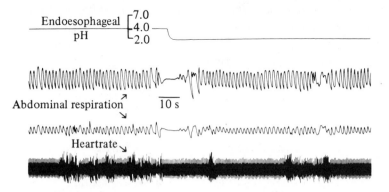

Figure 16.4 Simultaneous recording of endoesophageal pH, respiration and electrocardiogram (lead II) in a 9-month-old infant boy having esophageal reflux associated with apnea

Conclusion

Chronomedicine is evolving toward the use of ambulatory and home monitoring systems. This brief outline of some of the tests which are currently performed using polysomnography is far from a complete list. Continuous growth of this field combined with new technical advances is allowing more long-term evaluations of patients. The goals are earlier detection of disease and development of better therapeutic approaches. The state of alertness has a drastic impact on the entire neuronal network and the central control of all vital functions are constantly modified relative to the 24-hour rhythm and the sleep-wake and REM/NREM cycles. Chronomedicine focuses on understanding these changes and their impact on disease.

Acknowledgement

This research was supported in part by INSERM and by National Institutes of Health Grants RR–70 and RR–81 from the General Clinical Research Centers Program Division of Research Resources.

References

1 ANDERS, T., EMDE, R. and PARMELEE, A. (Editors) *A Manual of Standardized Terminology, Techniques and Criteria for the Scoring of States of Sleep and Wakefulness in Newborn Infants*, 39. Brain Information Service, University of California at Los Angeles, USA.

2 ASERINSKY, E. and KLEITMAN, N. Regularly occurring periods of eye motility and concomitant phenomena during sleep. *Science*, **118**, 273–274 (1953)

3 BAUST, W. and BOHNERT, B. The regulation of heart rate during sleep. *Experimental Brain Research*, **7**, 169–180 (1969)

4 COCCAGNA, G. and LUGARESI, E. Arterial blood gases and pulmonary and systemic arterial pressure during sleep in chronic obstructive pulmonary disease, *Sleep*, **1**, 117–124 (1978)

5 COCCAGNA, G., MANTOVANI, M., BRIGNAMI, F., MANZINI, A. and LUGARESI, E. Arterial pressure changes during spontaneous sleep in man. *Electroencephalography and Clinical Neurophysiology*, **31**, 277–281 (1971)

6 COCCAGNA, G., MANTOVANI, M., PARCHI, C., MIRONI, F. and LUGARESI, E. Alveolar hypoventilation and hypersomnia in myotonic dystrophy. *Journal of Neurology, Neurosurgery and Psychiatry*, **38,** 977–984 (1975)

7 DURON, B. and MARLOT, D. Intercostal and diaphragmatic electrical activity during wakefulness and sleep in normal unrestrained adult cats. *Sleep* (in press)

8 DURON, B. Postural and ventilatory functions of intercostal muscles. *Acta Neurobiologiae Experimentalis*, **33,** 355–380 (1973)

9 EULER, A. R. and AMENT, M. E. Detection of gastroesophageal reflux by Tuttle Test. *Pediatrics*, **60,** 65–70 (1977)

10 GALLAGHER, T. F., YOSHIDA, K., ROFFWARG, H. D., FUKUSHIMA, D. K., WEITZMAN, E. D. and HELLMAN, L. ACTH and cortisol secretory patterns in man. *Journal of Clinical Endocrinology and Metabolism*, **36,** 1058–1068 (1973)

11 GASTAUT, H., TASSINARI, C. A. and DURON, B. Etude polygraphique des manifestations épisodiques (hypniques et respiratoires) diurnes et nocturnes du syndrome de pickwick. *Revue Neurologique*, **112,** 573–579 (1965)

12 GUILLEMINAULT, C., CUMMISKEY, J., MOTTA, J. and LYNNE-DAVIES, P. Respiratory and hemodynamic study during wakefulness and sleep in myotonic dystrophy. *Sleep*, **1,** 19–31 (1978)

13 GUILLEMINAULT, C., CUMMISKEY, J. and MOTTA, J. Chronic obstructive air-flow disease, sleep apnea syndrome, and daytime somnolence. *American Review of Respiratory Disease*, **122,** 397–406 (1980)

14 GUILLEMINAULT, C. and DEMENT, W. C. (Editors) *Sleep Apnea Syndromes*, New York, Alan R. Liss, Inc. (1978)

15 GUILLEMINAULT, C., KURLAND, G., WINKLE, R. and MILES, L. Severe kyphoscoliosis, breathing and sleep (the Quasimodo syndrome during sleep). *Chest* (in press)

16 GUILLEMINAULT, C. and SOUQUET, M. Sleep states and related pathology. In *Advances in Perinatal Neurology*, **1,** edited by R. G. Korobkin and C. Guilleminault, 225–248. New York, Spectrum Inc. (1979)

17 HERBST, J. J., MINTON, S. D. and BOOK, L. S. Gastroesophageal reflux causing respiratory distress and apnea in newborn infants. *Journal of Pediatrics*, **95,** 763–768 (1979)

18 HILL, J. L., PELLAGRINI, C. A., BURRINGTON, J. D., REYES, H. M. and DeMEESTER, T. R. Technique and experience with 24 hour esophageal pH monitoring in children. *Journal of Pediatric Surgery*, **12,** 877–887 (1977)

19 JEFFERY, H. E., REID, I., RAHILLY, P. and READ, D. J. C. Gastroesophageal reflux in 'near-miss' sudden infant death infants in active but not quiet sleep. *Sleep* (in press)

20 JOUVET, M., The role of monoamines and acetylcholine-containing neurons in the regulation of the sleep-waking cycle. *Review of Physiology*, **64**, 166–307. New York, Springer-Verlag (1972)

21 KURTZ, D., BAPST-REITER, J., FLETTO, R., MICHELETTI, G., MEUNIER-CARUS, J., LONSDORFER, J. and LAMPERT-BENIGNUS, E. Les formes de transition du Syndrome Pickwickien. *Bulletin de Physio-pathologie Respiratoire*, **8**, 1115–1125 (1972)

22 LUGARESI, E., COCCAGNA, G., MANTOVANI, M. and CIRIGNOTTA, F. Snoring. *Electroencephalography and Clinical Neurophysiology*, **39**, 59–64 (1975)

23 METZ, J., PIVIK, R. T. and RECHTSCHAFFEN, A. Phasic facial and extra-ocular activity during sleep in cats and humans. In *Sleep Research*, **4**, edited by P. L. Walter, 33. Brain Information Service, University of California at Los Angeles (1975)

24 PARKER, D. C., ROSSMAN, L. G. and VANDERLAAN, E. F. Relation of sleep entrained human prolactin release to REM-nonREM cycles. *Journal of Clinical Endocrinology and Metabolism*, **38**, 646–651 (1974)

25 PHILLIPSON, E. A. Control of breathing during sleep. *American Review of Respiratory Diseases*, **118**, 909–939 (1978)

26 RECHTSCHAFFEN, A. Phasic EMG in human sleep, I. Relation of EMG to brainstem events. In *Sleep Research*, **7**, edited by M. H. Chase, M. M. Mitler and P. L. Walter, 56pp. Brain Information Service, University of California at Los Angeles (1978)

27 RECHTSCHAFFEN, A. and KALES, A. *A Manual of Standardized Terminology, Techniques, and Scoring System for Sleep Stages of Human Subjects*. Brain Information Service, University of California at Los Angeles (1968)

28 RUBIN, P., BLASCHKE, T. and GUILLEMINAULT, C. Effect of naloxone – a specific opioid inhibitor on blood pressure fall during sleep. *Circulation* (in press)

29 RUBIN, P., SWEZEY, S. and BLASCHKE, T. Naloxone lowers plasma prolactin in man. (Letter to the editor). *Lancet*, **1**, 1293 (1979)

30 SHANNON, D. C., MARSLAND, D. W., GOULD, J. B., CALLAHAN, B., TODRES, I. D. and DENNIS, J. Central hypoventilation during quiet sleep in two infants. *Pediatrics*, **57**, 342–346 (1976)

31 SORBINI, C. A., GRASSI, V. and SOLINAS, E.. Arterial oxygen tension in relation to age in healthy subjects. *Respiration*, **25**, 3–13 (1968)

32 SULLIVAN, C. E., MURPHY, E., KOZAR, F. and PHILLIPSON, E. A. Ventilatory responses to CO_2 and lung inflation in tonic versus phasic REM sleep. *Journal of Applied Physiology*, **47**, 1304–1310 (1979)

33 TAKAHASHI, Y., KIPNIS, D. M. and DAUGHADAY, W. H. Growth hormone secretion during sleep. *Journal of Clinical Investigation*, **47**, 2079–2090 (1968)

34 TUSIEWICZ, K., MOLKOFSKY, H., BRYAN, A. C. and BRYAN, M. H. Mechanics of the rib cage and diaphragm during sleep. *Journal of Applied Physiology*, **43**, 600–602 (1977)

35 TZIVONI, D. and STERN, S. Electrocardiographic patterns during sleep in healthy subjects and patients with ischemic heart disease. *Journal of Electrocardiology*, **6**, 225–299 (1973)

36 WILLIAMS, R. L. and KARACAN, I. (Editors), *Sleep Disorders: Diagnosis and Treatment*. New York, John Wiley and Sons (1978)

Index

405